Mitochondrial Metabolism Alterations in Health and Disease

Mitochondrial Metabolism Alterations in Health and Disease

Guest Editors

Graziantonio Lauria
Vincenza Dolce
Rosita Curcio

MDPI

Basel • Beijing • Wuhan • Barcelona • Belgrade • Novi Sad • Cluj • Manchester

Guest Editors

Graziantonio Lauria
Department of Pharmacy, Health and Nutritional Sciences
University of Calabria
Rende, CS
Italy

Vincenza Dolce
Department of Pharmacy, Health and Nutritional Sciences
University of Calabria
Rende, CS
Italy

Rosita Curcio
Department of Pharmacy, Health and Nutritional Sciences
University of Calabria
Rende, CS
Italy

Editorial Office
MDPI AG
Grosspeteranlage 5
4052 Basel, Switzerland

This is a reprint of the Special Issue, published open access by the journal *International Journal of Molecular Sciences* (ISSN 1422-0067), freely accessible at: https://www.mdpi.com/journal/ijms/special_issues/0R1K2T1C1F.

For citation purposes, cite each article independently as indicated on the article page online and as indicated below:

Lastname, A.A.; Lastname, B.B. Article Title. *Journal Name* **Year**, *Volume Number*, Page Range.

ISBN 978-3-7258-5107-2 (Hbk)
ISBN 978-3-7258-5108-9 (PDF)
https://doi.org/10.3390/books978-3-7258-5108-9

Contents

International Journal of *Molecular Sciences*

MDPI

Editorial

Special Issue "Mitochondrial Metabolism Alterations in Health and Disease"

Graziantonio Lauria * and Rosita Curcio *

Department of Pharmacy, Health and Nutritional Sciences, University of Calabria, Via P. Bucci, 87036 Rende, CS, Italy

* Correspondence: graziantonio.lauria@unical.it (G.L.); rosita.curcio@unical.it (R.C.); Tel.: +39-0984-493046 (G.L. & R.C.)

Mitochondria are central hubs of cellular metabolism and signaling that play key roles in stress response, inflammation, calcium homeostasis, mitochondrial quality control, and cell death, with mitochondrial impairment potentially being the underlying cause of several conditions, including metabolic, neurodegenerative, and cardiovascular diseases. Furthermore, mitochondrial dysfunction can contribute to the hallmarks of cancer, including sustained proliferative signaling, resistance to cell death, and altered cellular energetics. Therefore, analyzing the mechanisms underlying mitochondrial dysfunction and developing targeted therapies to restore mitochondrial function have become essential research areas. This Special Issue offers an outstanding collection of up-to-date reviews and research articles focusing on mitochondria and their potential for fighting human diseases.

The article by Chandrasekarant et al. demonstrates that AMP-activated protein kinase (AMPK) activators could have therapeutic potential for diabetic peripheral neuropathy (DPN) by modulating mitochondrial metabolism [1]. The authors investigated the effects of the AMPK activator 5-Aminoimidazole-4-carboxamide 1-β-D-ribofuranoside (AICAR) in mouse models of Type 1 and Type 2 diabetes, finding that AICAR had preventive and reversing effects on experimental DPN. AICAR treatment promoted mitochondrial homeostasis through AMPK phosphorylation and activation. The latter resulted in increased levels of the mitochondrial fission marker dynamin-related protein 1, augmented phosphorylation of the autophagy-activating kinase, and increased levels of the autophagosome marker LC3-II, suggesting improved mitochondrial turnover and mitophagy. In mitochondria isolated from dorsal root ganglion neurons of mice that were fed high-fat diets, AICAR treatment enhanced mitochondrial function by increasing ADP-stimulated state 3 respiration. Furthermore, AICAR treatment improved systemic metabolic parameters, such as insulin sensitivity and glycemic and lipid profiles. All of these findings suggest that AMPK activators may act as exercise mimetics and neuroprotective agents, with therapeutic potential for the treatment of DPN, although further clinical studies in humans are still needed.

Levitt et al. demonstrated that short-term and chronic binge alcohol (CBA) non-synergistically decreased the differentiation capacity of myoblasts from simian immunodeficiency virus-infected female macaques [2]. The authors proved that short-term alcohol treatment decreased myoblast differentiation capacity and impaired cell bioenergetics by decreasing glycolytic function, ATP production, mitochondrial membrane potential and pyruvate kinase activity, while increasing the mitochondrial production of reactive oxygen species (ROS) and aldolase activity. Conversely the activity of the latter enzyme was found to be decreased, in chronically alcohol-fed rats. This suggests possible alternative metabolic fates of glucose in alcohol misuse. Potentially different mechanisms could be responsible for the decreased myoblast differentiation capacity following short-term alcohol consumption and CBA, highlighting the need to clarify the impact of different types of alcohol misuse on myopathy. These findings might be useful for attenuating the negative effects of alcohol abuse on mitochondrial bioenergetics, as well as for improving skeletal muscle mass and quality of life in subjects with alcohol use disorders.

Mitochondrial dysfunction has emerged as a significant pathogenetic factor in post-viral fatigue syndrome (PVFS), a condition that leads to low-grade systemic inflammation and includes myalgic encephalomyelitis, also known as chronic fatigue syndrome, fibromyalgia (FM), and post-COVID-19 (long COVID) illness. Decreased ATP production, immune dysregulation, and increased oxidative stress have been observed in PVFS patients, but no FDA-approved treatment is currently available. In their review, Mantle et al. discussed the efficacy of CoQ10 supplementation to improve mitochondrial function, reduce oxidative stress, and alleviate fatigue in PVFS patients [3]. The ability of CoQ10 to ameliorate mitochondrial dysfunction stems from the key role it plays in mitochondria. It is an electron carrier in the mitochondrial respiratory chain that can restore electron flow and enhance ATP generation. Moreover, CoQ10 is a fat-soluble antioxidant that protects mitochondria from damage caused by free radical species generated during oxidative phosphorylation. Some clinical trials showed promising results, especially in FM patients, where CoQ10 supplementation reduced pain and fatigue and improved energy generation.

Several authors critically reviewed the involvement of mitochondrial dysfunction in the pathogenesis of neurodegenerative disorders, including Parkinson's disease (PD) and Alzheimer's disease (AD). Neuronal functionality and survival require high energy levels to ensure the proper functioning of mitochondria. The article by Uspalenko et al. highlighted the involvement of mitochondrial ATP-dependent potassium channels in the development of PD. These authors demonstrated the protective effect of uridine in an experimental rat model of PD, induced by the injection of the neurotoxin, 6-hydroxydopamine (6-OHDA), into the substantia nigra [4]. 6-OHDA was used because it can inhibit complex I of the respiratory chain, mimicking the process that occurs in PD patients, where a reduction in the activity of this complex was observed. 6-OHDA inhibition increased ROS generation in dopaminergic neurons, thus causing severe mitochondrial dysfunction and impairing neuronal function, which resulted in motor deficit. Uridine treatment was able to increase the concentration of uridine diphosphate, a natural activator of these channels, resulting in reduced oxidative stress and mitochondrial dysfunction. Based on these findings, uridine treatment could be useful for preventing the development of PD and/or to treat this disease in its early stages.

Mitochondrial dysfunction plays a crucial role in mediating the intercorrelation between PD and associated cardiac comorbidities. Although the mechanisms underlying the increased prevalence of cardiac dysfunction observed in PD patients are still unclear, Salis Torres et al. reviewed some shared pathways capable of impairing mitochondrial function in both cardiac and neuronal tissues [5]. These authors highlighted numerous common pathways, including compromised mitochondrial bioenergetics; alterations in mitochondrial biogenesis and dynamics; the dysregulation of the PINK1/PRKN-mediated mitophagy pathway; disrupted mitochondrial calcium handling with decreased ATP production and increased oxidative stress; and excessive ROS production and lipid peroxidation resulting in cellular damage, protein aggregation, and mitochondrial dysfunction. These pathways are all common hallmarks of cardiac and neurological diseases, as well as genetic susceptibility, since certain PD-associated genes (PRKN, PINK1, and PARK7) are also expressed in cardiac tissue and play critical roles in mitochondrial quality control. This review provides insights into future research directions, as studying the role of mitochondrial dysfunction as a link between cardiac dysfunction and PD may offer an opportunity to reveal common metabolic pathways, leading to promising opportunities in research areas that aim to identify relevant shared therapeutic targets.

The comprehensive review by Yu et al. highlighted the genetic, proteomic, and metabolic alterations in AD linked to mitochondrial one-carbon metabolism [6]. The latter is involved in several processes, such as mitochondrial function, nucleotide synthesis, amino acid metabolism, and epigenetic regulation. Furthermore, it plays a central role in replenishing pools of nucleotides to preserve substrate bioavailability, which is useful for DNA repair. The authors proposed that multiple AD hallmarks, such as Aβ accumulation, tau hyperphosphorylation, and genetic risk factors converge on mitochondrial dysfunction. They suggested that enhancing mitochondrial one-carbon metabolism could help neurons counteract damage and delay AD-related pathologies, emphasizing the role of folate and NAD+ in mitigating mitochondrial dysfunction. The folate one-carbon pathway is critical for cellular health, as it supplies purine biosynthesis, takes part in the reduction of the essential redox cofactor NAD(P)+ to NAD(P)H, and allows the biosynthesis of the main methylation factor, S-adenosylmethionine. In addition, NAD+ and NADP+ are crucial cofactors in electron transfer and redox reactions. Defects in the function of respiratory chain complex I and low levels of NAD+ have been found in AD patients. Furthermore, NAD+ levels are also reduced in animal models of AD. On this basis, attempts have been made to restore cellular NAD+ levels in animal models of neurodegeneration with promising results. These approaches are currently undergoing clinical trials.

Other authors pointed out the critical involvement of mitochondria in cancer and how this could be exploited for new potential anti-cancer strategies, as well as for improving the diagnosis and prognosis of certain cancer types.

The review by Moon provided an excellent overview of the role of ATP-sensitive potassium channels in cancer biology, highlighting their promising role as potential therapeutic targets in cancer treatment, as they modulate key cellular processes that are often dysregulated in cancer cells [7]. These channels are expressed in cell membranes, where they play a key role in linking cellular metabolism to electrical activity, as well as in mitochondria, where they modulate mitochondrial function, ATP generation, programmed cell death, and defense mechanisms against physiological stress. The structural features, regulation, mechanisms, expression, and mutations of these channels, as well as their role in modulating metabolic and ion balance, cell cycle progression, and proliferation in cancer cells are described in detail. Furthermore, the role of activators and inhibitors in cancer biology is extensively discussed. KATP channel activators, such as diazoxide, minoxidil, pinacidil, and cromakalim, can affect proliferation, invasion, drug delivery, and apoptosis in a context-dependent manner. In contrast, KATP channel inhibitors, particularly sulfonylurea drugs, such as glyburide, glipizide, and repaglinide, have shown promising anti-cancer properties, modulating signaling pathways involved in angiogenesis, cell cycle regulation, and cell death. According to the author, selectively disrupting the proliferation and survival of cancer cells requires a thorough understanding of the several roles that these channels play in different cancer cells, as their function can vary significantly depending on the environment and cancer cell type. Furthermore, a future challenge will be the design of potential drugs able to act specifically on mitochondrial channels without affecting those located in the plasma membrane.

The article by Frattaruolo et al. demonstrated the promising in vitro antitumor activity of some plant-derived flavanones in breast cancer cell lines [8]. The authors compared the selective and dose-dependent cytotoxic activity of three natural flavanones isolated from the leaves of Glycyrrhiza glabra—Glabranin, Pinocembrin, and Licoflavanone—in the breast cancer cell lines, MCF-7, MDA-MB-231, and MCF-10A. Licoflavanone exhibited the best cytotoxic and proapoptotic activity, along with the greatest ability to inhibit cell motility and reduce macrophage activation induced by breast-cancer-conditioned media. Furthermore, Licoflavanone treatment modulated breast cancer cell energy metabolism by decreasing the mitochondrial oxygen consumption rate linked to ATP production. Although all three tested compounds were able to inhibit the propagation and survival of cancer stem cells (CSCs) and reduce the expression of stemness markers in CSCs, Licoflavanone emerged as the most potent inhibitor. Notably, CSCs are a subpopulation of tumor cells with high metabolic flexibility, whose proliferation is largely dependent on mitochondrial function. These features increase their chemoresistance and ability to metastasize and relapse, and are often responsible for the failure of conventional therapeutic strategies. In this context, the study of molecules that are able to modulate mitochondrial bioenergetics could prove to be an opportunity for the development of basic research findings into possible future clinical applications, especially for those tumors that strictly depend on mitochondrial oxidative metabolism.

Nowadays, the diagnosis of thyroid cancer is mainly based on imaging techniques and cytological analysis. When the diagnosis is ambiguous, the quantification of molecular biomarkers is evaluated after cytological examination. Currently commercially available molecular tests are expensive and widely vary. Therefore, new molecular biomarkers with higher diagnostic reliability are being developed, as well as better classification of prognosis and recurrence. Current research has focused on different promising biomarkers for thyroid cancer. In this regard, the review by Cabané et al. provided a comprehensive overview of the current state of molecular markers for thyroid cancer diagnosis and prognosis, with a focus on emerging opportunities from non-coding RNAs and mitochondrial signatures [9]. Promising biomarkers related to non-coding genome include miRNAs, long non-coding RNAs, circular and double-stranded RNAs, while those related to mitochondria include mitochondrial DNA signatures, circulating cell-free mtDNA, and mitophagic gene signatures (expression of the mitophagic proteins FAM162A, NIX, and BNIP3). It is known that high mtDNA heteroplasmy results in increased ROS levels, which impairs mitochondrial bioenergetics and alters mitophagy, thus favoring the development of pathologies such as cancer. When mitochondrial stress and/or defective mitophagy occurs, mtDNA can escape from mitochondria and cells into the bloodstream, where it can be detected and measured. Therefore, the amount and features of circulating cell-free mtDNA represent useful parameters of mitochondrial dysfunction and disease.

Overall, this Special Issue of *IJMS* provides a collection of nine articles that discuss various aspects of mitochondrial involvement in human diseases, aiming to find new promising therapeutic strategies to treat, prevent, and/or diagnose them. Different authors pointed out that some treatments that are able to restore mitochondrial function were effective in counteracting DPN, PVFS, and altered myoblast differentiation following alcohol misuse. A group of articles shed light on the critical role of mitochondria and associated pathways in neurodegenerative diseases, focusing on the latest knowledge and emphasizing the importance of understanding and harnessing mitochondrial pathways to counteract mitochondrial dysfunction, which underlies many of the defects found in these diseases. Possible approaches should target mitochondrial dynamics and bioenergetics to alleviate symptoms and progression. Another group of articles helped pave the way for new research and possible therapeutic approaches in the fight against cancer, focusing on modulating mitochondrial function. In this context, one of the most important future challenges of personalized medicine will be the development of strategies capable of selectively targeting tumor cells while minimizing damage to healthy cells. In addition, the promising role of emerging biomarkers for improving the diagnosis and prognosis of thyroid cancer is discussed. All of this knowledge can provide new and valuable insights for future research directions.

Author Contributions: Conceptualization, R.C. and G.L.; data curation, G.L. and R.C.; writing and editing, R.C. and G.L. All authors have read and agreed to the published version of the manuscript.

Conflicts of Interest: The authors declare no conflicts of interest.

References

1. Chandrasekaran, K.; Choi, J.; Salimian, M.; Hedayat, A.F.; Russell, J.W. Administration of AICAR, an AMPK Activator, Prevents and Reverses Diabetic Polyneuropathy (DPN) by Regulating Mitophagy. *Int. J. Mol. Sci.* **2024**, *26*, 80. [CrossRef] [PubMed]
2. Levitt, D.E.; Bourgeois, B.L.; Rodríguez-Graciani, K.M.; Molina, P.E.; Simon, L. Alcohol Impairs Bioenergetics and Differentiation Capacity of Myoblasts from Simian Immunodeficiency Virus-Infected Female Macaques. *Int. J. Mol. Sci.* **2024**, *25*, 2448. [CrossRef] [PubMed]
3. Mantle, D.; Hargreaves, I.P.; Domingo, J.C.; Castro-Marrero, J. Mitochondrial Dysfunction and Coenzyme Q10 Supplementation in Post-Viral Fatigue Syndrome: An Overview. *Int. J. Mol. Sci.* **2024**, *25*, 574. [CrossRef] [PubMed]
4. Uspalenko, N.I.; Mosentsov, A.A.; Khmil, N.V.; Pavlik, L.L.; Belosludtseva, N.V.; Khunderyakova, N.V.; Shigaeva, M.I.; Medvedeva, V.P.; Malkov, A.E.; Kitchigina, V.F.; et al. Uridine as a Regulator of Functional and Ultrastructural Changes in the Brain of Rats in a Model of 6-OHDA-Induced Parkinson's Disease. *Int. J. Mol. Sci.* **2023**, *24*, 14304. [CrossRef] [PubMed]
5. Salis Torres, A.; Lee, J.E.; Caporali, A.; Semple, R.K.; Horrocks, M.H.; MacRae, V.E. Mitochondrial Dysfunction as a Potential Mechanism Mediating Cardiac Comorbidities in Parkinson's Disease. *Int. J. Mol. Sci.* **2024**, *25*, 10973. [CrossRef] [PubMed]
6. Yu, Y.; Martins, L.M. Mitochondrial One-Carbon Metabolism and Alzheimer's Disease. *Int. J. Mol. Sci.* **2024**, *25*, 6302. [CrossRef] [PubMed]
7. Moon, D.O. Exploring the Role of Surface and Mitochondrial ATP-Sensitive Potassium Channels in Cancer: From Cellular Functions to Therapeutic Potentials. *Int. J. Mol. Sci.* **2024**, *25*, 2129. [CrossRef]
8. Frattaruolo, L.; Lauria, G.; Aiello, F.; Carullo, G.; Curcio, R.; Fiorillo, M.; Campiani, G.; Dolce, V.; Cappello, A.R. Exploiting *Glycyrrhiza glabra* L. (Licorice) Flavanones: Licoflavanone's Impact on Breast Cancer Cell Bioenergetics. *Int. J. Mol. Sci.* **2024**, *25*, 7907. [CrossRef] [PubMed]
9. Cabané, P.; Correa, C.; Bode, I.; Aguilar, R.; Elorza, A.A. Biomarkers in Thyroid Cancer: Emerging Opportunities from Non-Coding RNAs and Mitochondrial Space. *Int. J. Mol. Sci.* **2024**, *25*, 6719. [CrossRef] [PubMed]

International Journal of *Molecular Sciences*

MDPI

Article

Administration of AICAR, an AMPK Activator, Prevents and Reverses Diabetic Polyneuropathy (DPN) by Regulating Mitophagy

Krish Chandrasekaran [1], Joungil Choi [1,2], Mohammad Salimian [1], Ahmad F. Hedayat [1] and James W. Russell [1,2,3,4,*]

1 Department of Neurology, University of Maryland School of Medicine, Baltimore, MD 21201, USA; krishchandra0630@gmail.com (K.C.); joungil.choi@va.gov (J.C.); mohammad.salimian@gmail.com (M.S.); fahim.hedayat@yahoo.com (A.F.H.)
2 Veterans Affairs Medical Center, Baltimore, MD 21201, USA
3 CAMC Department of Neurology, Institute for Academic Medicine, 415 Morris Street Suite 300, Charleston, WV 25301, USA
4 West Virginia University, Charleston, WV 25301, USA
* Correspondence: james.russell@camc.org or jrussell7092082@gmail.com

Abstract: Diabetic peripheral neuropathy (DPN) is a common complication of diabetes in both Type 1 (T1D) and Type 2 (T2D). While there are no specific medications to prevent or treat DPN, certain strategies can help halt its progression. In T1D, maintaining tight glycemic control through insulin therapy can effectively prevent or delay the onset of DPN. However, in T2D, overall glucose control may only have a moderate impact on DPN, although exercise is clearly beneficial. Unfortunately, optimal exercise may not be feasible for many patients with DPN because of neuropathic foot pain and poor balance. Exercise has several favorable effects on health parameters, including body weight, glycemic control, lipid profile, and blood pressure. We investigated the impact of an exercise mimetic, 5-aminoimidazole-4-carboxamide ribonucleotide (AICAR), on DPN. AICAR treatment prevented or reversed experimental DPN in mouse models of both T2D and T1D. AICAR in high-fat diet (HFD-fed) mice increased the phosphorylation of AMPK in DRG neuronal extracts, and the ratio of phosphorylated AMPK to total AMPK increased by 3-fold (HFD vs. HFD+AICAR; $p < 0.001$). Phospho AMP increased the levels of dynamin-related protein 1 (*DRP1*, a mitochondrial fission marker), increased phosphorylated autophagy activating kinase 1 (ULK1) at Serine-555, and increased microtubule-associated protein light chain 3-II (LC3-II, a marker for autophagosome assembly) by 2-fold. Mitochondria isolated from DRG neurons of HFD-fed had a decrease in ADP-stimulated state 3 respiration (120 $\pm$ 20 nmol O_2/min in HFD vs. 220 $\pm$ 20 nmol O_2/min in control diet (CD); $p < 0.001$. Mitochondria isolated from HFD+AICAR-treated mice had increased state 3 respiration (240 $\pm$ 30 nmol O_2/min in HFD+AICAR). However, AICAR's protection in DPN in T2D mice was also mediated by its effects on insulin sensitivity, glucose metabolism, and lipid metabolism. Drugs that enhance AMPK phosphorylation may be beneficial in the treatment of DPN.

Keywords: exercise mimetics; AICAR; AMPK; diabetic neuropathy; mitochondrial fission; mitochondrial biogenesis; lipid metabolism; glucose metabolism; nerve conduction; intraepidermal nerve fiber density

1. Introduction

While there is no specific treatment for diabetic peripheral neuropathy (DPN), aerobic exercise may slow the progression of neuropathy [1–4]. Aerobic (endurance) and resistance exercise play crucial roles in improving glycemic control and insulin sensitivity in individuals with diabetes [2,4–8]. However, some patients with type 2 diabetes may not participate in regular physical exercise therapy [9]. One of the critical obstacles in utilizing exercise therapy is the inability of those with DPN to participate fully in weight-bearing exercises due to discomfort and poor balance related to the neuropathy [2,3]. To address this problem, researchers have explored the concept of exercise mimetics—a substance that mimics the effects of exercise without the need for physical activity.

Exercise mediates its action via the AMP-activated protein kinase (AMPK) or 5′ AMP-activated protein kinase (EC 2.7.11.31) [10,11]. Exercise decreases the ATP/AMP ratio, leading to increased AMP levels. Increased AMP promotes the phosphorylation of AMPK. Phosphorylated AMPK then promotes adenosine triphosphate (ATP) production by inhibiting ATP-consumption pathways and accelerating ATP-generation pathways. AMPK is thus acting like a 'fuel gauge' [12,13]. When ATP levels are low (indicating energy deficiency), AMPK is activated. AMPK in turn increases the expression of the PPARγ-coactivator (PGC-1α), which has been shown to be protective in preventing DPN [14]. Increased expression of PGC-1α leads to downstream activation of pathways that are critical in regulating mitochondrial function that in turn protect against DPN [15–18]. PGC-1α also stimulates GLUT4 translocation to the plasma membrane, increases glucose uptake, and reduces fatty acid levels, which in turn improves glycemic control. AMP regulates various pathways related to lipid metabolism and mitochondrial function. Additionally, AMPK regulates mitochondrial dynamics (fission and fusion) and their function [10,19–21].

Some medications used for the treatment of diabetes, such as thiazolidinediones and metformin, are mild activators of AMPK. Metformin activates AMPK by inhibiting mitochondrial function [22,23]. In contrast, 5-aminoimidazole-4-carboxamide ribonucleotide (AICAR) is a potent AMP analog, produced naturally by the body. AICAR significantly improves metabolic control in obese Zucker rats [24] and mimics the effect of exercise in mice [25]. However, nothing is known about the effect of AICAR on neuropathy. By addressing multiple risk factors, including dyslipidemia, insulin sensitivity, and glycemic control, AICAR shows promise in ameliorating DPN. This research opens possibilities for novel treatments that harness the power of AMPK.

2. Results

2.1. A High-Fat Diet (HFD) Decreases Neuronal AMPK Phosphorylation and AICAR Increased AMPK Phosphorylation in HFD-Fed Mice

Our proposed working model is that administration of AICAR can ameliorate peripheral sensory neuropathy in both HFD-induced type 2 and streptozotocin (STZ)—induced type 1 diabetic mice by regulating mitochondrial function via AMPK phosphorylation in both neuronal and non-neuronal tissues, thereby alleviating a diabetes-induced energy metabolic failure (Figure 1). To test this, AICAR was administered to control diet (CD-fed) and HFD-fed mice for 4 months. AICAR was dissolved in DMSO (5%)/alcohol (5%)/saline (90%) and 100 μL of this solution was administered subcutaneously for 3 days in a week (Monday, Wednesday, and Friday) at a dose of 500 mg/kg. The vehicle, DMSO (5%)/alcohol (5%)/saline (90%) was administered to CD- and HFD-fed mice for 4 months. Thus, there were four groups, CD (4 months), CD+AICAR (4 months), HFD (4 months), and HFD+AICAR (4 months). Baseline nerve conduction studies (NCS) and Von Frey monofilament studies were not statistically different between the mice randomized to each of the groups. At the end of 4 months, NCS were performed, mice were euthanized, and blood chemistry was obtained in the four groups of mice. Dorsal root ganglion (DRG) neurons were harvested. Protein extracts from DRG neurons were prepared, and Western blots were completed. The effect of AICAR administration on the phosphorylation of AMPK is shown in Figure 1. The ratio of AMPK phosphorylated at threonine residue 172 to total AMPK was constant in DRG neuronal extracts from CD and CD+AICAR-treated mice. On the other hand, feeding mice with an HFD caused a decrease in phosphorylation of AMPK in DRG protein extracts (Figure 2). Administration of AICAR to HFD-fed mice increased the phosphorylation of AMPK, and the ratio of phosphorylated AMPK to total AMPK increased by 3-fold (HFD vs. HFD+AICAR; $p < 0.001$).

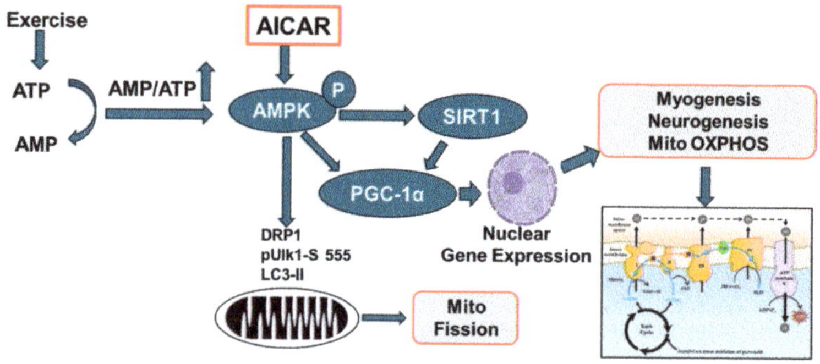

Figure 1. Exercise consumes a large amount of ATP, elevating the AMP-to-ATP ratio. Increased AMP binds to the enzyme AMPK and induces the phosphorylation of AMPK (Figure 1). On the other hand, **AICAR directly phosphorylates AMPK.** (1) Phosphorylated AMPK activates SIRT1/PGC1-α in the catabolic process of exercise (increased OXPHOS), resulting in decreased body weight, reduced triglycerides, improved HOMA-IR index and lower NEFA levels; (2) phosphorylated AMPK activates PGC-1α co-transcriptional complexes that initiate the overexpression of target genes to promote myogenesis, neurogenesis, and mitochondrial bioenergetics; and (3) phosphorylated AMPK led to phosphorylation of mitochondrial fission factor (MFF), recruitment of dynamin-like protein DRP1 to mitochondria, and activation of ULK1, an upstream kinase in autophagy and mitophagy. Mitochondrial fission allows damaged mitochondria to be selectively degraded through mitophagy pathways. The main points of this paper are boxed in red.

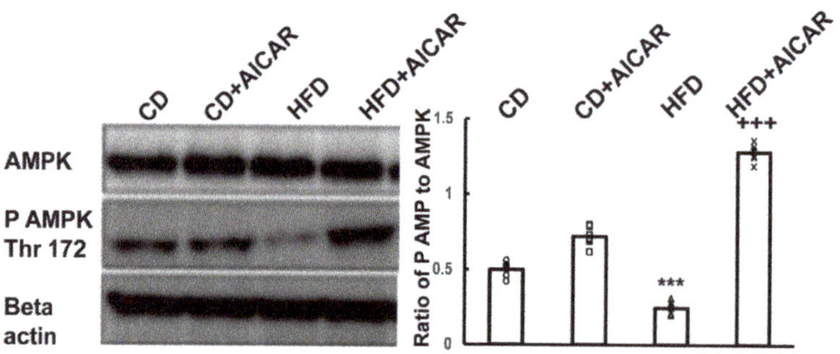

Figure 2. Western blot analysis of AMPK and quantification of phospho-AMPK to total AMPK (Figure 2). DRG neurons were isolated from CD (n = 6), CD+AICAR (n = 6), HFD (n = 6), and HFD+AICAR (n = 6) mice, and protein extracts were prepared. Antibodies recognize total AMPK, AMPK phosphorylated at the Thr 176 residue, and beta-actin. The levels of expression were quantified by the intensity of the bands. The ratio of pAMPK to total AMPK was calculated, and the values were analyzed by ANOVA. The significance is denoted by the following p-values: *** $p < 0.001$; CD or CD+AICARD vs. HFD, +++ $p < 0.001$; HFD vs. HFD+AICAR.

2.2. Phosphorylated AMPK Promoted Mitochondrial Turnover

To correlate how AMPK phosphorylation corresponds with mitochondrial function, mitochondria were isolated from small amounts of neuronal samples following the procedure described in the Materials and Methods section. Western blots were performed on mitochondrial protein extracts to quantify mitochondrial fission/fusion proteins. The results are shown in Figure 3. In AICAR-treated samples, there was a significant increase in the levels of dynamin-related protein 1 (*DRP1*, a mitochondrial fission marker), an increase in phosphorylated autophagy activating kinase 1 (ULK1) at Serine-555, and increased microtubule-associated protein, light chain 3-II (LC3-II, a marker for autophagosome assembly). There was also an increase in the levels of the same proteins in HFD-fed neuronal tissue samples. We interpret these results as suggesting that feeding mice with an HFD does induce a physiological response in neurons to eliminate damaged mitochondria via mitophagy. Furthermore, AICAR treatment enhances this effect to protect mitochondria against HFD-induced oxidative stress.

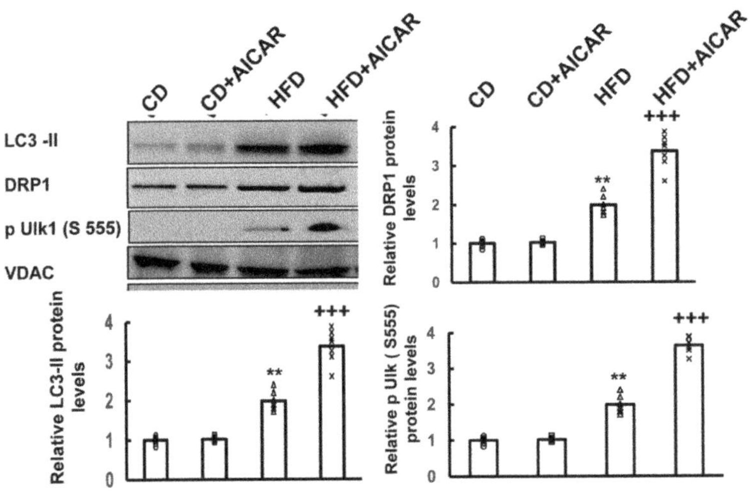

Figure 3. Western blot analysis of proteins involved in mitophagy in neuronal mitochondria isolated from CD (n = 6), CD+AICAR (n = 6), HFD (n = 6), and HFD+AICAR (n = 6) mice. Western blots were carried out on the protein extracts using anti-LC3, anti-DRP1, anti-phospho (S555) ULK1, and anti-VDAC. The levels of expression were quantified based on the intensity of the bands. The relative ratio was calculated, and the values were analyzed by ANOVA. The significance is denoted by the following p-values: ** $p < 0.01$ HFD vs. CD or CD+AICAR; +++ $p < 0.001$ HFD+AICAR vs. HFD.

2.3. AICAR Promoted Neuronal Mitochondrial State 3 Respiration

To determine if AICAR-induced mitochondrial fission in HFD-fed mice regulates mitochondrial respiration, we assessed the bioenergetics profile of mitochondria isolated from DRG neurons of CD, CD+AICAR, HFD, and HFD+AICAR mice. The oxygen consumption rate was measured using the Seahorse Biosciences analyzer (Figure 4). Basal, ADP-stimulated (state 3), and oligomycin-sensitive (state 4) respiration were measured with serial additions of 10 mM glutamate and 2 mM malate (state 2), 2.5 mM ADP (state 3), and 1.5 mM oligomycin (state 4_0). Respiratory control ratios (state 3 to state 4_0) were calculated. Ratios greater than 4 have been routinely observed in isolated neuronal mitochondria from WT mice. Exogenous cytochrome c did not enhance mitochondrial respiration in these preparations, indicating minimal damage to the outer mitochondrial membrane during isolation procedures. The results showed similar basal and state 4 respiration among the four samples (~53 ± 5 nmol O_2/min/mg protein). The significant difference that was observed was that an HFD caused a decrease in ADP-stimulated, state 3 respiration compared to the other three samples (120 ± 20 nmol O_2/min in HFD vs. 220 ± 20 nmol O_2/min in CD and CD+AICAR samples; $p < 0.001$). Mitochondria isolated from HFD+AICAR-treated mice had increased state 3 respiration (240 ± 30 nmol O_2/min in HFD+AICAR). This suggested that AICAR treatment in HFD-fed mice was able to couple the mitochondria to energy demand, namely ADP.

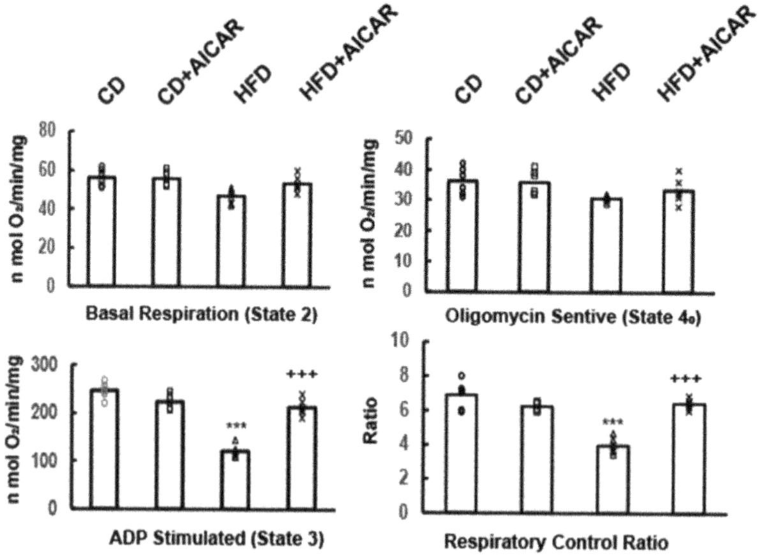

Figure 4. Impaired ADP-stimulated mitochondrial respiration in HFD mice was prevented by AICAR treatment. Oxygen consumption rate (OCR) was measured in the presence of complex I substrates (malate/glutamate) with the subsequent and sequential addition of ADP, oligomycin, and rotenone + antimycin A to mitochondria to measure state 2 (basal), state 3 (ADP-stimulated), state 4_0 (oligomycin-sensitive), and FCCP-induced respiration rates were measured. ADP-stimulated respiration was significantly decreased in neuronal mitochondria from HFD-fed mice compared to CD and CD+AICAR-treated mice. Administration of AICAR to HFD-fed mice significantly increased ADP-stimulated respiration. The respiratory control ratio (RCR) was calculated. *** $p < 0.001$ HFD vs. CD, CD+AICAR. +++ $p < 0.001$ HFD vs. HFD+AICAR.

2.4. Administration of AICAR Prevented HFD-Induced Increases in Body Weight Gain, Triglyceride, Homeostatic Model Assessment for Insulin Resistance (HOMA-IR) Index, and Non-Esterified Fatty Acids (NEFA) Levels in Mice

Several studies have shown that the main effects of AICAR occur in peripheral tissues, particularly in muscle. Muscles are a major consumer of glucose and regulator of lipid metabolism. To determine if AICAR treatment also altered glucose and lipid metabolism, body physiology and blood chemistry were completed in all four groups of mice. Significant changes were noted in the following parameters: AICAR administration to HFD-fed mice for 4 months caused a significant decrease in their body weight (from 50 ± 5 g to 42 ± 4.5 g; $p < 0.01$) and a significant decrease in triglycerides (1.4 ± 0.3 mmol/L in HFD-fed mice to 1.0 ± 0.1 mmol/L in HFD+AICAR mice; $p < 0.01$). The HFD-fed mice showed increased insulin resistance: the HOMA-IR index in HFD-fed mice was 10 ± 1 ($p < 0.001$) compared to CD-fed mice (5 ± 0.6) and to CD+AICAR-treated mice (5.1 ± 0.7). In the AICAR-treated HFD-fed mice, the HOMA-IR index was 7.3 ± 0.6; $p < 0.01$ compared to HFD-fed mice. AICAR treatment also decreased NEFA levels (HFD = 0.7 ± 0.08 mmol/L vs. HFD+AICAR = 0.4 ± 0.01 mmol/L; $p < 0.01$). The measurement of intraperitoneal-glucose tolerance test

(IP-GTT; $n = 6$) showed a significant increase in the area under the curve (AUC) in HFD mice compared to CD mice and CD+AICAR-treated mice. There was a significant decrease in AUC in HFD+AICAR-treated mice compared to HFD mice (Table 1). We suggest that some of the improvements in AICAR-treated HFD-fed mice are due to their effect on reducing lipid levels, decreasing insulin resistance, better glycemic control, and resistance to an increase in body weight.

Table 1. Metabolic end points in CD-fed and HFD-fed mice with and without AICAR treatment at 4 months.

Parameters	CD		HFD		Significance			
	($n = 6$) 1	+AICAR ($n = 6$) 2	($n = 6$) 3	+AICAR ($n = 6$) 4	1 vs. 2	1 vs. 3	2 vs. 4	3 vs. 4
Body Weight (g)	29 ± 3	28 ± 3	39 ± 5	29 ± 5	NS	<0.05	NS	<0.05
Plasma Glucose (mg/dL)	108 ± 20	111 ± 9	178 ± 9	138 ± 9	NS	<0.01	<0.05	<0.01
HbA1c%	5.4 ± 1	5 ± 0.6	6.8 ± 1	5.8 ± 0.9	NS	0.045	NS	<0.05
Insulin (ng/mL)	2.5 ± 0.2	2.3 ± 0.9	6.2 ± 1	3 ± 0.05	NS	<0.01	<0.05	<0.01
Total Cholesterol (mg/dL)	80 ± 4.2	78 ± 6.7	153 ± 9	133 ± 10	NS	<0.01	<0.01	<0.05
Triglycerides (mg/dL)	41 ± 6.1	39 ± 1.9	65 ± 5	46 ± 6	NS	<0.01	<0.05	<0.01
HDL Cholesterol (mg/dL)	70 ± 4	69 ± 5	143 ± 6	103 ± 5	NS	<0.01	<0.01	<0.05
HOMA-IR	5.0 ± 0.5	4.8 ± 0.4	10 ± 0.9	6.0 ± 0.6	NS	<0.001	<0.05	<0.001
NEFA (mM)	0.6 ± 0.06	0.6 ± 0.03	0.3 ± 0.03	0.2 ± 0.03	NS	<0.05	<0.01	<0.05
GTT-AUC (mg min/dL × 10^3)	3.6 ± 0.46	3 ± 0.29	6.1 ± 1	4.1 ± 0.5	NS	<0.01	<0.05	<0.05

GTT-AUC = glucose tolerance test-area under the curve; HDL = high-density lipoprotein; HOMA-IR = HOMA-IR—an index used to determine if insulin resistance is present. NEFA = non-esterified fatty acids; NS = not significant.

2.5. *Subcutaneous Administration of AICAR Prevented Peripheral Neuropathy Induced by HFD*

We tested if administration of AICAR would prevent HFD-induced peripheral neuropathy. AICAR was injected into HFD-fed mice for 4 months. After 4 months of HFD feeding ($n = 6$), C57BL6 mice showed a significant slowing of sciatic motor nerve conduction velocity (SMNCV, Figure 5) (from 41 ± 2 m/s with a CD to 29 ± 1.2 m/s with an HFD; $p < 0.001$), increased tail motor latency (TML, from 1.3 ± 0.07 ms in CD to 2.67 ± 0.3 ms; $p < 0.001$ with an HFD), and decreased tail sensory nerve conduction velocity (TSNCV, from 34.6 ± 0.9 m/s in CD to 29 ± 1.4 m/s in HFD; $p < 0.001$). These changes in nerve conduction velocity (NCV) in HFD-fed mice were consistent with the development of peripheral neuropathy. There was no statistically significant difference in the compound muscle action potential (CMAP) or sensory nerve action potential (SNAP) amplitudes compared between groups or compared at the start and end of the treatment. This is expected because of considerable variability in the CMAP and SNAP amplitudes obtained in nerve conduction studies (NCS) in both mice and humans, especially when interval repeat studies are performed [26–28]. The CMAP sciatic amplitudes (mV) after 4 months of treatment were as follows: CD: 7.28 ± 2.42 (SEM); CD+AICAR: 5.53 ± 1.65; HFD: 3.60 ± 0.98; HFD+AICAR: 3.602 ± 0.979. The CMAP tail amplitudes (mV) after 4 months of treatment were as follows: CD: 1.58 ± 0.15; CD+AICAR: 1.71 ± 0.09; HFD: 1.22 ± 0.18; HFD+AICAR: 1.57 ± 0.37. The SNAP tail amplitudes (μV) after 4 months of treatment were as follows: CD: 93.45 ± 9.20; CD+AICAR: 103.21 ± 15.01; HFD: 126.51 ± 26.39; HFD+AICAR: 95.18 ± 10.09.

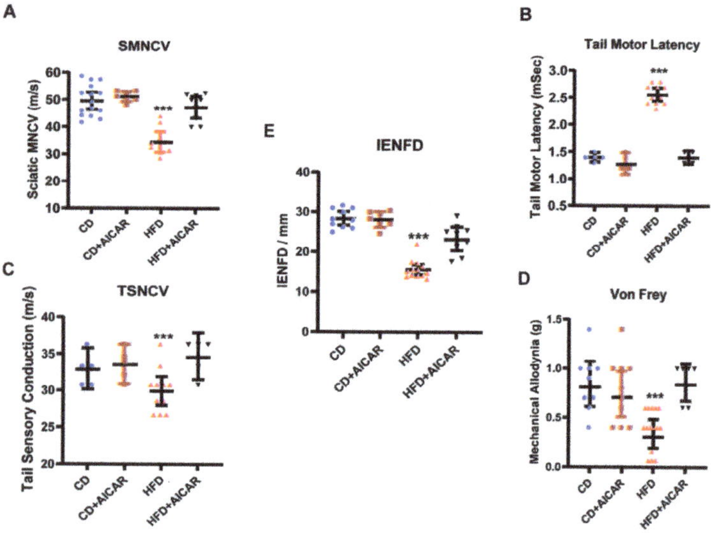

Figure 5. AICAR prevented HFD-induced neuropathy in C57Bl6 mice (n = 6 to 8 per group). WT C57BL6 mice were randomly assigned to four groups of six to eight mice per group. Group #1: CD; Group #2: CD+AICAR (500 mg/kg); Group #3: HFD; and Group #4: HFD+AICAR (500 mg/kg). Placebo or AICAR was administered for 4 months to CD and HFD mice. Mice were tested for the following parameters: SMNCV (**A**), TML (**B**), TSNCV (**C**), mechanical allodynia (MA) by Von Frey filament paw withdrawal threshold (**D**), and IENFD of the hind paw (**E**). Statistical comparisons were made among the 5 groups by ANOVA and post hoc Tukey test. *** $p < 0.001$; HFD, Group #3 at 4 months compared to all other groups in all the parameters.

After 4 months on an HFD, there was a significant decrease in the Von Frey paw withdrawal threshold in HFD compared to CD mice (CD = 1.42 ± 0.22 g vs. HFD = 0.64 ± 0.1 g; $p < 0.001$, consistent with the development of tactile allodynia). In contrast, the AICAR-injected HFD-fed mice had preserved NCVs, and the velocities were comparable to CD-fed mice (Figure 5). These findings are consistent with protection against peripheral neuropathy by the administration of AICAR. HFD+AICAR mice had normal tactile allodynia at 4 months compared to CD or CD+AICAR mice. Four months after feeding mice with either a CD or an HFD with and without AICAR treatment, the mice were euthanized, and paw skins were examined for IENFD (Figure 5). Skin biopsies showed a significant decrease in the IENFD of HFD mice (14.7 ± 2.35 fibers/mm) compared to CD mice (29 ± 4 fibers/mm; $p < 0.001$). On the other hand, in AICAR-treated mice fed with a CD or an HFD, the IENFD was the same as in CD mice (HFD+AICAR = 31 ± 3 fibers/mm). These results suggest that the administration of AICAR protected against HFD-induced peripheral neuropathy.

2.6. Subcutaneous Administration of AICAR Reversed HFD-Induced Peripheral Neuropathy in Mice

We tested whether the administration of AICAR could reverse DPN in an HFD-induced T2D model of peripheral neuropathy. C57BL6 mice (n = 8) were fed with an HFD for 2 months, and NCS were performed (Figure 6). After 2 months on an HFD, there was a significant decrease in the SMNCV, TSNCV, and Von Frey paw withdrawal threshold and an increase in the TML in the HFD mice compared to the CD mice that persisted up to 4 months and is consistent with developing DPN (Figure 6). At 2 months, AICAR was then administered to CD- and HFD-fed mice for an additional 2 months. At the end of 4 months, NCS were performed in all four groups. The results are shown in Figure 6. Administration of AICAR for a further 2 months in mice originally on an HFD alone for 2 months resulted in reversal of the NCVs and Von Frey thresholds, consistent with reversal of DPN (Figure 6). Four months after feeding mice with either a CD or an HFD, the mice were euthanized, and the paw skins were examined for the IENFD. Skin biopsies showed a significant decrease in the IENFD in the HFD mice (14.5 ± 2.5 fibers/mm) compared to the CD mice (29.6 ± 4.4 fibers/mm; $p < 0.001$). In contrast, in AICAR + HFD-fed mice, the IENFD were restored to CD mice levels (HFD+AICAR = 30.8 ± 3.2 fibers/mm). These results suggest that the administration of AICAR reversed the HFD-induced peripheral neuropathy.

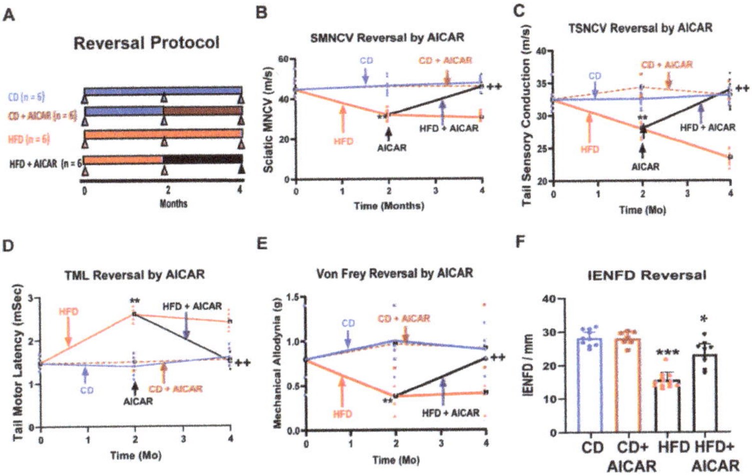

Figure 6. Two months of AICAR treatment reversed HFD-induced neuropathy in C57BL6 mice ($n = 6$/group). Three-month-old C57BL6 WT mice were fed with either a control diet (CD) or a high-fat diet (HFD). Baseline NCSs were completed at the beginning of the study. At 2 months, SMNCV, TML, TSNCV, and MA were measured in the mice fed a CD and the mice fed an HFD. After confirming that consumption of the HFD for 2 months induced development of peripheral neuropathy as observed by the changes in the NCSs and MA, AICAR was administered to the CD and HFD mice at a dose of 500 mg/kg for an additional 2 months. The vehicle was administered to CD and HFD mice. Nerve conduction studies were performed 2 months after administration of the AICAR or vehicle. The protocol is described in (**A**), the results of SMNCV (**B**), TSNCV (**C**), TML (**D**), MA using the Von Frey filament paw withdrawal threshold method (**E**), and intraepidermal fiber density (**F**) are shown. Statistical comparisons were made among the three groups with the ANOVA and post hoc Tukey test. * $p < 0.05$, ** $p < 0.01$, and *** $p < 0.001$; HFD mice at 2 months compared to 0-month-old HFD and CD mice in all parameters. $^{++}$ $p < 0.01$, HFD+AICAR mice at 4 months compared to HFD at 2 months in all parameters. The administration of AICAR reversed all the deficits of HFD-induced neuropathy. The administration of AICAR to non-diabetic mice had no significant effect. There was no statistically significant difference in CMAP or SNAP amplitudes compared between groups or compared at the start, during, and at the end of the treatment. The baseline (prior to starting any treatment) CMAP sciatic amplitude (mV) was 6.17 ± 0.78; CMAP tail amplitude (mV) was 3.050 ± 0.60, and SNAP tail amplitude (μV) was 51.92 ± 13.08. The CMAP sciatic amplitudes (mV) after 4 months of treatment were as follows: CD: 5.14 ± 0.99 (SEM); CD+AICAR: 5.70 ± 1.68; HFD: 8.31 ± 1.66; HFD+AICAR: 5.09 ± 0.76. The CMAP tail amplitudes (mV) after 4 months of treatment were as follows: CD: 1.24 ± 0.24; CD+AICAR: 2.16 ± 0.41; HFD: 2.96 ± 0.96; HFD+AICAR: 1.87 ± 0.70. The SNAP tail amplitudes (μV) after 4 months of treatment were as follows: CD: 102.48 ± 24.88; CD+AICAR: 126.77 ± 22.88; HFD: 56.21 ± 19.47; HFD+AICAR: 77.375 ± 19.46. There was no statistically significant difference in the CMAP or SNAP amplitudes during the reversal study, compared between groups or compared at the start and end of the treatment. This is as expected because of considerable variability in the CMAP and SNAP amplitudes [26–28].

2.7. Subcutaneous Administration of AICAR Reversed Type 1 Diabetic Peripheral Neuropathy Induced Via Streptozotocin (STZ) in Mice

In this experiment, we investigated whether AICAR would reverse DPN in a T1D model of STZ diabetic mice. To test this hypothesis, we purchased 3-month-old C57Bl6 STZ-induced diabetic mice (n = 20) and non-diabetic C57Bl6 mice (n = 12). Baseline neuropathy measurements were taken in non-diabetic and STZ-induced diabetic mice immediately after STZ induction (Figure 7, time point 0), and then all mice were fed a control diet (Harlan Teklad) for 1 month. At the end of 1 month, neuropathy measurements were made in all mice. Once neuropathy developed, based on measurements of the NCS, the diabetic mice were split into two groups: one group was administered AICAR in DMSO (5%)/alcohol (5%)/saline (90%) vehicle daily subcutaneously (*sc*) at a dose of 500 mg/kg for an additional 2 months (Group #4), and another group of diabetic mice was administered daily *sc* with the vehicle (Group #3) for an additional 2 months. Non-diabetic mice, likewise, were split into two groups. One group of mice was administered AICAR in vehicle (Group #2), and another group was administered the vehicle alone for 2 months (Group #1). At 3 months, nerve conduction studies and MA were measured in all four groups of mice. The results showed that at 1 month after STZ-induced diabetes, compared to the non-diabetic mice, the STZ mice had a significantly slower sciatic motor nerve conduction velocity (SMNCV) (from 43 ± 6 m/s in non-diabetic mice to 26.6 ± 7 m/s in the STZ mice; $p < 0.001$); an increased TML (from 1.12 ± 0.2 msec to 2.17 ± 0.09 msec; $p < 0.001$); decreased TSNCV (from 40.7 ± 2.6 m/s to 26.4 ± 3 m/s; $p < 0.001$), and had developed MA (Figure 6). However, the administration of AICAR to the STZ-induced diabetic mice for a further 2 months resulted in normal tactile allodynia at 3 months, while the von Frey paw withdrawal threshold was still decreased in the STZ mice (Figure 7). Hind paw skin biopsies at 3 months, showed that the intraepidermal nerve fiber density (IENFD) was significantly decreased in the STZ mice compared to the non-diabetic mice. In contrast, the IENFD was higher in the STZ + AICAR mice compared to the STZ mice (STZ = 11.5 ± 1.8 fibers/mm vs. STZ + AICAR = 25.1 ± 2.9 fibers/mm; $p < 0.001$). These findings show that the administration of AICAR could effectively reverse peripheral neuropathy in STZ-induced diabetic mice.

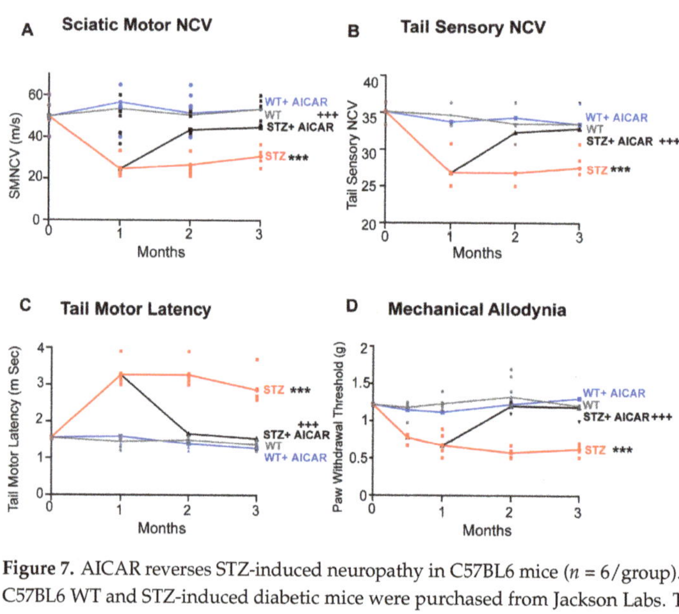

Figure 7. AICAR reverses STZ-induced neuropathy in C57BL6 mice (n = 6/group). Three-month-old C57BL6 WT and STZ-induced diabetic mice were purchased from Jackson Labs. The mice were fed

with a control diet for a month. Measurement of NCSs and MA after a month showed that the STZ mice had developed neuropathy. Some of the STZ mice were then administered AICAR at a dose of 500 mg/kg for an additional 2 months. NCSs were performed at 5 and 6 months of age, namely after 2 and 3 months of STZ-induced diabetes or after 1 or 2 months of AICAR treatment. The results are shown as follows: SMNCV (**A**), TSNCV (**B**), TML (**C**), and MA (**D**) using the Von Frey filament paw withdrawal threshold method. Statistical comparisons were made among the three groups with the ANOVA and post hoc Tukey test. *** $p < 0.001$; STZ at experimental time 3 months compared to 1 month in all parameters. $^{+++}$ $p < 0.001$, STZ+AICAR at experimental time 3 months compared to STZ at 1 month in all parameters. Thus, administration of AICAR reversed all the peripheral neuropathy deficits of STZ mice.

3. Discussion

3.1. DPN Affects Peripheral Neuronal Mitochondrial Metabolism

Mitochondria play a crucial role in providing energy (ATP) for maintaining membrane potential, supporting neuronal plasticity, and preventing neuropathy [16,29,30]. Several intersecting pathways can regulate mitochondrial function in DPN, including PGC-1α, TFAM, and SIRT1 [16–18]. Activation of AMPK acts as a common mechanism leading to an increase in SIRT1 and PGC-1α signaling with an improvement in mitochondrial function [14,31]. This study evaluated the potential of the exercise mimetic AICAR, an AMP analog, in promoting the elimination of dysfunctional mitochondria to prevent and reverse DPN.

3.2. Exercise Decreases Neuropathic Pain and Improves Cutaneous Nerve Fiber Branching in Diabetic Patients

Exercise plays a crucial role in reducing neuropathic pain and improving cutaneous nerve fiber branching in diabetic patients [2,4,6,32–35]. Moderately intense aerobic and resistance exercise has been shown to significantly reduce pain and neuropathic symptoms in people with DPN [4,6,33]. Moderate aerobic exercise benefits cutaneous regeneration capacity, even in patients with metabolic syndrome [8]. Both aerobic (endurance) and resistance exercise contribute to improved glycemic control and insulin sensitivity in individuals with diabetes [11,32,36]. Thus, a therapy, such as AICAR, that functions as an exercise mimetic would be expected to prevent or reverse DPN.

3.3. Exercise and AICAR Activate AMPK in Non-Neural Tissues

In response to exercise, the key molecule that modulates energy metabolism in muscle is AMP-activated protein kinase (AMPK) [10,37]. AMPK directly binds adenine nucleotides and senses the cellular energy status. When the ATP-to-ADP or ATP-to-AMP ratio changes, AMPK is activated through an allosteric mechanism, stimulating its kinase activity. AICAR, an AMP analog, binds to the same site as AMP and activates AMPK [10]. Once activated, AMPK orchestrates phosphorylation of key proteins in pathways related to lipid oxidation, glycolysis, and mitochondrial homeostasis [38–40]. In this study, compared to HFD mice, AICAR administration to HFD-fed mice over 4 months resulted in decreased body weight, reduced triglycerides, improvement in the HOMA-IR index, lower NEFA levels, and improved glycemic control (AUC in IP-GTT). The observed improvements in neuropathy measures in AICAR-treated HFD-fed mice could result from its effects on lipid reduction, decreased insulin resistance, better glycemic control, and resistance to weight gain [39,41–43]. This is supported by findings in non-neuronal tissue that show AMPK enhances the concentration of glucose transporters like GLUT 1 and GLUT 4, resulting in the lowering of blood glucose levels and the influx of blood glucose into cells [44]. Furthermore, AMPK increases insulin sensitivity and decreases insulin resistance. This was observed in primary Schwann cells treated with the saturated fatty acid palmitate to mimic prediabetic conditions to cause insulin resistance, which was reversed by AICAR [45].

3.4. AICAR Regulates Mitochondrial Homeostasis in DRG Neurons

Mitochondrial fission and fusion are important in maintaining both oxidative and reductive biosynthesis in response to a change in the availability of nutrients and bioenergetic demand [46]. Recent research has shown that there is specialization of mitochondria determined by the presence of cristae that promotes OXPHOS, while proline synthesis promotes mitochondria lacking in cristae. Thus, mitochondrial fission and fusion are important in maintaining both oxidative and reductive biosynthesis in response to changing nutrient availability and bioenergetic demand [46]. The primary effect of AICAR administration in high-fat diet (HFD)-fed mice was the regulation of mitochondrial homeostasis [10,19–22,47–52]. AICAR activated AMP-activated protein kinase (AMPK) in DRG neurons of HFD-fed mice (Figure 2). This activation led to phosphorylation of mitochondrial fission factor (MFF), recruitment of dynamin-like protein DRP1 to mitochondria, and activation of ULK1, an upstream kinase in autophagy and mitophagy. Mitochondrial fission is essential for mitophagy (Figure 3). It allows damaged mitochondria to be selectively degraded through mitophagy pathways. These findings are consistent with observations that AICAR treatment in primary myotubes increases FOXO3 expression and the expression of the mitochondrial E3 ligase Mul1 involved in mitochondrial mitophagy [51,53]. Furthermore, deacetylation of SIRT1 can induce mitophagy through the PINK1-Parkin pathway, while activation of the AMPK-mTOR-ULK complex induces autophagic cell death [54].

Importantly, AICAR also activates the mitochondrial biogenesis pathway [55–59]. This involves increasing the expression of PGC-1α and SIRT1 [56]. AICAR treatment brings about mitochondrial homeostasis by eliminating dysfunctional mitochondria and synthesizing new functional mitochondria. These effects occur in various peripheral tissues. Importantly, recent research reveals that DPN decreases SIRT1 expression in rodent skin [17]. Reduced SIRT1 leads to a decrease in brain-derived neurotrophic factor (BDNF). Loss of BDNF affects Meissner corpuscles, which are mechanoreceptors expressing the BDNF receptor TrkB. AICAR-induced overexpression of SIRT1 in skin promotes Meissner corpuscle reinnervation and regeneration. Consequently, this results in a significant improvement in diabetic MA.

3.5. AICAR for DPN

Metformin, in high doses, is an indirect activator of AMPK and currently serves as a first-line therapy for T2D [22,47,60–63]. Interestingly, it is also proposed as a potential therapeutic treatment for CNS neurological diseases. Metformin is a relatively weak activator of AMPK. Metformin would be expected to enhance neuronal bioenergetics, promote mitophagy, support nerve repair, and reduce toxic protein aggregates in neurological conditions. However, AICAR could be an even better therapeutic agent for neurological diseases. AICAR directly activates AMPK. It is transported into cells by the nucleoside transporter ENT1. AICAR increases the phosphorylation of AMPK only in HFD-fed mice and not in CD-fed mice (see Figure 2). Feeding with an HFD decreases AMPK phosphorylation, while AICAR reverses this process by binding to the AMP site on AMPK and inducing AMPK phosphorylation. Phosphorylated AMPK, in turn, promotes mitochondrial turnover to eliminate dysfunctional mitochondria, reduces mitochondrial oxidative stress, and contributes to its neuroprotective properties.

AICAR (acadesine) has been used in human studies. AICAR has been used to treat surgical ischemia to reduce post-perfusion myocardial infarction [64] and relapsing chronic leukemia [65]. In humans, doses up to 210 mg/kg IV are well tolerated [65]. At doses up to 100 mg/kg, only mild and transient side effects are reported equally in placebo and drug groups [66]. Thus, the dose used in this study in mice would fall well within the therapeutic human equivalent dose [67]. At doses greater than 200 mg/kg, adverse effects included hyperuricemia that occurred commonly but was not clinically significant and resolved with the administration of prophylactic allopurinol [65]. Other adverse events included transient anemia and/or thrombocytopenia (not clinically significant), renal impairment, and transient infusion-related hypotension (clinically significant) [65]. Furthermore, AICAR was well tolerated in more than 4000 cardiac patients [64,66,68–70]. Unfortunately, the energy-promoting effects of AICAR have led to abuse in human athletes and animals involved in sports [71]. To place this in context, AICAR is a normal cellular intermediate in the human body [72] at concentrations necessary for human cellular activity, is orally active [25], but bioavailability is poor [66]. Thus, at physiological concentrations, AICAR is non-toxic in the body. However, if AICAR is abused at high, sustained doses, it would be expected to be toxic. However, there is interest in developing direct AMPK activators that may be safer. For example, DW14006, administered at a dose of 15 or 30 mg/kg by i.p. injection for 4 weeks, has been shown to ameliorate DPN by regulating mitochondrial dysfunction, oxidative stress, and inflammation [73].

3.6. Potential Limitations of the Study

We did not address the combined effect of exercise and AICAR. This is because the premise in this study is that many patients with DPN cannot exercise due to significant neuropathic pain and poor balance and therefore need an alternative to exercise to reduce the effect of DPN. However, exercise has been tested in mice for running endurance. In sedentary mice, 4 weeks of AICAR treatment alone induced metabolic genes and enhanced running endurance by 44% [25]. However, it was also shown in the same study that AMPK activation and exercise training synergistically increased oxidative myofibers and running endurance in adult mice [25,74]. Other potential limitations of the study include no statistically significant difference in the compound CMAP or SNAP amplitudes compared between groups or compared at the start and end of the treatment. There were statistically significant differences in the motor and sensory conduction velocities and latencies as described in the results. The increased variances in the CMAP or SNAP amplitudes have been previously recognized [26–28]. Variances may have been improved by increasing the number of animals tested or the number of data points in each group. Furthermore, there were no measurements of the number of innervated Meissner's corpuscles in the paw pads. In a recent publication, we and colleagues showed that in both HFD and STZ mouse models of DPN, there was profound loss of Meissner corpuscles as well as degeneration or retraction of the Aβ sensory axons that innervate them [17].

4. Materials and Methods

4.1. CD and HFD

All animal protocols followed the National Institutes of Health (NIH) Guide for the Care and Use of Laboratory Animals and were approved by the Institutional Animal Care and Use Committee. To ensure that our results are robust, unbiased, and reproducible, the following was performed for all experiments: (1) random assignment of mice; (2) performance of behavioral studies by personnel blinded to the identity of the groups; (3) blind assessment of outcome measures; and (4) specific exclusion criteria identified prior to initiation of all experiments. Three-month-old, wild-type, C57BL6 mice were fed with a CD or an HFD. The CD (Harlan Teklad #2018) contained 6.2% fat (18% calories from fat), 18.6% protein (24% calories from protein), and 44.2% carbohydrate (58% calories from carbohydrate). The HFD (Bio-Serv #F3282) contained 36% fat (60% calories from fat),

20.5% protein (15% calories from protein), and 37.5% carbohydrate (26% calories from carbohydrate). In the prevention studies, NCS and Von Frey measurements were performed at baseline, and the animals were randomized into the treatment groups. We ensured that there was no difference between any of the test groups in the baseline measurements. Those performing the testing were blinded to the test group. Animals in the HFD group were treated with the HFD as described above for a period of 4 months. Animals treated with AICAR were given AICAR 500 mg/kg sc for the duration of the study as described in Section 4.2. NCS, Von Frey, IENFD, and tissues were collected at 4 months. In the reversal study, baseline studies were performed, and animals were randomized into the treatment groups. Baseline values were confirmed to not be statistically different between the treatment groups. Three-month-old male C57BL6 WT mice were fed with either a control diet (CD) or a high-fat diet (HFD) for 2 months. NCS and Von Frey testing was performed at baseline, 2 months, and 4 months. After confirming that consumption of the HFD for 2 months induced development of peripheral neuropathy as observed by the changes in the NCSs and MA, AICAR (as in Section 4.2 below) was administered to the CD and HFD mice at a dose of 500 mg/kg for an additional 2 months. The vehicle was administered to CD and HFD mice. NCS were performed 2 months after administration of the AICAR or the vehicle (4-month time point).

4.2. Diabetes Induction with STZ

Three-month-old male C57BL6 WT and streptozotocin (STZ)-induced diabetic mice were purchased from Jackson Labs. Six-week-old males were identified, weighed, and a baseline non-fasted glucose measurement was taken with a OneTouch Ultra2 or Ultra/Mini glucometer. Mice received daily IP injections of 50 mg STZ/kg body weight (C57BL/6J) for five consecutive days; age-matched controls received buffer injections. Mice were housed in disposable cages with absorbent bedding and ad libitum access to food and water while they metabolized STZ for at least 48 h after the final injection. After transfer to regular cages, mice were observed daily, then weighed and glucose-tested 7–14 days after the final injection. In addition, only healthy mice without significant changes in body weight were used.

Baseline neuropathy measurements were taken in both groups (time point 0), and then all mice were fed a control diet (Harlan Teklad #2018) for 1 month. Diabetic mice having a fasting blood glucose level of 300 mg/dL (11 mmol/L) were used (8 weeks old). At the end of the month of STZ diabetes, neuropathy measurements were performed in all mice. Once DPN developed, the diabetic mice were split into two groups: one group was administered AICAR, which was dissolved in DMSO (5%)/alcohol (5%)/saline (90%), and 100 μL of this solution was administered subcutaneously (*sc*) for 3 days in a week (Monday, Wednesday, and Friday) at a dose of 500 mg/kg for an additional 2 months (Group #4), and another group of diabetic mice were administered the vehicle, DMSO (5%)/alcohol (5%)/saline (90%) for an additional 2 months (Group #3). Non-diabetic mice, likewise, were divided into two groups. One group of mice was administered AICAR in the vehicle (Group #2), and another group was administered the vehicle alone for 2 months (Group #1). At 3 months, nerve conduction studies and MA were measured in all four groups of mice.

4.3. Western Blot Analysis

Mouse DRG neurons were collected, and proteins were extracted with an ice-cold extraction buffer with protease and phosphatase inhibitors [18,30]. Protein concentration was determined with a BCA kit (BCA Protein Assay Kit, P0010). Equal amounts of protein samples (30 μg) were electrophoresed on SDS-PAGE gels and transferred to PVDF membranes [30]. The membranes were blocked with 5% BSA in a TBST buffer and incubated overnight at 4°C with different primary antibodies: The sources of the various antibodies used in this study were: Cell Signaling: AMPKα Antibody #2532; Phospho-AMPKα (Thr172) Antibody #2531; β-Actin (13E5) Rabbit mAb #4970; LC3A/B (D3U4C) XP® Rabbit mAb #12741; DRP1 (D6C7) Rabbit mAb #8570; Phospho-ULK1 (Ser555) (D1H4) Rabbit mAb #5869; VDAC Antibody #4866; ENT1 Polyclonal Antibody, PA5-116468 (Invitrogen, Carlsbad, CA, USA). The intensity was normalized to β-actin or VDAC. After rinsing with TBST, the membranes were incubated with a secondary antibody, peroxidase-conjugated goat anti-rabbit IgG (H+L). The membranes were developed with an advanced reagent (Bio-Rad, Hercules, CA, USA), and the protein bands were visualized with an automatic chemiluminescence apparatus (Bio-Rad, USA). The densities of the bands were determined using the Bio-Rad software 2.4.

4.4. Isolation of Mitochondria

Dorsal root ganglion mitochondria from mouse brain were isolated using a Percoll (Amersham Biosciences, Piscataway, NJ, USA) gradient centrifugation as described previously [14]. Briefly, DRG neurons were homogenized in ice-cold mitochondria isolation buffer (225 mmol/L mannitol, 75 mmol/L sucrose, 5 mmol/L HEPES, 1 mmol/L EGTA, 1 mg/mL fatty-acid-free bovine serum albumin [BSA], pH 7.4 at 4°C). The homogenate was centrifuged at 1300× *g* for 3 min, and the pellet was resuspended and centrifuged again at 1300× *g* for 3 min. The pooled supernatants were centrifuged at 22,200× *g* for 8 min, the crude mitochondrial pellet was resuspended in 15% Percoll, and layered on a pre-formed gradient of 40% and 24% Percoll. After centrifugation at 31,700× *g* for 8 min, the mitochondria were collected from the interface of the lower two layers, diluted with isolation medium, and centrifuged at 16,700× *g* for 10 min. The mitochondrial pellet was then resuspended to a final volume of 1.5 mL of mitochondrial storage buffer (230 mM mannitol, 70 mM sucrose, 0.02 mM EGTA, 20 mM Tris-HCl, 5 mM K_2HPO_4, pH 7.4) and centrifuged at 22,000× *g* for 10 min at 4 °C in a microfuge. The resulting mitochondrial pellet was resuspended in the mitochondrial storage without EGTA. Protein concentrations were determined by the BCA method.

4.5. Mitochondrial Respiration

Isolated mitochondria were diluted in cold 1x respiration buffer (230 mM mannitol, 70 mM sucrose, 0.02 mM EDTA, 20 mM Tris-HCl, 5 mM K2HPO4 at pH 7.4, 37 °C) and transferred to a Seahorse 24-well plate (10 µg Mt in each well) and spun at 2000× *g* for 20 min to settle the mitochondria [75–77]. To assess complex I-mediated respiration, malate and pyruvate were used as substrates. State 3 respiration was initiated by the addition of 40 mM ADP. Approximately 2 min later, state 3 respiration was terminated, and state 4° respiration (resting) was initiated with the addition of 20 µM oligomycin, an inhibitor of the mitochondrial ATP synthase. The maximal rate of uncoupled respiration was subsequently measured by the addition of 40 µM carbonyl cyanide p-(trifluoromethoxy)phenylhydrazone (FCCP), which is a protonophore uncoupling molecule. Rates are an average of 4–6 independent experiments for complex I respiration.

4.6. Neuropathy Measurements

The guidelines of the European diabetic neuropathy study group of the EASD (Neurodiab) were used to test peripheral neuropathy [26]. Somedic von Frey monofilaments were used to assess MA [14,30]. Nerve conduction studies were performed as described [30]. The PGP9.5 antibody staining, in a blinded fashion, was used to measure the IENFD, as previously described [30]. The IENFD was calculated (as fibers/mm) by the number of complete baseline crossings of nerve fibers at the dermo–epidermal junction divided by the measured length of the epidermal surface using standardized validated methods [78,79].

4.7. Statistical Analysis

Variances from the mean in described data are standard errors of the mean (SEM) unless otherwise described. To determine the significance among the groups, the data were transformed using factorial ANOVA with a post hoc Tukey test, and then a comparison of dependent variables was performed. Individual comparisons were made using Student's t-test, assuming unequal variances as previously described [80]. The associations between mitochondrial function and measures of neuropathy (NCVs and MA) were evaluated using Spearman correlation statistics.

5. Conclusions

In summary, the administration of AICAR increased phosphorylation of AMPK. Phosphorylated AMPK, in turn, activated proteins involved in the segregation of mitochondria by promoting mitochondrial fission. Administration of AICAR also improved insulin sensitivity, glucose, and lipid metabolism. These metabolic effects, in turn, protected or reversed DPN in both T1D and T2D mouse models. Drugs targeting AMPK phosphorylation, such as AICAR, may function as exercise mimetics. Humans with DPN are often disabled and cannot exercise adequately. Thus, exercise mimetics could play a crucial role as therapy in DPN, but this would require further clinical trials in humans to assess this. AICAR directs AMPK activation and transport via ENT1 and makes it an intriguing candidate for further investigation to develop isoform-specific AMPK activators in the nervous system. The neuroprotective properties of AMPK activators could be utilized in DPN, but further studies are needed in humans.

Author Contributions: K.C., J.C. and J.W.R.; methodology, J.C., M.S. and A.F.H.; software and validation, K.C., J.C., A.F.H. and M.S.; formal analysis, J.C., M.S. and A.F.H.; investigation, K.C. and J.W.R.; resources, J.W.R.; writing—original draft preparation, K.C., J.C. and J.W.R.; writing—review and editing, K.C. and J.W.R.; project administration, K.C. and J.W.R.; funding acquisition, J.W.R. All authors have read and agreed to the published version of the manuscript.

Funding: This study was supported in part by the National Institute of Diabetes and Digestive and Kidney Diseases, National Institutes of Health 1R01DK107007-01A1, Office of Research Development, Department of Veterans Affairs (Biomedical and Laboratory Research Service and Rehabilitation Research and Development, 101RX001030), Diabetes Action Research and Education Foundation (J.W.R.), and the Atlantic Nutrition Obesity Research Center, grant P30 DK072488 from the National Institute of Diabetes and Digestive and Kidney Diseases, National Institutes of Health.

Institutional Review Board Statement: Approved by University of Maryland, Baltimore, Animal Welfare Assurance Committee. The approval numbers are 0421009 and 0518013.

Informed Consent Statement: Not applicable.

Data Availability Statement: Data are available on request.

Conflicts of Interest: The authors declare no conflicts of interest.

References

1. Smith, A.G.; Russell, J.W.; Feldman, E.L.; Goldstein, J.; Peltier, A.; Smith, S.; Hamwi, J.; Pollari, D.; Bixby, B.; Howard, J.; et al. Lifestyle intervention for prediabetic neuropathy. *Diabetes Care* **2006**, *29*, 1294–1299. [CrossRef]
2. Zilliox, L.A.; Russell, J.W. Physical activity and dietary interventions in diabetic neuropathy: A systematic review. *Clin. Auton. Res.* **2019**, *4*, 443–455. [CrossRef]
3. Feldman, E.L.; Callaghan, B.C.; Pop-Busui, R.; Zochodne, D.W.; Wright, D.E.; Bennett, D.L.; Bril, V.; Russell, J.W.; Viswanathan, V. Diabetic neuropathy. *Nat. Rev. Dis. Primers* **2019**, *5*, 41. [CrossRef]
4. Kluding, P.M.; Pasnoor, M.; Singh, R.; Jernigan, S.; Farmer, K.; Rucker, J.; Sharma, N.K.; Wright, D.E. The effect of exercise on neuropathic symptoms, nerve function, and cutaneous innervation in people with diabetic peripheral neuropathy. *J. Diabetes Complicat.* **2012**, *26*, 424–429. [CrossRef] [PubMed]

5. Balducci, S.; Iacobellis, G.; Parisi, L.; Di Biase, N.; Calandriello, E.; Leonetti, F.; Fallucca, F. Exercise training can modify the natural history of diabetic peripheral neuropathy. *J. Diabetes Complicat.* **2006**, *20*, 216–223. [CrossRef] [PubMed]
6. Knauf, M.T.; Koltyn, K.F. Exercise-induced modulation of pain in adults with and without painful diabetic neuropathy. *J. Pain* **2014**, *15*, 656–663. [CrossRef]
7. Nakagawa, N.; Yamamoto, S.; Hanai, A.; Oiwa, A.; Arao, H. Exercise intervention for the management of chemotherapy-induced peripheral neuropathy: A systematic review and network meta-analysis. *Front. Neurol.* **2024**, *15*, 1346099. [CrossRef] [PubMed]
8. Singleton, J.R.; Marcus, R.L.; Lessard, M.K.; Jackson, J.E.; Smith, A.G. Supervised exercise improves cutaneous reinnervation capacity in metabolic syndrome patients. *Ann. Neurol.* **2015**, *77*, 146–153. [CrossRef]
9. Nelson, K.M.; Reiber, G.; Boyko, E.J. Diet and exercise among adults with type 2 diabetes: Findings from the third national health and nutrition examination survey (NHANES III). *Diabetes Care* **2002**, *25*, 1722–1728. [CrossRef]
10. Herzig, S.; Shaw, R.J. AMPK: Guardian of metabolism and mitochondrial homeostasis. *Nat. Rev. Mol. Cell Biol.* **2018**, *19*, 121–135. [CrossRef]
11. O'Neill, H.M. AMPK and Exercise: Glucose Uptake and Insulin Sensitivity. *Diabetes Metab. J.* **2013**, *37*, 1–21. [CrossRef]
12. Viollet, B.; Mounier, R.; Leclerc, J.; Yazigi, A.; Foretz, M.; Andreelli, F. Targeting AMP-activated protein kinase as a novel therapeutic approach for the treatment of metabolic disorders. *Diabetes Metab.* **2007**, *33*, 395–402. [CrossRef]
13. Hardie, D.G. AMPK: A key regulator of energy balance in the single cell and the whole organism. *Int. J. Obes.* **2008**, *32* (Suppl. S4), S7–S12. [CrossRef] [PubMed]
14. Choi, J.; Chandrasekaran, K.; Inoue, T.; Muragundla, A.; Russell, J.W. PGC-1α regulation of mitochondrial degeneration in experimental diabetic neuropathy. *Neurobiol. Dis.* **2014**, *64*, 118–130. [CrossRef] [PubMed]
15. Chandrasekaran, K.; Najimi, N.; Sagi, A.R.; Yarlagadda, S.; Salimian, M.; Arvas, M.I.; Hedayat, A.F.; Kevas, Y.; Kadakia, A.; Russell, J.W. NAD$^+$ Precursors Repair Mitochondrial Function in Diabetes and Prevent Experimental Diabetic Neuropathy. *Int. J. Mol. Sci.* **2022**, *23*, 4887. [CrossRef] [PubMed]
16. Chandrasekaran, K.; Anjaneyulu, M.; Choi, J.; Kumar, P.; Salimian, M.; Ho, C.Y.; Russell, J.W. Role of mitochondria in diabetic peripheral neuropathy: Influencing the NAD$^+$-dependent SIRT1-PGC-1alpha-TFAM pathway. *Int. Rev. Neurobiol.* **2019**, *145*, 177–209. [CrossRef]
17. O'Brien, J.; Niehaus, P.; Chang, K.; Remark, J.; Barrett, J.; Dasgupta, A.; Adenegan, M.; Salimian, M.; Kevas, Y.; Chandrasekaran, K.; et al. Skin keratinocyte-derived SIRT1 and BDNF modulate mechanical allodynia in mouse models of diabetic neuropathy. *bioRxiv* **2024**, *147*, 3471–3486. [CrossRef] [PubMed]
18. Chandrasekaran, K.; Najimi, N.; Sagi, A.R.; Yarlagadda, S.; Salimian, M.; Arvas, M.I.; Hedayat, A.F.; Kevas, Y.; Kadakia, A.; Kristian, T.; et al. NAD$^+$ Precursors Reverse Experimental Diabetic Neuropathy in Mice. *Int. J. Mol. Sci.* **2024**, *25*, 1102. [CrossRef] [PubMed]
19. Laker, R.C.; Drake, J.C.; Wilson, R.J.; Lira, V.A.; Lewellen, B.M.; Ryall, K.A.; Fisher, C.C.; Zhang, M.; Saucerman, J.J.; Goodyear, L.J.; et al. Ampk phosphorylation of Ulk1 is required for targeting of mitochondria to lysosomes in exercise-induced mitophagy. *Nat. Commun.* **2017**, *8*, 548. [CrossRef] [PubMed]
20. Tian, W.; Li, W.; Chen, Y.; Yan, Z.; Huang, X.; Zhuang, H.; Zhong, W.; Chen, Y.; Wu, W.; Lin, C.; et al. Phosphorylation of ULK1 by AMPK regulates translocation of ULK1 to mitochondria and mitophagy. *FEBS Lett.* **2015**, *589*, 1847–1854. [CrossRef]
21. Seabright, A.P.; Lai, Y.C. Regulatory Roles of PINK1-Parkin and AMPK in Ubiquitin-Dependent Skeletal Muscle Mitophagy. *Front. Physiol.* **2020**, *11*, 608474. [CrossRef] [PubMed]
22. Zhang, Y.; Zhang, T.; Li, Y.; Guo, Y.; Liu, B.; Tian, Y.; Wu, P.; Shi, H. Metformin attenuates early brain injury after subarachnoid hemorrhage in rats via AMPK-dependent mitophagy. *Exp. Neurol.* **2022**, *353*, 114055. [CrossRef]
23. Li, W.; Gao, M.; Hu, C.; Chen, X.; Zhou, Y. NMNAT2: An important metabolic enzyme affecting the disease progression. *Biomed. Pharmacother.* **2023**, *158*, 114143. [CrossRef] [PubMed]
24. Buhl, E.S.; Jessen, N.; Pold, R.; Ledet, T.; Flyvbjerg, A.; Pedersen, S.B.; Pedersen, O.; Schmitz, O.; Lund, S. Long-term AICAR administration reduces metabolic disturbances and lowers blood pressure in rats displaying features of the insulin resistance syndrome. *Diabetes* **2002**, *51*, 2199–2206. [CrossRef] [PubMed]
25. Narkar, V.A.; Downes, M.; Yu, R.T.; Embler, E.; Wang, Y.X.; Banayo, E.; Mihaylova, M.M.; Nelson, M.C.; Zou, Y.; Juguilon, H.; et al. AMPK and PPARdelta agonists are exercise mimetics. *Cell* **2008**, *134*, 405–415. [CrossRef] [PubMed]
26. Biessels, G.J.; Bril, V.; Calcutt, N.A.; Cameron, N.E.; Cotter, M.A.; Dobrowsky, R.; Feldman, E.L.; Fernyhough, P.; Jakobsen, J.; Malik, R.A.; et al. Phenotyping animal models of diabetic neuropathy: A consensus statement of the diabetic neuropathy study group of the EASD (Neurodiab). *J. Peripher. Nerv. Syst.* **2014**, *19*, 77–87. [CrossRef]
27. Chaudhry, V.; Cornblath, D.R.; Mellits, E.D.; Avila, O.; Freimer, M.L.; Glass, J.D.; Reim, J.; Ronnett, G.V.; Quaskey, S.A.; Kuncl, R.W. Inter- and intra-examiner reliability of nerve conduction measurements in normal subjects. *Ann. Neurol.* **1991**, *30*, 841–843. [CrossRef] [PubMed]
28. Dyck, P.J.; Albers, J.W.; Wolfe, J.; Bolton, C.F.; Walsh, N.; Klein, C.J.; Zafft, A.J.; Russell, J.W.; Thomas, K.; Davies, J.L.; et al. A trial of proficiency of nerve conduction: Greater standardization still needed. *Muscle Nerve* **2013**, *48*, 369–374. [CrossRef]

29. Flatters, S.J. The contribution of mitochondria to sensory processing and pain. *Prog. Mol. Biol. Transl. Sci.* **2015**, *131*, 119–146. [CrossRef] [PubMed]
30. Chandrasekaran, K.; Salimian, M.; Konduru, S.R.; Choi, J.; Kumar, P.; Long, A.; Klimova, N.; Ho, C.Y.; Kristian, T.; Russell, J.W. Overexpression of Sirtuin 1 protein in neurons prevents and reverses experimental diabetic neuropathy. *Brain* **2019**, *142*, 3737–3752. [CrossRef]
31. Fakhri, S.; Moradi, S.Z.; Moradi, S.Y.; Piri, S.; Shiri Varnamkhasti, B.; Piri, S.; Khirehgesh, M.R.; Bishayee, A.; Casarcia, N.; Bishayee, A. Phytochemicals regulate cancer metabolism through modulation of the AMPK/PGC-1α signaling pathway. *BMC Cancer* **2024**, *24*, 1079. [CrossRef] [PubMed]
32. Groover, A.L.; Ryals, J.M.; Guilford, B.L.; Wilson, N.M.; Christianson, J.A.; Wright, D.E. Exercise-mediated improvements in painful neuropathy associated with prediabetes in mice. *Pain* **2013**, *154*, 2658–2667. [CrossRef]
33. Hernando-Garijo, I.; Medrano-de-la-Fuente, R.; Mingo-Gomez, M.T.; Lahuerta Martin, S.; Ceballos-Laita, L.; Jimenez-Del-Barrio, S. Effects of exercise therapy on diabetic neuropathy: A systematic review and meta-analysis. *Physiother. Theory Pract.* **2023**, *40*, 2116–2129. [CrossRef]
34. Tumusiime, D.K.; Stewart, A.; Venter, F.W.D.; Musenge, E. The effects of a physiotherapist-led exercise intervention on peripheral neuropathy among people living with HIV on antiretroviral therapy in Kigali, Rwanda. *S. Afr. J. Physiother.* **2019**, *75*, 1328. [CrossRef] [PubMed]
35. White, C.M.; Pritchard, J.; Turner-Stokes, L. Exercise for people with peripheral neuropathy. *Cochrane Database Syst. Rev.* **2004**, CD003904. [CrossRef]
36. Friedrichsen, M.; Mortensen, B.; Pehmoller, C.; Birk, J.B.; Wojtaszewski, J.F. Exercise-induced AMPK activity in skeletal muscle: Role in glucose uptake and insulin sensitivity. *Mol. Cell Endocrinol.* **2013**, *366*, 204–214. [CrossRef] [PubMed]
37. Jorgensen, S.B.; Rose, A.J. How is AMPK activity regulated in skeletal muscles during exercise? *Front. Biosci.* **2008**, *13*, 5589–5604. [CrossRef]
38. Shah, A.K.; Gupta, A.; Dey, C.S. AICAR induced AMPK activation potentiates neuronal insulin signaling and glucose uptake. *Arch. Biochem. Biophys.* **2011**, *509*, 142–146. [CrossRef]
39. Tukhovskaya, E.A.; Shaykhutdinova, E.R.; Pakhomova, I.A.; Slashcheva, G.A.; Goryacheva, N.A.; Sadovnikova, E.S.; Rasskazova, E.A.; Kazakov, V.A.; Dyachenko, I.A.; Frolova, A.A.; et al. AICAR Improves Outcomes of Metabolic Syndrome and Type 2 Diabetes Induced by High-Fat Diet in C57Bl/6 Male Mice. *Int. J. Mol. Sci.* **2022**, *23*, 15719. [CrossRef]
40. Wang, H.; Zheng, A.; Thorley, D.; Arias, E.B.; Cartee, G.D. Independent and combined effects of calorie restriction and AICAR on glucose uptake and insulin signaling in skeletal muscles from 24-month-old female and male rats. *Appl. Physiol. Nutr. Metab.* **2024**, *49*, 614–625. [CrossRef]
41. Borgeson, E.; Wallenius, V.; Syed, G.H.; Darshi, M.; Lantero Rodriguez, J.; Biorserud, C.; Ragnmark Ek, M.; Bjorklund, P.; Quiding-Jarbrink, M.; Fandriks, L.; et al. AICAR ameliorates high-fat diet-associated pathophysiology in mouse and ex vivo models, independent of adiponectin. *Diabetologia* **2017**, *60*, 729–739. [CrossRef]
42. Du, L.L.; Chai, D.M.; Zhao, L.N.; Li, X.H.; Zhang, F.C.; Zhang, H.B.; Liu, L.B.; Wu, K.; Liu, R.; Wang, J.Z.; et al. AMPK activation ameliorates Alzheimer's disease-like pathology and spatial memory impairment in a streptozotocin-induced Alzheimer's disease model in rats. *J. Alzheimers Dis.* **2015**, *43*, 775–784. [CrossRef] [PubMed]
43. Habib, S.L.; Yadav, A.; Kidane, D.; Weiss, R.H.; Liang, S. Novel protective mechanism of reducing renal cell damage in diabetes: Activation AMPK by AICAR increased NRF2/OGG1 proteins and reduced oxidative DNA damage. *Cell Cycle* **2016**, *15*, 3048–3059. [CrossRef] [PubMed]
44. Kakoti, B.B.; Alom, S.; Deka, K.; Halder, R.K. AMPK pathway: An emerging target to control diabetes mellitus and its related complications. *J. Diabetes Metab. Disord.* **2024**, *23*, 441–459. [CrossRef]
45. Eid, S.A.; Elzinga, S.E.; Kim, B.; Rumora, A.E.; Hayes, J.M.; Carter, A.; Pacut, C.; Allouch, A.M.; Koubek, E.J.; Feldman, E.L. High-Intensity Interval Training, Caloric Restriction, or Their Combination Have Beneficial Effects on Metabolically Acquired Peripheral Neuropathy. *Diabetes* **2024**, *73*, 1895–1907. [CrossRef] [PubMed]
46. Ryu, K.W.; Fung, T.S.; Baker, D.C.; Saoi, M.; Park, J.; Febres-Aldana, C.A.; Aly, R.G.; Cui, R.; Sharma, A.; Fu, Y.; et al. Cellular ATP demand creates metabolically distinct subpopulations of mitochondria. *Nature* **2024**, *635*, 746–754. [CrossRef] [PubMed]
47. Dombi, E.; Mortiboys, H.; Poulton, J. Modulating Mitophagy in Mitochondrial Disease. *Curr. Med. Chem.* **2018**, *25*, 5597–5612. [CrossRef] [PubMed]
48. Gao, J.; Yu, L.; Wang, Z.; Wang, R.; Liu, X. Induction of mitophagy in C2C12 cells by electrical pulse stimulation involves increasing the level of the mitochondrial receptor FUNDC1 through the AMPK-ULK1 pathway. *Am. J. Transl. Res.* **2020**, *12*, 6879–6894.
49. Garrido-Maraver, J.; Paz, M.V.; Cordero, M.D.; Bautista-Lorite, J.; Oropesa-Avila, M.; de la Mata, M.; Pavon, A.D.; de Lavera, I.; Alcocer-Gomez, E.; Galan, F.; et al. Critical role of AMP-activated protein kinase in the balance between mitophagy and mitochondrial biogenesis in MELAS disease. *Biochim. Biophys. Acta* **2015**, *1852*, 2535–2553. [CrossRef] [PubMed]

50. Villanueva Paz, M.; Cotan, D.; Garrido-Maraver, J.; Cordero, M.D.; Oropesa-Avila, M.; de La Mata, M.; Delgado Pavon, A.; de Lavera, I.; Alcocer-Gomez, E.; Sanchez-Alcazar, J.A. Targeting autophagy and mitophagy for mitochondrial diseases treatment. *Expert. Opin. Ther. Targets* **2016**, *20*, 487–500. [CrossRef] [PubMed]
51. Wu, B.; Chen, Y.; Clarke, R.; Akala, E.; Yang, P.; He, B.; Gao, H. AMPK Signaling Regulates Mitophagy and Mitochondrial ATP Production in Human Trophoblast Cell Line BeWo. *Front. Biosci.* **2022**, *27*, 118. [CrossRef] [PubMed]
52. Iorio, R.; Celenza, G.; Petricca, S. Mitophagy: Molecular Mechanisms, New Concepts on Parkin Activation and the Emerging Role of AMPK/ULK1 Axis. *Cells* **2021**, *11*, 30. [CrossRef] [PubMed]
53. Sanchez, A.M.J.; Candau, R.; Bernardi, H. AMP-activated protein kinase stabilizes FOXO3 in primary myotubes. *Biochem. Biophys. Res. Commun.* **2018**, *499*, 493–498. [CrossRef] [PubMed]
54. Yao, Z.Q.; Zhang, X.; Zhen, Y.; He, X.Y.; Zhao, S.; Li, X.F.; Yang, B.; Gao, F.; Guo, F.Y.; Fu, L.; et al. A novel small-molecule activator of Sirtuin-1 induces autophagic cell death/mitophagy as a potential therapeutic strategy in glioblastoma. *Cell Death Dis.* **2018**, *9*, 767. [CrossRef] [PubMed]
55. Chowdhury, S.K.; Dobrowsky, R.T.; Fernyhough, P. Nutrient excess and altered mitochondrial proteome and function contribute to neurodegeneration in diabetes. *Mitochondrion* **2011**, *11*, 845–854. [CrossRef]
56. Higashida, K.; Kim, S.H.; Jung, S.R.; Asaka, M.; Holloszy, J.O.; Han, D.H. Effects of resveratrol and SIRT1 on PGC-1α activity and mitochondrial biogenesis: A reevaluation. *PLoS Biol.* **2013**, *11*, e1001603. [CrossRef] [PubMed]
57. Lempiainen, J.; Finckenberg, P.; Levijoki, J.; Mervaala, E. AMPK activator AICAR ameliorates ischaemia reperfusion injury in the rat kidney. *Br. J. Pharmacol.* **2012**, *166*, 1905–1915. [CrossRef] [PubMed]
58. Li, J.; Liu, Y.; Liu, B.; Li, F.; Hu, J.; Wang, Q.; Li, M.; Lou, S. Mechanisms of Aerobic Exercise Upregulating the Expression of Hippocampal Synaptic Plasticity-Associated Proteins in Diabetic Rats. *Neural Plast.* **2019**, *2019*, 7920540. [CrossRef]
59. Price, N.L.; Gomes, A.P.; Ling, A.J.; Duarte, F.V.; Martin-Montalvo, A.; North, B.J.; Agarwal, B.; Ye, L.; Ramadori, G.; Teodoro, J.S.; et al. SIRT1 is required for AMPK activation and the beneficial effects of resveratrol on mitochondrial function. *Cell Metab.* **2012**, *15*, 675–690. [CrossRef] [PubMed]
60. Demare, S.; Kothari, A.; Calcutt, N.A.; Fernyhough, P. Metformin as a potential therapeutic for neurological disease: Mobilizing AMPK to repair the nervous system. *Expert Rev. Neurother.* **2021**, *21*, 45–63. [CrossRef] [PubMed]
61. Guo, Y.; Jiang, H.; Wang, M.; Ma, Y.; Zhang, J.; Jing, L. Metformin alleviates cerebral ischemia/reperfusion injury aggravated by hyperglycemia via regulating AMPK/ULK1/PINK1/Parkin pathway-mediated mitophagy and apoptosis. *Chem. Biol. Interact.* **2023**, *384*, 110723. [CrossRef]
62. Menassol, J.B.; Tautou, C.; Collet, A.; Chesneau, D.; Lomet, D.; Dupont, J.; Malpaux, B.; Scaramuzzi, R.J. The effect of an intracerebroventricular injection of metformin or AICAR on the plasma concentrations of melatonin in the ewe: Potential involvement of AMPK? *BMC Neurosci.* **2011**, *12*, 76. [CrossRef] [PubMed]
63. Williams, T.; Courchet, J.; Viollet, B.; Brenman, J.E.; Polleux, F. AMP-activated protein kinase (AMPK) activity is not required for neuronal development but regulates axogenesis during metabolic stress. *Proc. Natl. Acad. Sci. USA* **2011**, *108*, 5849–5854. [CrossRef] [PubMed]
64. Mangano, D.T.; Miao, Y.; Tudor, I.C.; Dietzel, C.; Investigators of the Multicenter Study of Perioperative Ischemia (McSPI) Research Group; Ischemia Research and Education Foundation (IREF). Post-reperfusion myocardial infarction: Long-term survival improvement using adenosine regulation with acadesine. *J. Am. Coll. Cardiol.* **2006**, *48*, 206–214. [CrossRef] [PubMed]
65. Van Den Neste, E.; Cazin, B.; Janssens, A.; Gonzalez-Barca, E.; Terol, M.J.; Levy, V.; Perez de Oteyza, J.; Zachee, P.; Saunders, A.; de Frias, M.; et al. Acadesine for patients with relapsed/refractory chronic lymphocytic leukemia (CLL): A multicenter phase I/II study. *Cancer Chemother. Pharmacol.* **2013**, *71*, 581–591. [CrossRef]
66. Dixon, R.; Gourzis, J.; McDermott, D.; Fujitaki, J.; Dewland, P.; Gruber, H. AICA-riboside: Safety, tolerance, and pharmacokinetics of a novel adenosine-regulating agent. *J. Clin. Pharmacol.* **1991**, *31*, 342–347. [CrossRef]
67. Nair, A.B.; Jacob, S. A simple practice guide for dose conversion between animals and human. *J. Basic Clin. Pharm.* **2016**, *7*, 27–31. [CrossRef] [PubMed]
68. Mangano, D.T. Effects of acadesine on myocardial infarction, stroke, and death following surgery. A meta-analysis of the 5 international randomized trials. The Multicenter Study of Perioperative Ischemia (McSPI) Research Group. *JAMA* **1997**, *277*, 325–332. [CrossRef] [PubMed]
69. Drew, B.G.; Kingwell, B.A. Acadesine, an adenosine-regulating agent with the potential for widespread indications. *Expert Opin. Pharmacother.* **2008**, *9*, 2137–2144. [CrossRef]
70. Mahaffey, K.W.; Puma, J.A.; Barbagelata, N.A.; DiCarli, M.F.; Leesar, M.A.; Browne, K.F.; Eisenberg, P.R.; Bolli, R.; Casas, A.C.; Molina-Viamonte, V.; et al. Adenosine as an adjunct to thrombolytic therapy for acute myocardial infarction: Results of a multicenter, randomized, placebo-controlled trial: The Acute Myocardial Infarction STudy of ADenosine (AMISTAD) trial. *J. Am. Coll. Cardiol.* **1999**, *34*, 1711–1720. [CrossRef]

71. Pokrywka, A.; Cholbinski, P.; Kaliszewski, P.; Kowalczyk, K.; Konczak, D.; Zembron-Lacny, A. Metabolic modulators of the exercise response: Doping control analysis of an agonist of the peroxisome proliferator-activated receptor delta (GW501516) and 5-aminoimidazole-4-carboxamide ribonucleotide (AICAR). *J. Physiol. Pharmacol.* **2014**, *65*, 469–476. [PubMed]
72. Visnjic, D.; Lalic, H.; Dembitz, V.; Tomic, B.; Smoljo, T. AICAr, a Widely Used AMPK Activator with Important AMPK-Independent Effects: A Systematic Review. *Cells* **2021**, *10*, 1095. [CrossRef] [PubMed]
73. Xu, X.; Wang, W.; Wang, Z.; Lv, J.; Xu, X.; Xu, J.; Yang, J.; Zhu, X.; Lu, Y.; Duan, W.; et al. DW14006 as a Direct AMPKα Activator Ameliorates Diabetic Peripheral Neuropathy in Mice. *Diabetes* **2020**, *69*, 1974–1988. [CrossRef] [PubMed]
74. Richter, E.A.; Kiens, B.; Wojtaszewski, J.F. Can exercise mimetics substitute for exercise? *Cell Metab.* **2008**, *8*, 96–98. [CrossRef] [PubMed]
75. Kristian, T.; Balan, I.S.; Schuh, R.A.; Onken, M. Mitochondrial dysfunction and NAD+ catabolism as mechanisms of cell death and promising targets for neuroprotection. *J. Neurosci. Res.* **2011**, *89*, 1946–1955. [CrossRef]
76. Long, A.N.; Owens, K.; Schlappal, A.E.; Kristian, T.; Fishman, P.S.; Schuh, R.A. Effect of nicotinamide mononucleotide on brain mitochondrial respiratory deficits in an Alzheimer's disease-relevant murine model. *BMC Neurol.* **2015**, *15*, 19. [CrossRef]
77. Owens, K.; Park, J.H.; Schuh, R.; Kristian, T. Mitochondrial dysfunction and NAD(+) metabolism alterations in the pathophysiology of acute brain injury. *Transl. Stroke Res.* **2013**, *4*, 618–634. [CrossRef]
78. Lauria, G.; Hsieh, S.T.; Johansson, O.; Kennedy, W.R.; Leger, J.M.; Mellgren, S.I.; Nolano, M.; Merkies, I.S.; Polydefkis, M.; Smith, A.G.; et al. European Federation of Neurological Societies/Peripheral Nerve Society Guideline on the use of skin biopsy in the diagnosis of small fiber neuropathy. Report of a joint task force of the European Federation of Neurological Societies and the Peripheral Nerve Society. *Eur. J. Neurol.* **2010**, *17*, 903–912. [CrossRef] [PubMed]
79. Lauria, G.; Cornblath, D.R.; Johansson, O.; McArthur, J.C.; Mellgren, S.I.; Nolano, M.; Rosenberg, N.; Sommer, C. EFNS guidelines on the use of skin biopsy in the diagnosis of peripheral neuropathy. *Eur. J. Neurol.* **2005**, *12*, 747–758. [CrossRef]
80. Russell, J.W.; Berent-Spillson, A.; Vincent, A.M.; Freimann, C.L.; Sullivan, K.A.; Feldman, E.L. Oxidative injury and neuropathy in diabetes and impaired glucose tolerance. *Neurobiol. Dis.* **2008**, *30*, 420–429. [CrossRef]

International Journal of
Molecular Sciences

MDPI

Article

Alcohol Impairs Bioenergetics and Differentiation Capacity of Myoblasts from Simian Immunodeficiency Virus-Infected Female Macaques

Danielle E. Levitt [1,2,3], Brianna L. Bourgeois [1,2], Keishla M. Rodríguez-Graciani [1,2], Patricia E. Molina [1,2] and Liz Simon [1,2,*]

1 Department of Physiology, School of Medicine, Louisiana State University Health Sciences Center, New Orleans, LA 70112, USA; danielle.levitt@ttu.edu (D.E.L.); bbou11@lsuhsc.edu (B.L.B.); krodr7@lsuhsc.edu (K.M.R.-G.); pmolin@lsuhsc.edu (P.E.M.)

2 Comprehensive Alcohol-HIV/AIDS Research Center, Louisiana State University Health Sciences Center, New Orleans, LA 70112, USA

3 Department of Kinesiology and Sport Management, Texas Tech University, Lubbock, TX 79409, USA

* Correspondence: lsimo2@lsuhsc.edu; Tel.: +1-(504)-568-3395

Abstract: Alcohol misuse and HIV independently induce myopathy. We previously showed that chronic binge alcohol (CBA) administration, with or without simian immunodeficiency virus (SIV), decreases differentiation capacity of male rhesus macaque myoblasts. We hypothesized that short-term alcohol and CBA/SIV would synergistically decrease differentiation capacity and impair bioenergetic parameters in female macaque myoblasts. Myoblasts from naïve (CBA^-/SIV^-), vehicle [VEH]/SIV, and CBA/SIV (N = 4–6/group) groups were proliferated (3 days) and differentiated (5 days) with 0 or 50 mM ethanol (short-term). CBA/SIV decreased differentiation and increased non-mitochondrial oxygen consumption rate (OCR) versus naïve and/or VEH/SIV. Short-term alcohol decreased differentiation; increased maximal and non-mitochondrial OCR, mitochondrial reactive oxygen species (ROS) production, and aldolase activity; and decreased glycolytic measures, ATP production, mitochondrial membrane potential ($\Delta\Psi m$), and pyruvate kinase activity. Mitochondrial ROS production was closely associated with mitochondrial network volume, and differentiation indices were closely associated with key bioenergetic health and function parameters. Results indicate that short-term alcohol and CBA non-synergistically decrease myoblast differentiation capacity. Short-term alcohol impaired myoblast glycolytic function, driving the bioenergetic deficit. Results suggest potentially differing mechanisms underlying decreased differentiation capacity with short-term alcohol and CBA, highlighting the need to elucidate the impact of different alcohol use patterns on myopathy.

Keywords: alcohol use disorder; glycolysis; mitochondria; ethanol; antiretroviral therapy; HIV; myopathy; skeletal muscle; satellite cell

1. Introduction

Approximately one-quarter to one-third of adults in the United States report past-month alcohol misuse (i.e., binge or heavy drinking) [1,2] and an estimated 28.5 million (~15% of adults) have an alcohol use disorder (AUD) [3]. Globally, the prevalence of AUD is more than double among people with HIV (PWH) [4] compared to the general population [5]. Alcohol misuse has multisystemic adverse consequences [6,7] and may be especially harmful for PWH [8]. Myopathy, or decreased skeletal muscle (SKM) mass and function, affects nearly half of those with AUD [9] and has a high prevalence among PWH [10,11]. Myopathy, in turn, is associated with increased mortality in several clinical conditions [12], highlighting the importance of maintaining SKM mass and function.

Although SKM has emerged as a key tissue impacted by alcohol use [9,13–15], the underlying mechanisms of alcohol-associated myopathy and whether these differ among

PWH remain to be completely elucidated. Muscle precursor cells (myoblasts) are critical for the maintenance and regeneration of muscle mass [16,17], and their bioenergetic state supports their myogenic progression [18–20]. Therefore, bioenergetic dyshomeostasis in SKM and myoblasts may contribute to alcohol-associated myopathy with or without HIV. Among PWH, we found that alcohol misuse was associated with poorer myoblast bioenergetic health and altered SKM mitochondrial gene expression [21]. Using a highly relevant preclinical model of HIV pathogenesis and associated comorbidities, we also have previously shown that myoblasts from chronic binge alcohol (CBA)-administered, SIV-infected, antiretroviral therapy (ART)-treated male rhesus macaques had decreased maximal mitochondrial respiration compared to those from alcohol- and SIV-naïve macaques despite myoblast expansion in the absence of alcohol [22]. At higher alcohol concentrations (100 mM), mitochondrial bioenergetic function in C2C12 myotubes was also impaired [23]. At lower concentrations (50 mM), we observed a shift in bioenergetic function away from glycolysis and toward mitochondrial metabolism in myoblasts from alcohol- and SIV-naïve macaques [24]. However, specific contributions of each bioenergetic system and potential impairments in mitochondrial and glycolytic measures that may have been impacted remain unknown. Moreover, direct comparison of different alcohol exposure paradigms, reflecting different alcohol use patterns, has not been performed.

Findings from CBA-administered animals allow for the assessment of lasting effects of chronic alcohol misuse (i.e., after a period of abstinence) since myoblasts are cultured in the absence of alcohol. On the other hand, treating myoblasts with alcohol in vitro in the short-term (i.e., alcohol in cell culture removed $\leq$1 h prior to assay or harvest) reflects impacts of recent alcohol use, which may or may not extend to longer-term effects. Our previous work has used only one of the alcohol administration paradigms (i.e., CBA or short-term in vitro alcohol); however, we have not directly compared the effects of both or examined them in combination. The combination allows for modeling continued alcohol use in someone with a history of misuse, and short-term use could accentuate chronic effects. Since myopathy can result from short-term and chronic alcohol misuse, examining how these different patterns of alcohol misuse may contribute to the development of myopathy is critical for appropriate early intervention [25].

Data on the impact of alcohol and HIV infection are particularly sparse for females even though people assigned female at birth comprise more than 20% of PWH [26]. Based on our previous work in SIV-infected male macaques and SIV-naïve male and female macaques, we hypothesized that short-term alcohol and CBA/SIV would decrease differentiation capacity and impair multiple bioenergetic functional parameters, and that the effects would be additive with the combination of short-term alcohol treatment (mimicking acute, recent exposure) and chronic in vivo binge alcohol administration (CBA/SIV). Myoblasts rely heavily on anaerobic glycolysis during proliferation and early differentiation [18,27], and differential reliance on distinct metabolic pathways during myogenic progression appears critical for terminal fusion [28–30]. Moreover, we previously found that exposing proliferating myoblasts from naïve macaques to short-term alcohol treatment shifted their bioenergetic phenotype away from glycolysis in association with decreased differentiation [24]. Therefore, we aimed to further dissect this bioenergetic impairment during proliferation as a potential contributing factor to decreased myoblast differentiation.

2. Results

2.1. Myoblast Differentiation Indices

Myoblasts were isolated from *vastus lateralis* muscle of naïve macaques (no SIV or CBA exposure) and SIV-infected macaques administered a water vehicle (VEH/SIV) or CBA (CBA/SIV) for 14.5 months. Myoblasts at P4 were proliferated for 3 days and differentiated for 5 days in 0 or 50 mM ethanol (EtOH). Myoblasts from each macaque were grown in both short-term EtOH conditions. To quantify differentiation capacity, myoblasts were methanol-fixed and stained using HEMA3 stains. We assessed myotube differentiation indices from each short-term EtOH condition and in vivo treatment group (naïve, VEH/SIV, CBA/SIV) at differentiation day 5.

For fused nuclei (Figure 1A), there was a main effect of short-term EtOH ($p = 0.02$, $\eta^2 = 0.40$, large). Across all groups, short-term 50 mM EtOH treatment decreased fused nuclei (d = 0.8, large) compared to 0 mM EtOH. There was also a main effect of group ($p < 0.01$, $\eta^2 = 0.68$, large). Regardless of short-term EtOH, there were fewer fused nuclei in the CBA/SIV vs. naïve group ($p < 0.01$, d = 2.1, large) and in the CBA/SIV vs. VEH/SIV group ($p < 0.001$, d = 3.1, large). No EtOH × group interaction effect was observed for fused nuclei.

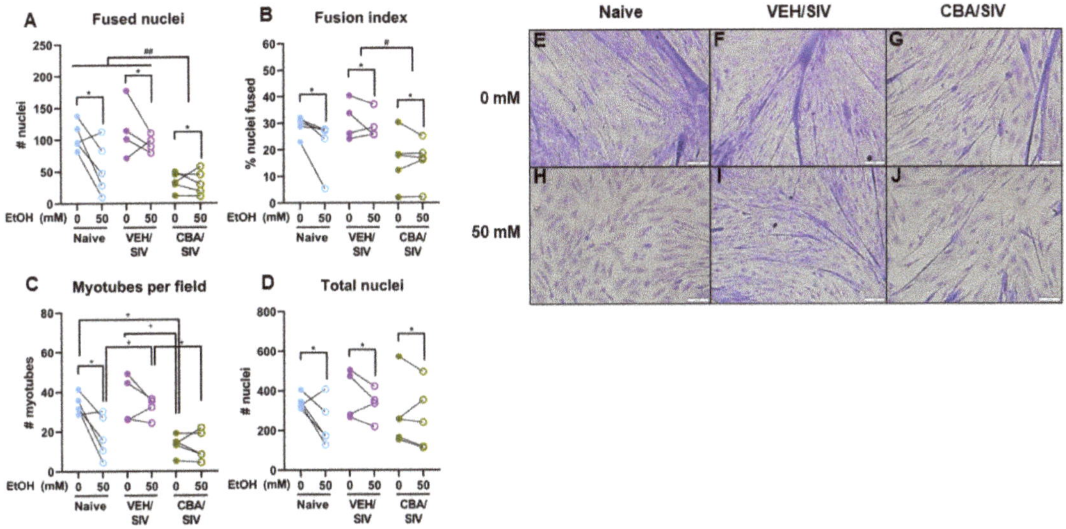

Figure 1. Quantification of myotube differentiation indices. Fused nuclei (**A**), fusion index (**B**), myotubes per field (**C**), and total nuclei (**D**) after 3 days of proliferation plus 5 days of differentiation with representative images (20×) of myoblasts from macaques in the naïve (N = 5), vehicle (VEH)/simian immunodeficiency virus (SIV)(N = 4), and chronic binge alcohol (CBA)/SIV (N = 5) groups cultured with 0 mM (**E–G**) or 50 mM (**H–J**) EtOH. Scale bars (lower right in each image) indicate 50 µm. Main effects of short-term EtOH, * $p < 0.05$; main effect of group (naïve, VEH/SIV, CBA/SIV) with post-hoc pairwise comparisons, # $p < 0.05$, ## $p < 0.01$; short-term EtOH × group (naïve, VEH/SIV, CBA/SIV) interaction effect with post-hoc pairwise comparisons, + $p < 0.05$. Lengths of bracket legs indicate direction of differences.

For the fusion index (Figure 1B), there was a main effect of short-term EtOH ($p = 0.05$, $\eta^2 = 0.30$, large). Across all groups, short-term 50 mM EtOH treatment decreased the fusion index (d = 0.4, medium) compared to 0 mM EtOH. There was also a main effect of group ($p = 0.04$, $\eta^2 = 0.44$, large). Regardless of short-term EtOH, the fusion index was decreased in the CBA/SIV vs VEH/SIV group ($p = 0.02$, d = 1.9, large). No EtOH × group interaction effect was observed for the fusion index.

For myotubes per field, there was a significant short-term EtOH x group interaction effect ($p = 0.05$, $\eta^2 = 0.42$, large; Figure 1C). For cells treated with 0 mM EtOH, there were fewer myotubes per field in the CBA/SIV vs naïve group ($p < 0.01$, d = 4.1, large) and the CBA/SIV vs. VEH/SIV group ($p < 0.001$, d = 2.5, large). For cells treated with 50 mM EtOH, there were fewer myotubes per field in the naïve vs VEH/SIV group ($p = 0.03$, d = 1.7, large) and in the CBA/SIV vs. VEH/SIV group ($p < 0.01$, d = 3.0, large). Compared with 0 mM, 50 mM EtOH significantly decreased myotubes per field in the naïve group ($p < 0.01$, d = 1.9, large) but not in the VEH/SIV or CBA/SIV groups.

For total nuclei (Figure 1D), there was a main effect of short-term EtOH ($p = 0.03$, $\eta^2 = 0.36$, large). Regardless of group, short-term 50 mM EtOH treatment decreased total nuclei (d = 0.5, medium) compared to 0 mM EtOH. No main effect of group or EtOH × group interaction effect was observed for total nuclei. Representative images of myotubes from each EtOH condition and group are shown in Figure 1E–J.

2.2. Mitochondrial Stress Test

We performed a Mito Stress Test to examine mitochondrial function under resting and stressed conditions using myoblasts isolated from each group (naïve, VEH/SIV, and CBA/SIV) treated with 0 or 50 mM EtOH for 3 days. We measured basal oxygen consumption rate (OCR; Figure 2A), ATP-linked OCR (quantified after ATP synthase inhibition with oligomycin) (Figure 2B), and coupling efficiency (calculated as the percentage of basal OCR attributable to ATP production) (Figure 2C). No main effect of short-term EtOH, group (naïve, VEH/SIV, CBA/SIV), or short-term EtOH × group interaction effect was observed for these measures. After the addition of carbonyl cyanide-p-trifluoromethoxyphenylhydrazone (FCCP) to uncouple the inner mitochondrial membrane, main effects of short-term EtOH were observed for maximal oxygen consumption ($p = 0.05$, $\eta^2 = 0.31$, large, Figure 2D) and spare capacity ($p = 0.02$, $\eta^2 = 0.43$, large, Figure 2E). Regardless of group, short-term 50 mM EtOH treatment increased these measures (maximal oxygen consumption: d = 0.4, small; spare capacity: d = 0.5, medium) compared to 0 mM EtOH. After adding rotenone and antimycin A to inhibit electron transport chain complexes I and III to quantify negative indicators of bioenergetic health (non-mitochondrial OCR and proton leak-linked OCR), main effects of short-term EtOH ($p = 0.01$, $\eta^2 = 0.44$, large) and group ($p = 0.04$, $\eta^2 = 0.45$, large) were observed for non-mitochondrial OCR (Figure 2F). Regardless of group, short-term 50 mM EtOH treatment increased non-mitochondrial OCR (d = 0.7, medium) compared to 0 mM EtOH. Regardless of short-term EtOH, non-mitochondrial OCR was greater in the CBA/SIV vs VEH/SIV group ($p = 0.01$, d = 2.0, large). No differences were observed for proton leak (Figure 2G). A schematic diagram of an OCR trace for the Mito Stress Test and the resulting parameters reported herein is available in Figure S1 (Supplementary Materials).

To determine the overall bioenergetic phenotype, extracellular acidification rate (ECAR; indicative of glycolytic function) and the OCR/ECAR ratio (indicative of mitochondrial vs glycolytic function) at baseline and after ATP synthase inhibition were used. Main effects of short-term EtOH were observed for ECAR at baseline ($p < 0.001$, $\eta^2 = 0.85$, large, Figure 3A) and after ATP synthase inhibition ($p < 0.001$, $\eta^2 = 0.87$, large, Figure 3B), and for the ratio of OCR to ECAR at baseline ($p < 0.001$, $\eta^2 = 0.76$, large, Figure 3C) and after ATP synthase inhibition ($p < 0.001$, $\eta^2 = 0.81$, large, Figure 3D). Regardless of group, short-term 50 mM EtOH treatment decreased each of these measures (baseline ECAR: d = 1.2, large; ECAR after ATP synthase inhibition: d = 1.3, large; baseline OCR/ECAR: d = 1.2, large; OCR/ECAR after ATP synthase inhibition: d = 1.5, large) compared to 0 mM EtOH. No main effect of group (naïve, VEH/SIV, CBA/SIV) or EtOH × group interaction effect was observed for bioenergetic phenotype. The OCR and ECAR traces throughout the assay are shown by group in Figure 3E,F.

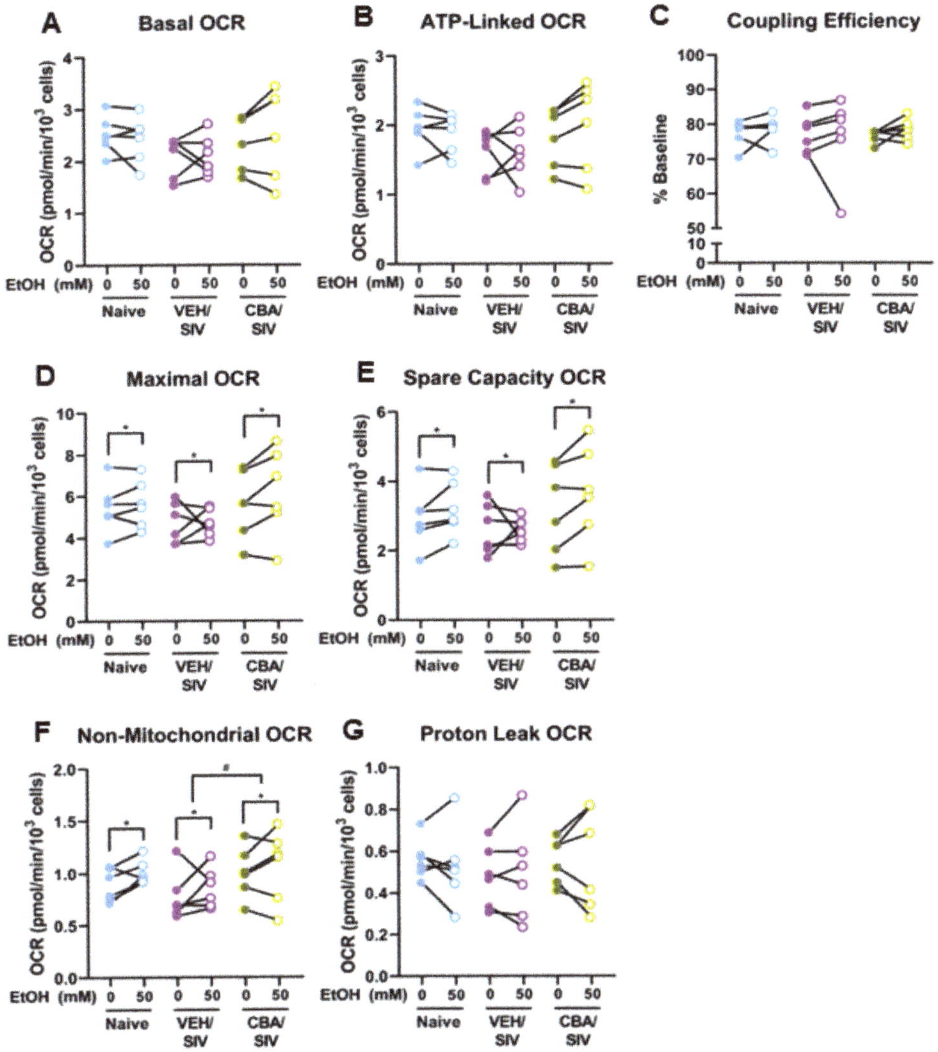

Figure 2. Mito Stress Test parameters. Basal (**A**) and ATP-linked (**B**) oxygen consumption rate (OCR) and coupling efficiency (**C**); ATP-linked OCR/baseline OCR × 100), maximal OCR (**D**) and spare capacity (**E**), non-mitochondrial OCR (**F**), and proton leak-linked OCR (**G**). Myoblasts from macaques in the naïve (N = 6), vehicle (VEH)/simian immunodeficiency virus (SIV) (N = 6), and chronic binge alcohol (CBA)/SIV (N = 6) groups were proliferated for 3 days with 0 mM or 50 mM EtOH. Main effects of short-term EtOH, * $p < 0.05$; main effect of group (naïve, VEH/SIV, CBA/SIV) with post-hoc pairwise comparisons, # $p < 0.05$. Lengths of bracket legs indicate direction of differences.

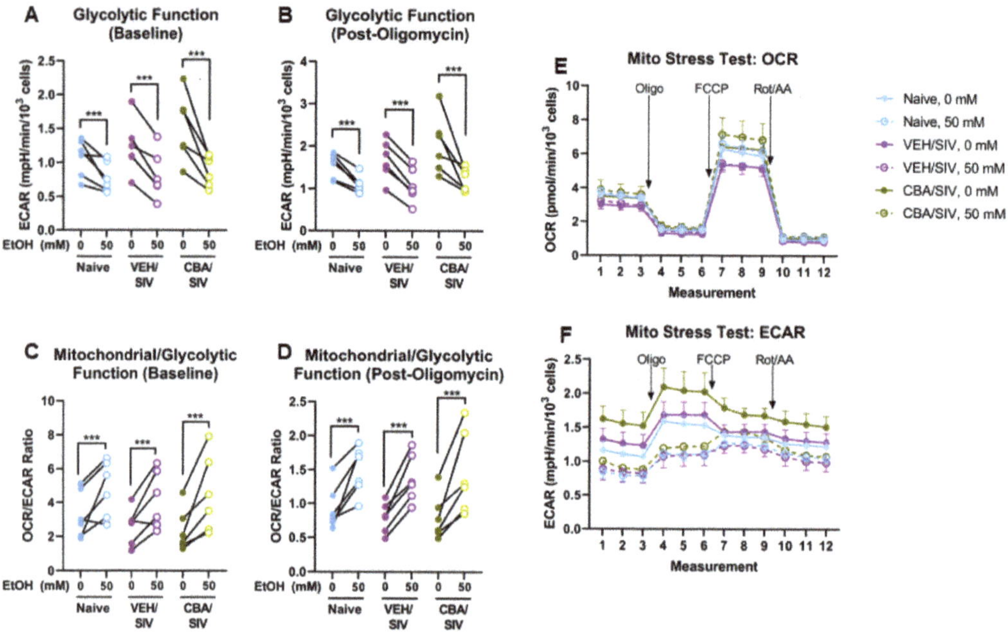

Figure 3. Bioenergetic phenotype indices. Glycolytic function measured as extracellular acidification rate (ECAR) at baseline (**A**) and after oligomycin administration (**B**), the relative ratio or mitochondrial to glycolytic function quantified as the ratio of oxygen consumption (OCR) to extracellular acidification (ECAR) rates at baseline (**C**) and after oligomycin administration (**D**), and OCR (**E**) and ECAR (**F**) throughout the assay with indications for injections of oligomycin (Oligo), carbonyl cyanide-p-trifluoromethoxyphenylhydrazone (FCCP), and rotenone/antimycin A (Rot/AA). Myoblasts from macaques in the naïve (N = 6), vehicle (VEH)/simian immunodeficiency virus (SIV) (N = 6), and chronic binge alcohol (CBA)/SIV (N = 6) groups were proliferated for 3 days with 0 mM or 50 mM EtOH. Main effects of short-term EtOH, *** $p < 0.001$. Lengths of bracket legs indicate direction of differences.

2.3. Glycolysis Stress Test

A glycolysis stress test was used to identify specific changes in glycolytic measures using myoblasts isolated from each group (naïve, VEH/SIV, and CBA/SIV) treated with 0 or 50 mM EtOH for 3 days. Main effects of short-term EtOH were observed for non-glycolytic acidification ($p = 0.02$, $\eta^2 = 0.42$, large, Figure 4A), baseline glycolysis ($p < 0.001$, $\eta^2 = 0.76$, large, Figure 4B), glycolytic capacity ($p < 0.001$, $\eta^2 = 0.80$, large, Figure 4C), and glycolytic reserve ($p < 0.001$, $\eta^2 = 0.66$, large, Figure 4D). Regardless of group (naïve, VEH/SIV, CBA/SIV), short-term 50 mM EtOH treatment decreased non-glycolytic acidification (d = 0.4, small), baseline glycolysis (d = 1.1, large), glycolytic capacity (d = 1.4, large), and glycolytic reserve (d = 1.3, large) compared to 0 mM EtOH. No main effects of group or EtOH × group interaction were observed for glycolysis stress test outcomes. The ECAR traces throughout the assay are shown by group in Figure 4E. A schematic diagram of an ECAR trace for the Glycolysis Stress Test and the resulting parameters reported herein are available in Figure S2 (Supplementary Materials).

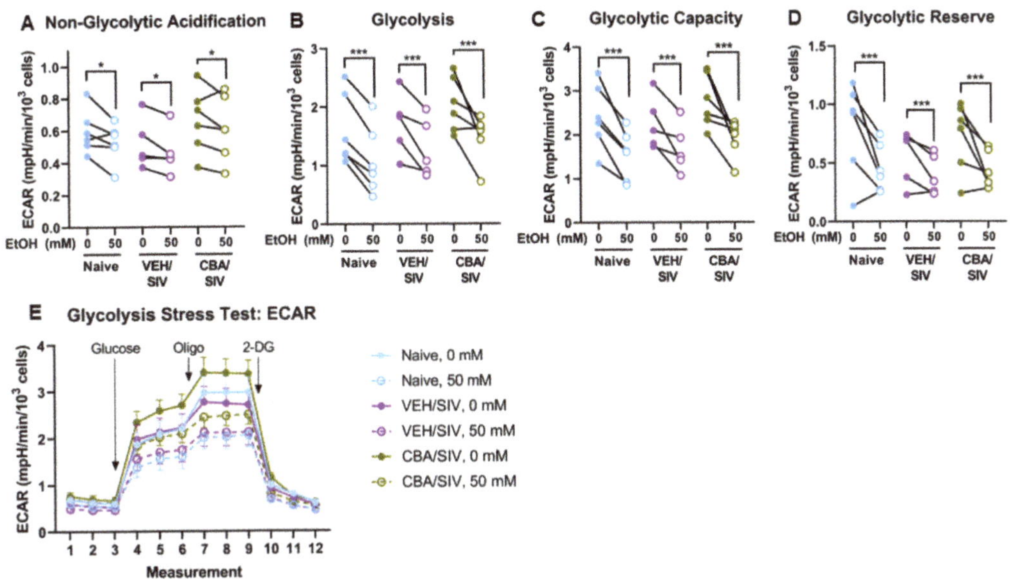

Figure 4. Glycolysis stress test parameters. Non-glycolytic acidification (**A**), basal glycolysis (**B**), glycolytic capacity (**C**), and glycolytic reserve (**D**) measured as extracellular acidification rates (ECAR) and ECAR traces throughout the assay (**E**) with indications for injections of glucose, oligomycin (Oligo), and 2-deoxyglucose (2-DG). Myoblasts from macaques in the naïve (N = 6), vehicle (VEH)/simian immunodeficiency virus (SIV) (N = 5), and chronic binge alcohol (CBA)/SIV (N = 6) groups were proliferated for 3 days with 0 mM or 50 mM EtOH. Main effects of short-term EtOH, * $p < 0.05$; *** $p < 0.001$. Lengths of bracket legs indicate direction of differences.

2.4. ATP Production Rates

To dissect differences in ATP production attributable to mitochondrial and glycolytic pathways, an ATP rate assay was performed using myoblasts isolated from each group (naïve, VEH/SIV, and CBA/SIV) treated with 0 or 50 mM EtOH for 3 days. Main effects of short-term EtOH were observed for total ATP production rate ($p < 0.001$, $\eta^2 = 0.76$, large, Figure 5A), ATP produced via mitochondrial ($p = 0.04$, $\eta^2 = 0.34$, large, Figure 5B) and glycolytic ($p < 0.001$, $\eta^2 = 0.65$, large, Figure 5C) metabolism. Short-term 50 mM EtOH treatment decreased the total ATP production rate (d = 1.3, large), glycolysis-derived ATP (d = 1.0, large), and mitochondrial-derived ATP (d = 0.5, medium) compared to 0 mM EtOH. No main effect of group (naïve, VEH/SIV, CBA/SIV) or short-term EtOH × group interaction was observed for ATP production rate outcomes. The OCR and ECAR traces throughout the assay are shown by group in Figure 5D,E.

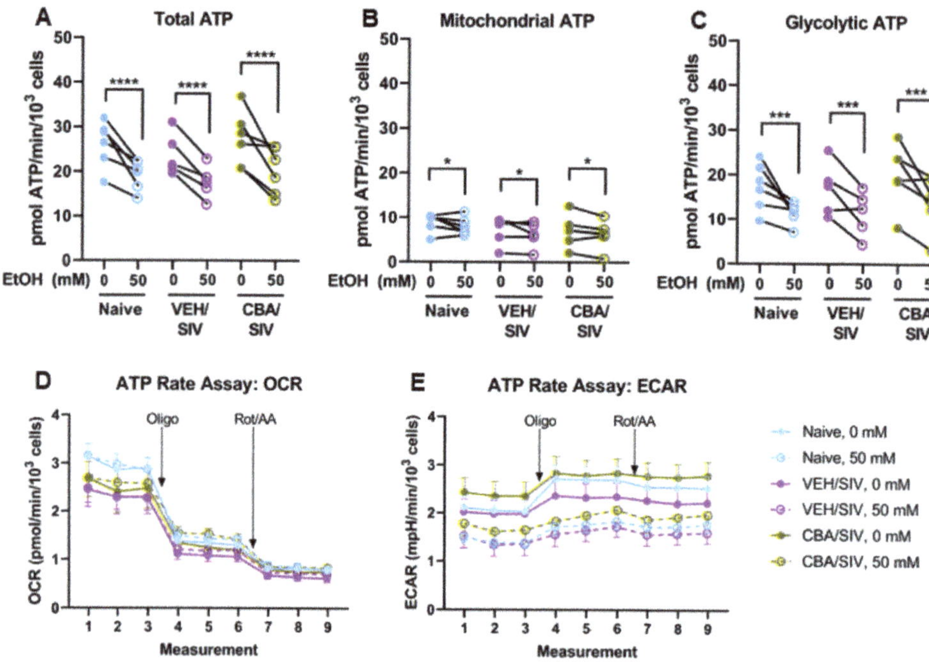

Figure 5. ATP rate assay parameters. Total ATP (**A**), ATP derived from mitochondrial metabolism (**B**) and anaerobic glycolysis (**C**), and oxygen consumption ((**D**); OCR) and extracellular acidification ((**E**); ECAR) rates throughout the assay, with indications for injections of oligomycin (Oligo) and rotenone/antimycin A (Rot/AA). Myoblasts from macaques in the naïve (N = 6), vehicle (VEH)/simian immunodeficiency virus (SIV) (N = 5), and chronic binge alcohol (CBA)/SIV (N = 6) groups were proliferated for 3 days with 0 mM or 50 mM EtOH. Main effects of short-term EtOH; * $p < 0.05$; *** $p < 0.001$; **** $p < 0.0001$. Lengths of bracket legs indicate direction of differences.

2.5. Mitochondrial Health

We used flow cytometric analyses to evaluate mitochondrial membrane potential (ΔΨm), reactive oxygen species (ROS) production, and network volume to assess the health of the myoblast mitochondrial network in myoblasts isolated from each group (naïve, VEH/SIV, and CBA/SIV) treated with 0 or 50 mM EtOH. MitoSOX mean fluorescence intensity (MFI) was below the detectable limit in four samples; these values were set to zero. Main effects of short-term EtOH were observed for ΔΨm ($p < 0.001$, $\eta^2 = 0.66$, large, Figure 6A) and ROS ($p = 0.034$, $\eta^2 = 0.63$, large, Figure 6B) but not mitochondrial network volume (Figure 6C). Regardless of group (naïve, VEH/SIV, CBA/SIV), short-term 50 mM EtOH treatment decreased ΔΨm (d = 1.0, large) and increased ROS production (d = 0.7, medium). Main effects of group were observed for mitochondrial ROS ($p = 0.02$, $\eta^2 = 0.54$, large, Figure 6B) and network volume ($p < 0.05$, $\eta^2 = 0.63$, large, Figure 6C) but not ΔΨm. Regardless of short-term EtOH treatment, mitochondrial ROS production (d = 4.8, large) and network volume (d = 4.8, large) were greater in the VEH/SIV group compared to the naïve group. No short-term EtOH × group interaction effects were observed for these mitochondrial health measures. Across all samples, there was a significant, positive association between mitochondrial network volume and ROS ($p < 0.001$, $\varrho = 0.87$, large, Figure 6D).

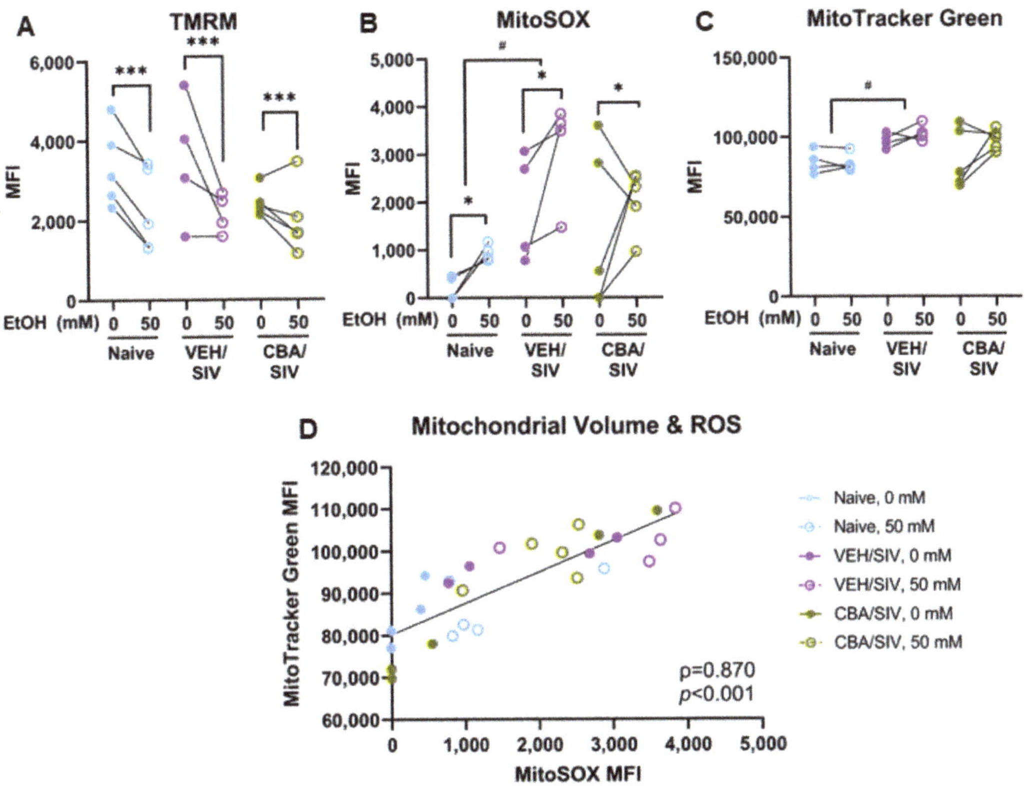

Figure 6. Mitochondrial health parameters. Mean fluorescence intensity (MFI) of tetramethylrhodamine methyl ester (TMRM) for mitochondrial membrane potential ($\Delta\Psi m$; (**A**)), MitoSOX for mitochondrial reactive oxygen species (ROS; (**B**)), and MitoTracker Green for mitochondrial network volume (**C**) measured using flow cytometry. Mitochondrial network volume was significantly associated with ROS (**D**). Myoblasts from macaques in the naïve (N = 5 [**A**] or 4 [**B–D**]), vehicle (VEH)/simian immunodeficiency virus (SIV) (N = 4), and chronic binge alcohol (CBA)/SIV (N = 5) groups were proliferated for 3 days with 0 mM or 50 mM EtOH. Main effects of EtOH, * $p < 0.05$, ***' $p < 0.001$, main effect of group with post-hoc pairwise comparisons, # $p < 0.05$. Lengths of bracket legs indicate direction of differences.

2.6. Glycolytic Enzyme Activity

To identify whether alterations in glycolytic enzyme activity could have had a role in the substantial decrease in glycolytic function observed, we measured the activity of two glycolytic enzymes in myoblasts isolated from each group (naïve, VEH/SIV, and CBA/SIV) treated with 0 or 50 mM EtOH for 3 days of proliferation (differentiation day 0) and 5 days of differentiation. Main effects of short-term EtOH were observed for aldolase activity at differentiation day 0 ($p = 0.04$, $\eta^2 = 0.34$, large, Figure 7A) and day 5 ($p = 0.01$, $\eta^2 = 0.46$, large, Figure 7B). Regardless of group (naïve, VEH/SIV, CBA/SIV), short-term 50 mM EtOH treatment increased aldolase activity at both time points (d = 0.6, medium, for both) vs 0 mM EtOH. Main effects of short-term EtOH were also observed for pyruvate kinase activity at differentiation day 0 ($p = 0.01$, $\eta^2 = 0.45$, large, Figure 7C) and day 5 ($p < 0.001$, $\eta^2 = 0.78$, large, Figure 7D). Regardless of group, short-term 50 mM EtOH treatment decreased pyruvate kinase activity at both time points (day 0: d = 0.7, medium; day 5: d = 0.8, large) compared to 0 mM EtOH. No main effect of group (naïve, VEH/SIV, CBA/SIV) or EtOH × group interaction was observed for glycolytic enzyme activity. A diagram showing the glycolytic steps catalyzed by aldolase and pyruvate kinase is shown in Figure 7E.

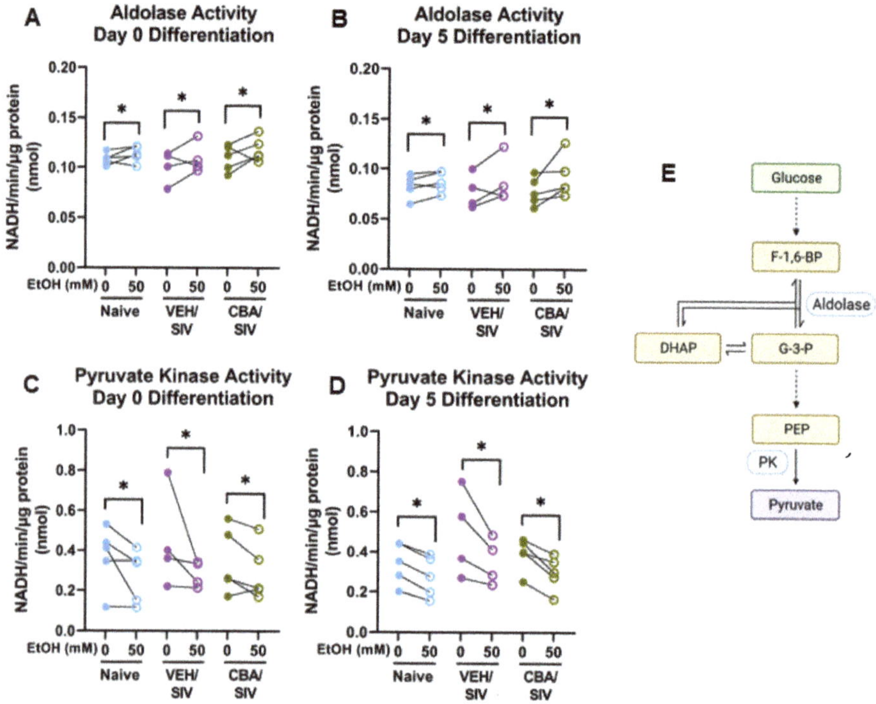

Figure 7. Activity of select glycolytic enzymes. Aldolase (**A**,**B**) and pyruvate kinase (**C**,**D**) activity in myoblasts from macaques in the naïve (N = 5), vehicle (VEH)/simian immunodeficiency virus (SIV) (N = 4), and chronic binge alcohol (CBA)/SIV (N = 5) groups after 3 days of proliferation (day 0 differentiation, (**A**,**C**)) and 5 days of differentiation (**B**,**D**) with 0 mM or 50 mM EtOH. Simplified schematic of the first 10 steps of anaerobic glycolysis (**E**) showing steps catalyzed by aldolase and pyruvate kinase (PK). Fructose-1,6-bisphosphate (F-1,6-BP); dihydroxyacetone phosphate (DHAP); glyceraldehyde-3-phosphate (G3P); phosphoenolpyruvate (PEP); dashed arrows indicate multiple steps between glycolysis intermediates. Main effects of short-term EtOH, * $p < 0.05$. Lengths of bracket legs indicate direction of differences.

2.7. Correlations between Differentiation Indices and Bioenergetics Parameters

To uncover potential explanatory mechanisms for the observed effects, we examined the relationships between key differentiation indices and key bioenergetic parameters by Spearman correlations (Figure 8). All samples were analyzed together to determine factors that may have contributed to impaired differentiation capacity regardless of EtOH exposure paradigm. Significant correlations were observed between myotubes per field and spare capacity ($p = 0.05$, $\varrho = -0.38$, medium), non-mitochondrial OCR ($p < 0.01$, $\varrho = -0.53$, large), and aldolase activity at differentiation day 0 ($p = 0.02$, $\varrho = -0.44$, medium); between fusion index and non-glycolytic acidification ($p = 0.02$, $\varrho = -0.44$, medium), mitochondrial ATP production ($p = 0.02$, $\varrho = 0.44$, medium), and $\Delta\Psi m$ ($p = 0.04$, $\varrho = 0.43$, medium); and between total nuclei and basal OCR ($p < 0.01$, $\varrho = -0.56$, large), proton leak ($p < 0.001$, $\varrho = -0.60$, large), non-mitochondrial OCR ($p < 0.001$, $\varrho = -0.66$, large), ATP-linked OCR ($p < 0.01$, $\varrho = -0.55$, large), aldolase activity at differentiation day 5 ($p < 0.001$, $\varrho = -0.61$, large), and pyruvate kinase activity at differentiation day 0 ($p < 0.01$, $\varrho = 0.54$, large).

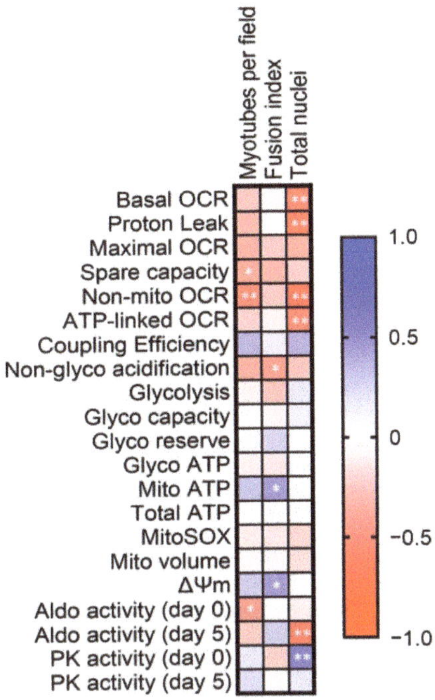

Figure 8. Associations between differentiation indices and bioenergetics parameters. Spearman correlations were run between raw values for key differentiation indices and bioenergetics parameters for samples collected from all groups and conditions. Oxygen consumption rate (OCR); pyruvate kinase (PK). * $p < 0.05$, ** $p < 0.01$.

3. Discussion

Herein, we report for the first time that CBA (reflecting the lasting effects of alcohol) and short-term in vitro alcohol (reflecting current or recent alcohol use) non-synergistically decrease differentiation capacity of myoblasts from SIV-infected female macaques. However, only short-term in vitro alcohol decreased myoblast glycolytic function, mitochondrial membrane potential, and mitochondrial ROS. This differential response suggests potentially divergent mechanisms of alcohol-mediated decreased differentiation capacity. These data further our understanding of decreased myogenic differentiation with alcohol misuse and provide evidence to support critical examination of the underlying mechanisms with different alcohol use paradigms. Understanding such mechanisms would help improve alcohol-mediated myopathy, characterized by SKM weakness, injury, and atrophy, since myoblast differentiation and fusion supports muscle repair after injury [31] and rebuilding after atrophy [32].

3.1. Differentiation Indices

Short-term alcohol and CBA/SIV independently decreased measures of myoblast fusion into myotubes. The finding that myoblast fusion index was lower in CBA/SIV versus VEH/SIV groups suggests that chronic alcohol and not SIV and ART negatively impacts fusion. These findings are consistent with our previous reports of decreased fusion index with short-term alcohol in myoblasts from alcohol- and SIV-naïve male and female macaques [24] and CBA in SIV-naïve male macaques [33]. Total nuclei were decreased with short-term alcohol. This decrease could have been due to increased cell death, decreased proliferation since proliferating myoblasts rely heavily on anaerobic glycolysis [28,34], or a combination of these factors. Dissecting this finding is the subject of ongoing experiments.

However, there was no decrease in total nuclei with CBA/SIV alone, and the magnitude of the decrease with short-term EtOH was not sufficient to fully explain the decreased fusion observed since the fusion index corrects for total nuclei.

Although not measured in vivo after short-term EtOH, the findings are consistent with reports of decreased expression of myogenic genes in whole SKM after chronic in vivo EtOH [35]. However, the results contrast with our findings from SIV-infected males, where myotube density, an additional differentiation index, was decreased in VEH and CBA-administered macaques compared to SIV-naïve controls [36]. Sex differences in decreased SKM mass with HIV serostatus have previously been reported [37], where males but not females had lower SKM mass versus seronegative controls after adjusting for lifestyle factors, including alcohol use. It is possible that exposure to female sex hormones, including estrogen, could provide sufficient protection against HIV-related muscle loss, especially with less myotoxic ART drugs such as emtricitabine or tenofovir [38], whereas alcohol could be a more potent stimulus for decreased differentiation capacity and muscle mass regardless of sex.

3.2. Bioenergetic Health and Function

Bioenergetic function supports myogenic progression, where myoblasts rely heavily on anaerobic glycolysis during proliferation and early differentiation [18]. The results of the present study show that short-term alcohol decreased all measures of glycolysis in proliferating myoblasts regardless of CBA and SIV. Moreover, the total rate of basal ATP production was decreased with short-term alcohol. Although a small yet significant decrease in mitochondrial ATP production was observed, there was a much more substantial decrease in the rate of glycolytic ATP production, suggesting that the bioenergetic deficit observed with short-term alcohol was primarily driven by decreased glycolytic function. Glycolytic capacity and reserve were also decreased with short-term alcohol, indicating a decreased ability for myoblasts to increase glycolytic function with increased demand for anaerobic energy production [28,34,39].

Although there was a decrease in basal mitochondrial ATP production rate with short-term alcohol, maximal mitochondrial respiration increased. These findings are aligned with previous results from our laboratory [24] and suggest a mitohormetic effect with short-term alcohol at a concentration of 50 mM, a physiologically relevant dose [40]. This could allow myotubes to rely more heavily on mitochondrial metabolism during times of increased energetic demands, which is particularly important given impaired glycolytic capacity and reserve. Given glycolytic deficits together with apparent mitohormesis and little evidence of decreased mitochondrial bioenergetic function despite indicators of impaired mitochondrial network health, there may be differences in fuel substrate preference with short-term EtOH. This will be the subject of future investigations. Mitohormesis with acute alcohol could be due to an altered redox state [41] requiring an adaptive increase in NAD^+ levels [42–44] and mitochondrial content [21,45], as observed in various cell types. This is in contrast to decreased maximal respiration in myotubes treated with 100 mM EtOH [23], which likely induces greater oxidative stress (e.g., an approximately 3-fold increase in mitochondrial superoxide versus less than double with 50 mM EtOH in the present study) such that the mitochondria can no longer adapt. Maximal respiration was also decreased in myoblasts from CBA/SIV male macaques versus naïve male controls [22], but similar effects were not observed in female macaques in the present study. This suggests a possible sex difference in myotube mitochondrial resilience to CBA and SIV. These findings add an additional layer of complexity to the concept of sex dimorphism in SKM mitochondria [46–48].

Although myoblast bioenergetic functional changes were primarily due to short-term alcohol in the present study, increased non-mitochondrial oxygen consumption was observed following short-term alcohol and in myoblasts from CBA/SIV animals, suggesting immediate and lasting poorer bioenergetic health with alcohol [49]. This finding is supported by increased non-mitochondrial oxygen consumption in myoblasts from PWH with alcohol misuse [21]. Increased ROS production and decreased ΔΨm with short-term alcohol in the present study likely contributed to the observed increased non-mitochondrial oxygen consumption, findings supported by prior work [23]. ROS production was closely associated with increased mitochondrial volume, suggesting a larger, less healthy mitochondrial network. Although we did not observe increased mitochondrial ROS production with chronic alcohol and SIV in the present study, the increased non-mitochondrial OCR could have originated from ROS outside the mitochondria. Additionally, MitoSOX specifically detects mitochondrial superoxide, and in the CBA/SIV condition, superoxide may have been converted to hydrogen peroxide since increased mitochondrial superoxide dismutase has been observed with chronic alcohol and with 100 mM EtOH in vitro [23,45,50]. A sustained increase in whole-cell ROS with chronic alcohol may have mitigated any myoblast mitohormetic adaptations observed with short-term alcohol.

3.3. Glycolytic Enzyme Activity

Given the substantial decreases in myoblast glycolytic parameters, the activity of glycolytic enzymes previously reported to be decreased with alcohol feeding in rodent SKM were assessed [51]. Contrary to findings in chronic alcohol-fed rats, aldolase activity was increased with short-term alcohol. As shown in the schematic provided in Figure 7E, aldolase catalyzes the cleavage of fructose 1,6-bisphosphate into dihydroxyacetone phosphate (DHAP) and glyceraldehyde 3-phosphate (G-3-P). In the canonical glycolytic pathway, DHAP is converted to an additional G-3-P molecule, and both are finally converted to pyruvate via pyruvate kinase. Alternatively, DHAP [52] and G-3-P [53] serve as precursors for triacylglycerol synthesis. Given the decreased pyruvate kinase activity with short-term alcohol that was consistent with decreased glycolysis, the increased aldolase activity observed could potentially be related to increased triacylglycerol synthesis. This hypothesis is supported by population-based studies showing greater circulating triacylglycerol among people with high levels of alcohol intake [54,55]. Such effects of alcohol on triacylglycerol synthesis in myoblasts will be the subject of future investigations. Pyruvate kinase serves as a rate-limiting enzyme, and its knockdown (M2 isoform) substantially decreases glycolytic function in H1299 and HepG2 cells [56]. As pyruvate is required for conversion to lactate, it is possible that decreased pyruvate kinase activity contributed to decreased glycolytic function, capacity, and reserve. An additional fate of pyruvate is entry into the mitochondria for oxidation. It is possible that decreased pyruvate availability from the lower pyruvate kinase activity could have contributed to the decreased mitochondrial ATP production rate; however, alternative fuel sources available for use could have limited the magnitude of this decrease.

3.4. Associations between Differentiation Indices and Bioenergetics Parameters

Basal and ATP-linked oxygen consumption (indicating mitochondrial function), proton leak and non-mitochondrial oxygen consumption (indicating cell stress), and aldolase activity were negatively associated with total nuclei, whereas pyruvate kinase activity was positively associated with total nuclei. Total nuclei depend, in part, on myoblast proliferation. Therefore, it appears that regardless of condition, lower cellular stress and more pyruvate kinase activity are likely to support myoblast proliferation. Although the relationships were weaker, we noted inverse relationships between differentiation and spare capacity, non-mitochondrial oxygen consumption, non-glycolytic acidification, and aldolase activity at differentiation day 0. Conversely, mitochondrial ATP production and ΔΨm were positively associated with differentiation. Although no substantial relationships between glycolytic parameters and differentiation were observed, samples from all groups were analyzed together and CBA/SIV independently decreased differentiation without a concomitant decrease in glycolysis. However, there was a non-significant pattern that we speculate may reflect adaptation in the bioenergetic phenotype toward glycolysis with chronic alcohol. This may have obscured relationships between glycolytic function and decreased differentiation capacity with short-term alcohol, and we propose that there may be divergent mechanisms underlying decreased myoblast differentiation capacity with short-term and chronic alcohol. Whereas short-term alcohol impairs glycolytic function, which is critical for proliferation and early differentiation [24,39], CBA-mediated decreased differentiation could be regulated by other pathways such as decreased miR-206 and an increase in one of its targets, histone deacetylase 4 [33,36,57].

3.5. Limitations

Although the experiments performed in the present study provide critical evidence, several limitations should be considered. We did not have a CBA group without SIV and ART. Therefore, although SIV and ART alone did not appear to decrease SKM differentiation capacity in females, it is possible that chronic alcohol could impact differentiation capacity differently in SIV and ART-naïve SKM. Although determining bioenergetics differences during differentiation is warranted, the purpose of the present study was to determine whether bioenergetic changes during the proliferative phase (i.e., changes preceding differentiation) could contribute to the impaired differentiation capacity. Pyruvate kinase activity was decreased at both 0 and 5 days of differentiation, suggesting that these bioenergetic changes likely persist throughout differentiation. Additionally, we did not measure whole-cell ROS production, mitochondrial biogenesis, or cell death. However, we did not previously observe differences in mitochondrial DNA quantity with short-term alcohol treatment [24] or CBA/SIV [22]. Finally, the majority of bioenergetic effects were observed with short-term alcohol performed using ex vivo studies rather than lasting effects of CBA/SIV after cell expansion in the absence of alcohol, although differentiation decreased similarly with both in vivo and in vitro treatments. Whether the same metabolic changes would be observed in the skeletal muscle precursor cell niche in vivo after short-term alcohol remains to be measured.

4. Materials and Methods

Muscle samples used to isolate myoblasts were derived from a previously described parent longitudinal study [58]. All animal experiments were approved by the Institutional Animal Care and Use Committee at Louisiana State University Health Sciences Center (LSUHSC) in New Orleans, Louisiana, and adhered to the National Institutes of Health guidelines for the care and use of experimental animals, and the methods and results are described in accordance with the ARRIVE guidelines 2.0. Adult (6–9 years old) female rhesus macaques (Macaca mulatta) were maintained on a standard chow diet before undergoing a baseline (i.e., alcohol- and SIV-naïve) vastus lateralis muscle biopsy, followed by randomization to receive chronic binge alcohol (CBA) or isovolumetric water vehicle (VEH) 5 days per week. In the CBA group, macaques were administered ethanol (30% *w/v*) in water over a 30 min intragastric infusion for a peak blood alcohol concentration (BAC) of 50–60 mM (approximately 0.23 g/dL) at 2 h after the start of the infusion. Three months after the initiation of CBA/VEH, macaques were intravaginally infected with SIV_{mac251}. Upon reaching viral set-point 2.5 months after SIV infection, macaques were initiated on an effective daily antiretroviral therapy (ART) regimen [59] consisting of emtricitabine (FTC, 30 mg/kg) and tenofovir (20 mg/kg) subcutaneously. ART medications were provided by Gilead Sciences (Foster City, CA, USA). In the parent study, half of the macaques received ovariectomy surgery one month after ART initiation; samples from macaques post-ovariectomy were not included in the present study. Nine months after ART initiation, animals were euthanized after an overnight fast at the study endpoint according to the guidelines set forth by the American Veterinary Medical Association. SKM samples (vastus lateralis) collected at baseline and at the study endpoint were used for myoblast isolation. The total duration of CBA or VEH administration was 14.5 months (see Figure 9 for study design). Myoblasts will be referred to as "naïve" if they were derived from muscle samples collected before CBA/VEH initiation and "VEH/SIV" or "CBA/SIV" if they were derived from the study endpoint from macaques who received VEH or CBA, respectively. Myoblasts were isolated from ~50 mg of vastus lateralis tissue of 6 female macaques per group (18 total), and cells from 4–6 macaques/group were used in each experiment in the present study. Samples were labeled with IDs and group assignments were masked for experiments.

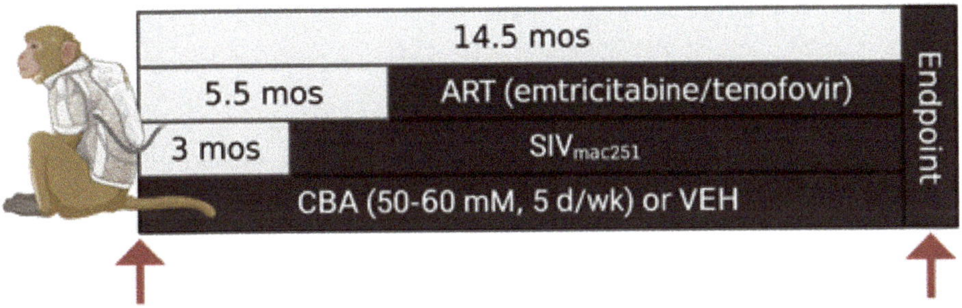

Figure 9. Non-human primate study design. Arrows indicate timing of muscle sampling. The first arrow indicates vastus lateralis muscle biopsy for the naïve group before initiation of CBA or VEH. The second arrow indicates muscle collection at the study endpoint for the CBA/SIV and VEH/SIV groups. Chronic binge alcohol (CBA); vehicle (isovolumetric water; VEH); simian immunodeficiency virus (SIV); antiretroviral therapy (daily subcutaneous injections; ART).

4.1. Myoblast Isolation and Expansion

Primary myoblasts were isolated according to previously published methods [60]. Briefly, excess fat and blood was quickly removed from fresh muscle samples (~50 mg), and samples were minced in trypsin-EDTA (0.25%; Gibco, ThermoFisher Scientific, Waltham, MA, USA) 1:4 in Ham's F-12 (Cytiva, Fisher Scientific, Pittsburgh, PA, USA) and agitated twice for 45 min each in 10 mL total (5 mL per agitation) of the trypsin-EDTA/Ham's F12 mixture at room temperature. After adding 2 mL of fetal bovine serum (FBS, MilliporeSigma, Burlington, MA, USA), the mixture was centrifuged (500× *g*, 5 min, room temperature), supernatant was separated, and the cell tissue mixture was resuspended in growth medium containing 10% FBS in Ham's F-12 with 2.5 ng/mL fibroblast growth factor (FGF, 233-FB, R&D systems, Bio-Techne, Minneapolis, MN, USA), 1× penicillin streptomycin (1% of final volume; Gibco, ThermoFisher Scientific, Waltham, MA, USA), and 4 mM L-glutamine (Gibco, ThermoFisher Scientific, Waltham, MA, USA). The cells were incubated overnight (37 °C, 5% CO_2) before moving to a new culture dish to remove fibroblasts. The growth medium was changed every other day. The cells were grown to approximately 40–50% confluence for passage (P)0 with dense (~100% confluent) individual colonies and 80–90% confluence for subsequent passages. Experiments were performed with myoblasts at P4.

4.2. Short-Term In Vitro Ethanol Treatment and HEMA3 Staining

Myoblasts at P4 from each group (naïve, VEH/SIV, CBA/SIV) were seeded at 70,000 cells/well in 6-well plates and cultured (37 °C, 5% CO_2) in growth media (2 mL/well) containing 0 or 50 mM ethanol (EtOH; 2.92 µL of 200-proof EtOH per 1.00 mL of media) for 3 days. Then, growth medium was replaced with differentiation medium (2% horse serum in Ham's F-12 with 4 mM L-glutamine) containing 0 or 50 mM ethanol (EtOH) for 5 days for fusion into myotubes. This EtOH concentration is physiologically relevant [61–64] and equivalent to the peak blood EtOH level achieved daily in our in vivo model. Myoblasts from each macaque were grown in control media (0 mM EtOH) and media containing 50 mM EtOH. In both phases, EtOH-exposed cells (50 mM) were grown in an incubator containing 75 mM EtOH in the water bath to maintain the media EtOH concentration at 50 mM. This design required the experimenter to be aware of EtOH condition only during short-term EtOH treatments; however, the procedures were planned in detail a priori to minimize risk of bias. At the end of the 5-day differentiation period, myotubes were fixed in ice-cold methanol for 10 min at room temperature and stained with HEMA 3 stains according to previously published methods [60]. Briefly, 1.5 mL of HEMA 3 Solution I (Fisher Scientific, Pittsburgh, PA, USA) were added to cover cells in each well and gently agitated for 10 min at room temperature. After two washes in 1.5 mL distilled water, 1.5 mL of HEMA 3 Solution II (Fisher Scientific, Pittsburgh, PA, USA) were added to cover cells and gently agitated for 10 min at room temperature. After two further washes in 1.5 mL distilled water, the wells were dried and stored at room temperature for imaging.

4.3. Differentiation Indices

HEMA 3-stained cells (naïve, N = 5; VEH/SIV, N = 4; CBA/SIV, N = 5) were imaged at 20× magnification (7–8 images per well) and differentiation indices were determined as previously described [24,60]. For each image, total nuclei, total number of nuclei fused into myotubes (2+ nuclei in one cell), and number of myotubes were counted using ImageJ (https://imagej.net/ij/, accessed on 14 January 2024, National Institutes of Health, Bethesda, MD, USA) by trained investigators not involved with the study to minimize risk of bias. From these counts, myotubes per field, fused nuclei per field, and fusion index (fused nuclei/total nuclei × 100) were calculated as differentiation indices. Total nuclei were also retained as an index of proliferation.

4.4. Mitochondrial Stress Test

Mitochondrial function was assessed using a Mito Stress Test (Agilent Technologies, Santa Clara, CA, USA) [24]. Myoblasts at P4 (naïve, VEH/SIV, CBA/SIV; N = 6/group) were proliferated for 2 days with 0 or 50 mM EtOH under standard cell culture conditions (5% CO_2, 37 °C). They were then transferred to a collagen-coated 96-well Seahorse plate and seeded in triplicate at a density of 30,000 cells/well with 0 or 50 mM EtOH and maintained under standard cell culture conditions overnight. The growth media was then replaced with EtOH-free RPMI (pH 7.4 without sodium bicarbonate or phenol red; Agilent Technologies, Santa Clara, CA, USA) supplemented with sodium pyruvate (1 mM; Agilent Technologies), L-glutamine (2 mM; Agilent Technologies) and glucose (10 mM; Agilent Technologies, Santa Clara, CA, USA). The cells were incubated at 37 °C without CO_2 for 1 h before measuring the myoblast respiratory parameters with an XFe96 Extracellular Flux Analyzer (Agilent Technologies, Santa Clara, CA, USA) according to the manufacturer's instructions. The oxygen consumption rate (OCR) and extracellular acidification rate (ECAR) were simultaneously measured at baseline and after the sequential addition of oligomycin (1.5 μM; Agilent Technologies, Santa Clara, CA, USA), carbonyl cyanide-p-trifluoromethoxyphenylhydrazone (FCCP; 2 μM; Agilent Technologies, Santa Clara, CA, USA), and rotenone/antimycin A (0.5 μM; Agilent Technologies, Santa Clara, CA, USA). The nuclei were stained with Hoechst dye (4 μM; ThermoFisher Scientific, Waltham, MA, USA) and cell counts were captured by visualization on a BioTek Cytation 1 cell imaging multi-mode reader (BioTek, Winooski, VT, USA). Data were normalized to the cell count. Figure S1 (Supplementary Materials) shows an example OCR trace and the graphical portion associated with each parameter.

4.5. Glycolysis Stress Test

Glycolytic function was assessed using a Glycolysis Stress Test (Agilent Technologies, Santa Clara, CA, USA) [65]. Myoblasts at P4 (naïve, VEH/SIV, CBA/SIV; N = 6/group) were grown for 2 days and seeded in triplicate on collagen-coated 96-well Seahorse plates with 0 or 50 mM EtOH overnight as described above. The growth media was then replaced with EtOH-free, glucose-free, pyruvate-free RPMI (pH 7.4 without sodium bicarbonate or phenol red, Agilent Technologies, Santa Clara, CA, USA) supplemented with L-glutamine (2 mM). The cells were incubated at 37 °C without CO_2 for 1 h before measuring the glycolytic parameters with an XFe96 Extracellular Flux Analyzer (Agilent Technologies, Santa Clara, CA, USA) according to the manufacturer's instructions. The extracellular acidification rate (ECAR) was measured at baseline and after the sequential addition of glucose (10 mM; Agilent Technologies, Santa Clara, CA, USA), oligomycin (1.5 μM; Agilent Technologies,

Santa Clara, CA, USA), and 2-deoxyglucose (2-DG; 50 mM; Agilent Technologies, Santa Clara, CA, USA). The nuclei were stained with Hoechst dye (ThermoFisher Scientific, Waltham, MA, USA) and the cells were counted as described above. Data were normalized to the cell count. Figure S2 (Supplementary Materials) shows an example ECAR trace and the graphical portion associated with each parameter.

4.6. *ATP Production Rates*

Total ATP production rates and the contribution of mitochondrial and glycolytic pathways were assessed using an ATP Rate Assay (Agilent Technologies, Santa Clara, CA, USA) [66]. Myoblasts at P4 (naïve, N = 6; VEH/SIV, N = 5; CBA/SIV, N = 6) were grown for 2 days and seeded in triplicate on collagen-coated 96-well Seahorse plates with 0 or 50 mM EtOH overnight as described above. The growth media was then replaced with EtOH-free RPMI (pH 7.4 without sodium bicarbonate or phenol red; Agilent Technologies, Santa Clara, CA, USA) supplemented with sodium pyruvate (1 mM; Agilent Technologies, Santa Clara, CA, USA), L-glutamine (2 mM; Agilent Technologies), and glucose (10 mM; Agilent Technologies, Santa Clara, CA, USA). The cells were incubated at 37 °C without CO_2 for 1 h before measuring the glycolytic parameters with an XFe96 Extracellular Flux Analyzer (Agilent Technologies, Santa Clara, CA, USA) according to the manufacturer's instructions. The oxygen consumption rate (OCR) and ECAR were simultaneously measured, and the proton efflux rate was calculated at baseline and after the sequential addition of oligomycin (1.5 µM, Agilent Technologies, Santa Clara, CA, USA) and rotenone/antimycin A (0.5 µM, Agilent Technologies, Santa Clara, CA, USA). The nuclei were stained with Hoechst dye (ThermoFisher Scientific, Waltham, MA, USA) and the cells were counted as described above. Data were normalized to the cell count.

4.7. *Mitochondrial Health*

Commercially available probes and flow cytometry were used to assess mitochondrial membrane potential ($\Delta\Psi m$) and mitochondrial reactive oxygen species (ROS) as important indicators of mitochondrial health, and to assess mitochondrial network volume to better understand adaptation during cell stress [67,68]. Myoblasts at P4 from each group were proliferated for 3 days with 0 or 50 mM EtOH and evaluated for mitochondrial membrane potential ($\Delta\Psi m$) by incubating cells (naïve, N = 5; VEH/SIV, N = 4; CBA/SIV, N = 5) with tetramethylrhodamine methyl ester (TMRM, 0.1 µM, T668, ThermoFisher Scientific, Waltham, MA, USA) for 30 min at 37 °C. Separately, cells (naïve, N = 4; VEH/SIV, N = 4; CBA/SIV, N = 5) were analyzed simultaneously for mitochondrial reactive oxygen species (ROS) generation using MitoSOX Red (0.5 µM, M36008, ThermoFisher Scientific Waltham, MA, USA) and mitochondrial network volume using MitoTracker Green (0.2 µM, M7514, ThermoFisher Scientific Waltham, MA, USA) for 1 h at 37 °C. Live and dead cells were distinguished using eFluor780 (Invitrogen, Waltham, MA, USA) for all flow cytometry experiments and only results from live cells were considered for analyses. Fifty thousand events per sample were acquired on an 8-color flow cytometer (FACSCANTOII, Becton Dickinson, Franklin Lakes, NJ, USA) and the results were processed using FACSDIVA software (ver. 8.0.1 Becton Dickinson, Franklin Lakes, NJ, USA). Flow cytometry gates were defined based on fluorescence minus one (FMO) controls and are shown in Figure S3 (Supplementary Materials).

4.8. *Glycolytic Enzyme Activity*

Commercially available assays were used to determine the activity of aldolase (MAK223, MilliporeSigma, Burlington, MA, USA) [69] and pyruvate kinase (MAK072, MilliporeSigma, Burlington, MA, USA) [70] in primary macaque myoblasts and myotubes in the naïve (N = 5), VEH/SIV (N = 4) and CBA/SIV (N = 5) groups treated in vitro with 0 or 50 mM EtOH. These enzymes were selected because of previously observed effects of chronic alcohol on their activity in SKM [51,71]. Cells were harvested for analysis after 3 days of proliferation (differentiation day 0) and differentiation day 5. The cells were lysed in the appropriate assay buffer for each kit and protein was quantified using the Pierce BCA Protein Assay Kit (ThermoFisher Scientific, Waltham, MA, USA). Samples were assayed in duplicate with 10 μg (aldolase) or 1 μg (pyruvate kinase) of protein per well. Enzyme activity was calculated according to the manufacturer's guidelines. Values are expressed as activity per μg of protein.

4.9. Statistical Analyses

Data were checked for the assumption of normality using the Shapiro–Wilk test and Q-Q plots. Where normality was not met, data were $\log_{10}$-transformed to correct for this violation [72]. These transformed variables were coupling efficiency, maximal OCR, spare capacity, non-mitochondrial OCR, proton leak, ECAR at baseline and after oligomycin, and the baseline OCR/ECAR ratio. For differentiation indices and bioenergetic health and function measures, data were analyzed using a 2 (short-term EtOH) × 3 (group) analysis of variance with repeated measures on EtOH because cells from each animal were exposed to both EtOH concentrations (0 and 50 mM) for each experiment. Group (naïve, VEH/SIV, or CBA/SIV) was a between-subjects factor because all samples were derived from different macaques. For glycolytic enzyme activity, a 2 (short-term EtOH) × 3 (group) analysis of variance with repeated measures on EtOH was used to analyze data at each time point (differentiation day 0 and day 5). Because the "group" factor had 3 levels, Tukey's HSD was used to detect the location of any main group effects. To minimize risk of bias, levels of each factor were numerically coded during analysis. Fisher's LSD post hoc pairwise analysis was used to detect the location of any short-term EtOH × group interaction effects. Eta squared (η^2) effect sizes were calculated for any main or interaction effects and Cohen's d effect sizes were calculated for any pairwise differences. Data are presented as individual data points with a line connecting results from myoblasts isolated from a single individual in the control treatment (0 mM EtOH) and exposed to short-term EtOH (50 mM). Then, Spearman correlations were used to assess relationships between mitochondrial ROS and network volume and between differentiation indices and key bioenergetics parameters. For correlations, Spearman's rho (ϱ) was used as the measure of effect size. All effect size interpretations are provided in accordance with Cohen's guidelines [73]. The alpha level of significance was set to $p \leq 0.05$. Statistical analyses were performed using SPSS Statistics (version 29, IBM Corporation, Armonk, NY, USA).

5. Conclusions

The results of the present study reveal for the first time that short-term and chronic alcohol non-synergistically decrease the differentiation capacity of myoblasts from female macaques. Moreover, bioenergetic function was impaired with short-term alcohol, with a deficit in ATP production driven largely by decreased glycolytic function. Short-term in vitro alcohol treatment increased maximal mitochondrial oxygen consumption and decreased glycolytic capacity and reserve. Finally, short-term alcohol decreased pyruvate kinase activity, mitochondrial membrane potential, and mitochondrial ROS production and increased aldolase activity, suggesting possible alternative glucose fates with alcohol misuse. Although further mechanistic data are needed for confirmation, these data suggest possible divergent mechanisms underlying differentiation capacity with short-term and chronic alcohol. These findings support future investigations to examine potential therapeutic or lifestyle interventions to mitigate the adverse effects of alcohol misuse on bioenergetic function and muscle differentiation capacity, and identify targets that effectively improve functional SKM mass and quality of life in people with AUD.

Supplementary Materials: The following supporting information can be downloaded at: https://www.mdpi.com/article/10.3390/ijms25042448/s1.

Author Contributions: Study conceptualization and methodology: D.E.L., P.E.M. and L.S., resources: P.E.M. and L.S., experimentation: D.E.L., B.L.B., K.M.R.-G. and L.S., validation and formal analyses: D.E.L., B.L.B. and K.M.R.-G., interpretation of results: D.E.L., K.M.R.-G., P.E.M. and L.S., figure preparation: D.E.L., manuscript drafting: D.E.L., manuscript editing and revision: B.L.B., K.M.R.-G.,

P.E.M. and L.S., approval of final manuscript version: D.E.L., B.L.B., K.M.R.-G., P.E.M. and L.S. All authors have read and agreed to the published version of the manuscript.

Funding: This work was supported by grants from the NIH/NIAAA: P60AA009803 (PEM), F32AA027982 (DEL), T32AA007577 (PEM), and K01AA024494 (LS).

Institutional Review Board Statement: This study was fully approved by the Institutional Animal Care and Use Committee (IACUC) at Louisiana State University Health Sciences Center (LSUHSC), New Orleans, LA, USA.

Informed Consent Statement: Not applicable.

Data Availability Statement: The data presented in this study are available on reasonable request from the corresponding author.

Acknowledgments: The authors would like to acknowledge Gregory Bagby and Steve Nelson for their support and design of the original animal study, Jeffrey Schumacher and Leslie Birke for their veterinary expertise, Patrick McTernan and Robert Siggins for their scientific and flow cytometry expertise, and the excellent veterinary and animal care from Larry Coleman and Heather McGarrah. The authors are grateful for the technical support of LSUHSC research associates Bryant Autin and Curtis Vande Stouwe, and for the assistance of Texas Tech University students Colby Newman, Chelsea Daniels, Matthew DiLeo, Rylea Helmberger, Connor Mills, Laiza Que, Ashley Williams, and Kaitlyn Zamagni. We would like to acknowledge the Cellular Immunology and Immune Metabolism Core at the Louisiana Cancer Research Center (Grant 5P30GM114732-05 NIH/NIGMS) for access to the Seahorse XFe96 Extracellular Flux Analyzer, and give thanks to Dorota Wyczechowska and Jay Dunn for technical support.

Conflicts of Interest: The authors declare no conflicts of interest.

References

1. SAMHSA, Center for Behavioral Health Statistics and Quality. *2021 National Survey on Drug Use and Health, Table 2.28B—Binge Alcohol Use in Past Month: Among People Aged 12 or Older; by Age Group and Demographic Characteristics, Percentages*; SAMHSA: Rockville, MD, USA, 2021.
2. SAMHSA, Center for Behavioral Health Statistics and Quality. *2021 National Survey on Drug Use and Health, Table 2.29B—Heavy Alcohol Use in Past Month: Among People Aged 12 or Older; by Age Group and Demographic Characteristics, Percentages*; SAMHSA: Rockville, MD, USA, 2021.
3. SAMHSA, Center for Behavioral Health Statistics and Quality. *2021 National Survey on Drug Use and Health, Table 5.6A—Alcohol Use Disorder in Past Year: Among People Aged 12 or Older; by Age Group and Demographic Characteristics, Numbers in Thousands;* SAMHSA: Rockville, MD, USA, 2021.
4. Duko, B.; Ayalew, M.; Ayano, G. The Prevalence of Alcohol Use Disorders among People Living with HIV/AIDS: A Systematic Review and Meta-Analysis. *Subst. Abus. Treat. Prev. Policy* **2019**, *14*, 52. [CrossRef]
5. Glantz, M.D.; Bharat, C.; Degenhardt, L.; Sampson, N.A.; Scott, K.M.; Lim, C.C.W.; Al-Hamzawi, A.; Alonso, J.; Andrade, L.H.; Cardoso, G.; et al. The Epidemiology of Alcohol Use Disorders Cross-Nationally: Findings from the World Mental Health Surveys. *Addict. Behav.* **2020**, *102*, 106128. [CrossRef] [PubMed]
6. Crotty, K.; Anton, P.; Coleman, L.G.; Morris, N.L.; Lewis, S.A.; Samuelson, D.R.; McMahan, R.H.; Hartmann, P.; Kim, A.; Ratna, A.; et al. A Critical Review of Recent Knowledge of Alcohol's Effects on the Immunological Response in Different Tissues. *Alcohol Clin. Exp. Res.* **2023**, *47*, 36–44. [CrossRef] [PubMed]
7. Olesen, M.A.; Quintanilla, R.A. The Effects of Alcohol Abuse against the Mitochondria: Functional Consequences for Liver, Muscle, and the Brain. In *Mitochondrial Intoxication;* Elsevier: Amsterdam, The Netherlands, 2023; pp. 181–204. ISBN 978-0-323-88462-4.
8. Molina, P.E.; Simon, L.; Amedee, A.M.; Welsh, D.A.; Ferguson, T.F. Impact of Alcohol on HIV Disease Pathogenesis, Comorbidities and Aging: Integrating Preclinical and Clinical Findings. *Alcohol Alcohol.* **2018**, *53*, 439–447. [CrossRef] [PubMed]
9. Estruch, R.; Nicolás, J.M.; Villegas, E.; Junqué, A.; Urbano-Márquez, A. Relationship between Ethanol-Related Diseases and Nutritional Status in Chronically Alcoholic Men. *Alcohol Alcohol.* **1993**, *28*, 543–550. [PubMed]
10. Richert, L.; Dehail, P.; Mercié, P.; Dauchy, F.-A.; Bruyand, M.; Greib, C.; Dabis, F.; Bonnet, F.; Chêne, G.; Groupe d'Epidémiologie Clinique du SIDA en Aquitaine (GECSA). High Frequency of Poor Locomotor Performance in HIV-Infected Patients. *AIDS* **2011**, *25*, 797–805. [CrossRef] [PubMed]
11. Echeverría, P.; Bonjoch, A.; Puig, J.; Estany, C.; Ornelas, A.; Clotet, B.; Negredo, E. High Prevalence of Sarcopenia in HIV-Infected Individuals. *BioMed Res. Int.* **2018**, *2018*, 5074923. [CrossRef] [PubMed]
12. Koon-Yee Lee, G.; Chun-Ming Au, P.; Hoi-Yee Li, G.; Chan, M.; Li, H.-L.; Man-Yung Cheung, B.; Chi-Kei Wong, I.; Ho-Fun Lee, V.; Mok, J.; Hon-Kei Yip, B.; et al. Sarcopenia and Mortality in Different Clinical Conditions: A Meta-Analysis. *Osteoporos. Sarcopenia* **2021**, *7*, S19–S27. [CrossRef] [PubMed]

13. Cáceres-Ayala, C.; Mira, R.G.; Acuña, M.J.; Brandan, E.; Cerpa, W.; Rebolledo, D.L. Episodic Binge-like Ethanol Reduces Skeletal Muscle Strength Associated with Atrophy, Fibrosis, and Inflammation in Young Rats. *Int. J. Mol. Sci.* **2023**, *24*, 1655. [CrossRef]
14. Steiner, J.L.; Lang, C.H. Dysregulation of Skeletal Muscle Protein Metabolism by Alcohol. *Am. J. Physiol. Endocrinol. Metab.* **2015**, *308*, E699–E712. [CrossRef]
15. Preedy, V.R.; Ohlendieck, K.; Adachi, J.; Koll, M.; Sneddon, A.; Hunter, R.; Rajendram, R.; Mantle, D.; Peters, T.J. The Importance of Alcohol-Induced Muscle Disease. *J. Muscle Res. Cell. Motil.* **2003**, *24*, 55–63. [CrossRef]
16. Chen, B.; Shan, T. The Role of Satellite and Other Functional Cell Types in Muscle Repair and Regeneration. *J. Muscle Res. Cell Motil.* **2019**, *40*, 1–8. [CrossRef]
17. Schmidt, M.; Schüler, S.C.; Hüttner, S.S.; von Eyss, B.; von Maltzahn, J. Adult Stem Cells at Work: Regenerating Skeletal Muscle. *Cell Mol. Life Sci.* **2019**, *76*, 2559–2570. [CrossRef]
18. Bhattacharya, D.; Scimè, A. Mitochondrial Function in Muscle Stem Cell Fates. *Front. Cell Dev. Biol.* **2020**, *8*, 480. [CrossRef]
19. Tang, A.H.; Rando, T.A. Induction of Autophagy Supports the Bioenergetic Demands of Quiescent Muscle Stem Cell Activation. *EMBO J.* **2014**, *33*, 2782–2797. [CrossRef] [PubMed]
20. Abreu, P.; Garay, B.I.; Nemkov, T.; Yamashita, A.M.S.; Perlingeiro, R.C.R. Metabolic Changes during In Vivo Maturation of PSC-Derived Skeletal Myogenic Progenitors. *Cells* **2023**, *13*, 76. [CrossRef]
21. Levitt, D.E.; Ferguson, T.F.; Primeaux, S.D.; Zavala, J.A.; Ahmed, J.; Marshall, R.H.; Simon, L.; Molina, P.E. Skeletal Muscle Bioenergetic Health and Function in People Living with HIV: Association with Glucose Tolerance and Alcohol Use. *Am. J. Physiol. Regul. Integr. Comp. Physiol.* **2021**, *321*, R781–R790. [CrossRef] [PubMed]
22. Duplanty, A.A.; Siggins, R.W.; Allerton, T.; Simon, L.; Molina, P.E. Myoblast Mitochondrial Respiration Is Decreased in Chronic Binge Alcohol Administered Simian Immunodeficiency Virus-Infected Antiretroviral-Treated Rhesus Macaques. *Physiol. Rep.* **2018**, *6*, e13625. [CrossRef] [PubMed]
23. Kumar, A.; Davuluri, G.; Welch, N.; Kim, A.; Gangadhariah, M.; Allawy, A.; Priyadarshini, A.; McMullen, M.R.; Sandlers, Y.; Willard, B.; et al. Oxidative Stress Mediates Ethanol-Induced Skeletal Muscle Mitochondrial Dysfunction and Dysregulated Protein Synthesis and Autophagy. *Free Radic. Biol. Med.* **2019**, *145*, 284–299. [CrossRef]
24. Levitt, D.E.; Chalapati, N.; Prendergast, M.J.; Simon, L.; Molina, P.E. Ethanol-Impaired Myogenic Differentiation Is Associated With Decreased Myoblast Glycolytic Function. *Alcohol. Clin. Exp. Res.* **2020**, *44*, 2166–2176. [CrossRef]
25. Ganjayi, M.S.; Brown, A.M.; Baumann, C.W. Longitudinal Assessment of Strength and Body Composition in Mice Subjected to Chronic Ethanol Consumption. *Alcohol* **2023**, *Ahead of Print*, 1–12. [CrossRef]
26. Centers for Disease Control and Prevention. Estimated HIV Incidence and Prevalence in the United States, 2015–2019. *HIV Surveill. Suppl. Rep.* **2021**, *26*, 1.
27. Zhang, Z.; Luo, W.; Chen, G.; Chen, J.; Lin, S.; Ren, T.; Lin, Z.; Zhao, C.; Wen, H.; Nie, Q.; et al. Chicken Muscle Antibody Array Reveals the Regulations of LDHA on Myoblast Differentiation through Energy Metabolism. *Int. J. Biol. Macromol.* **2024**, *254*, 127629. [CrossRef]
28. Tixier, V.; Bataillé, L.; Etard, C.; Jagla, T.; Weger, M.; Daponte, J.P.; Strähle, U.; Dickmeis, T.; Jagla, K. Glycolysis Supports Embryonic Muscle Growth by Promoting Myoblast Fusion. *Proc. Natl. Acad. Sci. USA* **2013**, *110*, 18982–18987. [CrossRef] [PubMed]
29. Sin, J.; Andres, A.M.; Taylor, D.J.R.; Weston, T.; Hiraumi, Y.; Stotland, A.; Kim, B.J.; Huang, C.; Doran, K.S.; Gottlieb, R.A. Mitophagy Is Required for Mitochondrial Biogenesis and Myogenic Differentiation of C2C12 Myoblasts. *Autophagy* **2016**, *12*, 369–380. [CrossRef]
30. Fortini, P.; Ferretti, C.; Iorio, E.; Cagnin, M.; Garribba, L.; Pietraforte, D.; Falchi, M.; Pascucci, B.; Baccarini, S.; Morani, F.; et al. The Fine Tuning of Metabolism, Autophagy and Differentiation during in Vitro Myogenesis. *Cell Death Dis.* **2016**, *7*, e2168. [CrossRef]
31. Roman, W.; Pinheiro, H.; Pimentel, M.R.; Segalés, J.; Oliveira, L.M.; García-Domínguez, E.; Gómez-Cabrera, M.C.; Serrano, A.L.; Gomes, E.R.; Muñoz-Cánoves, P. Muscle Repair after Physiological Damage Relies on Nuclear Migration for Cellular Reconstruction. *Science* **2021**, *374*, 355–359. [CrossRef] [PubMed]
32. Radugina, E.A.; Almeida, E.A.C.; Blaber, E.; Poplinskaya, V.A.; Markitantova, Y.V.; Grigoryan, E.N. Exposure to Microgravity for 30 Days Onboard Bion M1 Caused Muscle Atrophy and Impaired Regeneration in Murine Femoral Quadriceps. *Life Sci. Space Res.* **2018**, *16*, 18–25. [CrossRef]
33. Simon, L.; LeCapitaine, N.; Berner, P.; Vande Stouwe, C.; Mussell, J.C.; Allerton, T.; Primeaux, S.D.; Dufour, J.; Nelson, S.; Bagby, G.J.; et al. Chronic Binge Alcohol Consumption Alters Myogenic Gene Expression and Reduces in Vitro Myogenic Differentiation Potential of Myoblasts from Rhesus Macaques. *Am. J. Physiol. Regul. Integr. Comp. Physiol.* **2014**, *306*, R837–R844. [CrossRef]
34. Webster, K.A.; Gunning, P.; Hardeman, E.; Wallace, D.C.; Kedes, L. Coordinate Reciprocal Trends in Glycolytic and Mitochondrial Transcript Accumulations during the in Vitro Differentiation of Human Myoblasts. *J. Cell. Physiol.* **1990**, *142*, 566–573. [CrossRef]
35. Levitt, D.E.; Yeh, A.Y.; Prendergast, M.J.; Jr, R.G.B.; Adler, K.A.; Cook, G.; Molina, P.E.; Simon, L. Chronic Alcohol Dysregulates Skeletal Muscle Myogenic Gene Expression after Hind Limb Immobilization in Female Rats. *Biomolecules* **2020**, *10*, 441. [CrossRef] [PubMed]
36. Simon, L.; Ford, S.M.; Song, K.; Berner, P.; Vande Stouwe, C.; Nelson, S.; Bagby, G.J.; Molina, P.E. Decreased Myoblast Differentiation in Chronic Binge Alcohol-Administered Simian Immunodeficiency Virus-Infected Male Macaques: Role of Decreased miR-206. *Am. J. Physiol. Regul. Integr. Comp. Physiol.* **2017**, *313*, R240–R250. [CrossRef] [PubMed]

37. Yarasheski, K.E.; Scherzer, R.; Kotler, D.P.; Dobs, A.S.; Tien, P.C.; Lewis, C.E.; Kronmal, R.A.; Heymsfield, S.B.; Bacchetti, P.; Grunfeld, C.; et al. Age-Related Skeletal Muscle Decline Is Similar in HIV-Infected and Uninfected Individuals. *J. Gerontol. A Biol. Sci. Med. Sci.* **2011**, *66*, 332–340. [CrossRef] [PubMed]
38. Margolis, A.M.; Heverling, H.; Pham, P.A.; Stolbach, A. A Review of the Toxicity of HIV Medications. *J. Med. Toxicol.* **2014**, *10*, 26–39. [CrossRef] [PubMed]
39. Pala, F.; Di Girolamo, D.; Mella, S.; Yennek, S.; Chatre, L.; Ricchetti, M.; Tajbakhsh, S. Distinct Metabolic States Govern Skeletal Muscle Stem Cell Fates during Prenatal and Postnatal Myogenesis. *J. Cell. Sci.* **2018**, *131*, jcs212977. [CrossRef] [PubMed]
40. Olson, K.N.; Smith, S.W.; Kloss, J.S.; Ho, J.D.; Apple, F.S. Relationship Between Blood Alcohol Concentration and Observable Symptoms of Intoxication in Patients Presenting to an Emergency Department. *Alcohol Alcohol.* **2013**, *48*, 386–389. [CrossRef]
41. Liang, Y.; Harris, F.L.; Jones, D.P.; Brown, L.A.S. Alcohol Induces Mitochondrial Redox Imbalance in Alveolar Macrophages. *Free Radic. Biol. Med.* **2013**, *65*, 1427–1434. [CrossRef]
42. Han, D.; Ybanez, M.D.; Johnson, H.S.; McDonald, J.N.; Mesropyan, L.; Sancheti, H.; Martin, G.; Martin, A.; Lim, A.M.; Dara, L.; et al. Dynamic Adaptation of Liver Mitochondria to Chronic Alcohol Feeding in Mice: Biogenesis, Remodeling, and Functional Alterations. *J. Biol. Chem.* **2012**, *287*, 42165–42179. [CrossRef]
43. Han, D.; Johnson, H.S.; Rao, M.P.; Martin, G.; Sancheti, H.; Silkwood, K.H.; Decker, C.W.; Nguyen, K.T.; Casian, J.G.; Cadenas, E.; et al. Mitochondrial Remodeling in the Liver Following Chronic Alcohol Feeding to Rats. *Free Radic. Biol. Med.* **2017**, *102*, 100–110. [CrossRef]
44. Tice, A.L.; Laudato, J.A.; Fadool, D.A.; Gordon, B.S.; Steiner, J.L. Acute Binge Alcohol Alters Whole Body Metabolism and the Time-Dependent Expression of Skeletal Muscle-Specific Metabolic Markers for Multiple Days in Mice. *Am. J. Physiol.-Endocrinol. Metab.* **2022**, *323*, E215–E230. [CrossRef] [PubMed]
45. Keen, C.; Tamura, T.; Lönnerdal, B.; Hurley, L.; Halsted, C. Changes in Hepatic Superoxide Dismutase Activity in Alcoholic Monkeys. *Am. J. Clin. Nutr.* **1985**, *41*, 929–932. [CrossRef]
46. Nye, G.A.; Sakellariou, G.K.; Degens, H.; Lightfoot, A.P. Muscling in on Mitochondrial Sexual Dimorphism; Role of Mitochondrial Dimorphism in Skeletal Muscle Health and Disease. *Clin. Sci. (Lond.)* **2017**, *131*, 1919–1922. [CrossRef]
47. Colom, B.; Alcolea, M.; Valle, A.; Oliver, J.; Roca, P.; García-Palmer, F. Skeletal Muscle of Female Rats Exhibit Higher Mitochondrial Mass and Oxidative-Phosphorylative Capacities Compared to Males. *Cell Physiol. Biochem.* **2007**, *19*, 205–212. [CrossRef] [PubMed]
48. Miotto, P.M.; McGlory, C.; Holloway, T.M.; Phillips, S.M.; Holloway, G.P. Sex Differences in Mitochondrial Respiratory Function in Human Skeletal Muscle. *Am. J. Physiol. Regul. Integr. Comp. Physiol.* **2018**, *314*, R909–R915. [CrossRef] [PubMed]
49. Chacko, B.K.; Kramer, P.A.; Ravi, S.; Benavides, G.A.; Mitchell, T.; Dranka, B.P.; Ferrick, D.; Singal, A.K.; Ballinger, S.W.; Bailey, S.M.; et al. The Bioenergetic Health Index: A New Concept in Mitochondrial Translational Research. *Clin. Sci.* **2014**, *127*, 367–373. [CrossRef] [PubMed]
50. Thome, J.; Foley, P.; Gsell, W.; Davids, E.; Wodarz, N.; Wiesbeck, G.A.; Böning, J.; Riederer, P. Increased Concentrations of Manganese Superoxide Dismutase in Serum of Alcohol-Dependent Patients. *Alcohol Alcohol.* **1997**, *32*, 65–69. [CrossRef] [PubMed]
51. Trounce, I.; Byrne, E.; Dennett, X. Biochemical and Morphological Studies of Skeletal Muscle in Experimental Chronic Alcoholic Myopathy. *Acta Neurol. Scand.* **1990**, *82*, 386–391. [CrossRef] [PubMed]
52. Hajra, A.K.; Larkins, L.K.; Das, A.K.; Hemati, N.; Erickson, R.L.; MacDougald, O.A. Induction of the Peroxisomal Glycerolipid-Synthesizing Enzymes during Differentiation of 3T3-L1 Adipocytes. Role in Triacylglycerol Synthesis. *J. Biol. Chem.* **2000**, *275*, 9441–9446. [CrossRef] [PubMed]
53. Smith, S.B.; Lin, K.C.; Wilson, J.J.; Lunt, D.K.; Cross, H.R. Starvation Depresses Acylglycerol Biosynthesis in Bovine Subcutaneous but Not Intramuscular Adipose Tissue Homogenates. *Comp. Biochem. Physiol. B Biochem. Mol. Biol.* **1998**, *120*, 165–174. [CrossRef]
54. Whitfield, J.B.; Heath, A.C.; Madden, P.A.F.; Pergadia, M.L.; Montgomery, G.W.; Martin, N.G. Metabolic and Biochemical Effects of Low-to-Moderate Alcohol Consumption. *Alcohol. Clin. Exp. Res.* **2013**, *37*, 575–586. [CrossRef]
55. Foerster, M.; Marques-Vidal, P.; Gmel, G.; Daeppen, J.-B.; Cornuz, J.; Hayoz, D.; Pécoud, A.; Mooser, V.; Waeber, G.; Vollenweider, P.; et al. Alcohol Drinking and Cardiovascular Risk in a Population with High Mean Alcohol Consumption. *Am. J. Cardiol.* **2009**, *103*, 361–368. [CrossRef] [PubMed]
56. Li, T.; Han, J.; Jia, L.; Hu, X.; Chen, L.; Wang, Y. PKM2 Coordinates Glycolysis with Mitochondrial Fusion and Oxidative Phosphorylation. *Protein Cell* **2019**, *10*, 583–594. [CrossRef] [PubMed]
57. Adler, K.; Molina, P.E.; Simon, L. Epigenomic Mechanisms of Alcohol-Induced Impaired Differentiation of Skeletal Muscle Stem Cells; Role of Class IIA Histone Deacetylases. *Physiol. Genom.* **2019**, *51*, 471–479. [CrossRef] [PubMed]
58. Simon, L.; Torres, D.; Saravia, A.; Levitt, D.E.; Vande Stouwe, C.; McGarrah, H.; Coleman, L.; Dufour, J.P.; Amedee, A.M.; Molina, P.E. Chronic Binge Alcohol and Ovariectomy-Mediated Impaired Insulin Responsiveness in SIV-Infected Female Rhesus Macaques. *Am. J. Physiol. Regul. Integr. Comp. Physiol.* **2021**, *321*, R699–R711. [CrossRef] [PubMed]
59. Molina, P.E.; Amedee, A.M.; Veazey, R.; Dufour, J.; Volaufova, J.; Bagby, G.J.; Nelson, S. Chronic Binge Alcohol Consumption Does Not Diminish Effectiveness of Continuous Antiretroviral Suppression of Viral Load in Simian Immunodeficiency Virus-Infected Macaques. *Alcohol. Clin. Exp. Res.* **2014**, *38*, 2335–2344. [CrossRef] [PubMed]
60. Levitt, D.E.; Adler, K.A.; Simon, L. HEMA 3 Staining: A Simple Alternative for the Assessment of Myoblast Differentiation. *Curr. Protoc. Stem Cell Biol.* **2019**, *51*, e101. [CrossRef] [PubMed]
61. Honkanen, R.; Visuri, T. Blood Alcohol Levels in a Series of Injured Patients with Special Reference to Accident and Type of Injury. *Ann. Chir. Gynaecol.* **1976**, *65*, 287–294.

62. Perry, P.J.; Argo, T.R.; Barnett, M.J.; Liesveld, J.L.; Liskow, B.; Hernan, J.M.; Trnka, M.G.; Brabson, M.A. The Association of Alcohol-Induced Blackouts and Grayouts to Blood Alcohol Concentrations. *J. Forensic Sci.* **2006**, *51*, 896–899. [CrossRef]
63. Kenna, G.A.; Haass-Koffler, C.L.; Zywiak, W.H.; Edwards, S.M.; Brickley, M.B.; Swift, R.M.; Leggio, L. Role of the A1 Blocker Doxazosin in Alcoholism: A Proof-of-Concept Randomized Controlled Trial. *Addict. Biol.* **2016**, *21*, 904–914. [CrossRef]
64. Grant, K.A.; Leng, X.; Green, H.L.; Szeliga, K.T.; Rogers, L.S.M.; Gonzales, S.W. Drinking Typography Established by Scheduled Induction Predicts Chronic Heavy Drinking in a Monkey Model of Ethanol Self-Administration. *Alcohol. Clin. Exp. Res.* **2008**, *32*, 1824–1838. [CrossRef]
65. TeSlaa, T.; Teitell, M.A. Techniques to Monitor Glycolysis. In *Methods in Enzymology*; Elsevier: Amsterdam, The Netherlands, 2014; Volume 542, pp. 91–114. ISBN 978-0-12-416618-9.
66. Desousa, B.R.; Kim, K.K.; Jones, A.E.; Ball, A.B.; Hsieh, W.Y.; Swain, P.; Morrow, D.H.; Brownstein, A.J.; Ferrick, D.A.; Shirihai, O.S.; et al. Calculation of ATP Production Rates Using the Seahorse XF Analyzer. *EMBO Rep.* **2023**, *24*, e56380. [CrossRef] [PubMed]
67. Kuznetsov, A.V.; Kehrer, I.; Kozlov, A.V.; Haller, M.; Redl, H.; Hermann, M.; Grimm, M.; Troppmair, J. Mitochondrial ROS Production under Cellular Stress: Comparison of Different Detection Methods. *Anal. Bioanal. Chem.* **2011**, *400*, 2383–2390. [CrossRef] [PubMed]
68. Gilkerson, R.; De La Torre, P.; St. Vallier, S. Mitochondrial OMA1 and OPA1 as Gatekeepers of Organellar Structure/Function and Cellular Stress Response. *Front. Cell Dev. Biol.* **2021**, *9*, 626117. [CrossRef]
69. Guo, Z.; Pan, F.; Peng, L.; Tian, S.; Jiao, J.; Liao, L.; Lu, C.; Zhai, G.; Wu, Z.; Dong, H.; et al. Systematic Proteome and Lysine Succinylome Analysis Reveals Enhanced Cell Migration by Hyposuccinylation in Esophageal Squamous Cell Carcinoma. *Mol. Cell. Proteom.* **2021**, *20*, 100053. [CrossRef] [PubMed]
70. Coassolo, S.; Davidson, G.; Negroni, L.; Gambi, G.; Daujat, S.; Romier, C.; Davidson, I. Citrullination of Pyruvate Kinase M2 by PADI1 and PADI3 Regulates Glycolysis and Cancer Cell Proliferation. *Nat. Commun.* **2021**, *12*, 1718. [CrossRef]
71. Trounce, I.; Byrne, E.; Dennett, X.; Santamaria, J.; Doery, J.; Peppard, R. Chronic Alcoholic Proximal Wasting: Physiological, Morphological and Biochemical Studies in Skeletal Muscle. *Aust. N. Z. J. Med.* **1987**, *17*, 413–419. [CrossRef]
72. Pek, J.; Wong, O.; Wong, A.C.M. How to Address Non-Normality: A Taxonomy of Approaches, Reviewed, and Illustrated. *Front. Psychol.* **2018**, *9*, 2104. [CrossRef]
73. Cohen, J. *Statistical Power Analysis for the Behavioral Sciences*, 2nd ed.; Erlbaum: Hillsdale, NJ, USA, 1988.

International Journal of *Molecular Sciences*

MDPI

Review

Mitochondrial Dysfunction and Coenzyme Q10 Supplementation in Post-Viral Fatigue Syndrome: An Overview

David Mantle [1,*,†], Iain Parry Hargreaves [2], Joan Carles Domingo [3] and Jesus Castro-Marrero [4,*,†]

1 Pharma Nord (UK) Ltd., Morpeth, Northumberland NE61 2DB, UK
2 School of Pharmacy and Biomolecular Sciences, Liverpool John Moores University, Liverpool L3 3AF, UK; i.hargreaves@acl.ac.uk
3 Department of Biochemistry and Molecular Biomedicine, Faculty of Biology, University of Barcelona, 08028 Barcelona, Spain; jcdomingo@ub.edu
4 Research Unit in ME/CFS and Long COVID, Rheumatology Division, Vall d'Hebron Research Institute, Universitat Autònoma de Barcelona, 08035 Barcelona, Spain
* Correspondence: dmantle@pharmanord.com (D.M.); jesus.castro@vhir.org (J.C.-M.)
† These authors contributed equally to this work.

Abstract: Post-viral fatigue syndrome (PVFS) encompasses a wide range of complex neuroimmune disorders of unknown causes characterised by disabling post-exertional fatigue, myalgia and joint pain, cognitive impairments, unrefreshing sleep, autonomic dysfunction, and neuropsychiatric symptoms. It includes myalgic encephalomyelitis, also known as chronic fatigue syndrome (ME/CFS); fibromyalgia (FM); and more recently post-COVID-19 condition (long COVID). To date, there are no definitive clinical case criteria and no FDA-approved pharmacological therapies for PVFS. Given the current lack of effective treatments, there is a need to develop novel therapeutic strategies for these disorders. Mitochondria, the cellular organelles responsible for tissue energy production, have recently garnered attention in research into PVFS due to their crucial role in cellular bioenergetic metabolism in these conditions. The accumulating literature has identified a link between mitochondrial dysfunction and low-grade systemic inflammation in ME/CFS, FM, and long COVID. To address this issue, this article aims to critically review the evidence relating to mitochondrial dysfunction in the pathogenesis of these disorders; in particular, it aims to evaluate the effectiveness of coenzyme Q10 supplementation on chronic fatigue and pain symptoms as a novel therapeutic strategy for the treatment of PVFS.

Keywords: chronic fatigue syndrome; coenzyme Q10; fibromyalgia; long COVID; mitochondrial dysfunction; myalgic encephalomyelitis; post-viral fatigue syndrome

1. Introduction

Post-viral fatigue syndrome (PVFS) comprises common neuroimmune conditions of unknown aetiology based on the updated WHO International Classification of Diseases for Mortality and Morbidity Statistics (https://icd.who.int/browse11/l-m/en, accessed on 15 September 2023). PVFS includes myalgic encephalomyelitis/chronic fatigue syndrome (ME/CFS), fibromyalgia (FM), and recently post-COVID-19 condition (long COVID). PVFS is characterised by prolonged post-exertional fatigue as the hallmark symptom, which worsens with minimal physical and mental exertions, along with myalgia and joint pain; cognitive impairments; unrefreshing sleep; dysautonomia; and neuropsychiatric symptoms, such as emotional lability, anxiety/depression, and apathy, which typically occur following repeated viral infections. Although PVFS is not a generally recognised disorder, it has recently become increasingly associated with the post-COVID-19 condition [1,2].

There are over 65 million people worldwide suffering from chronic disabling disorders who are diagnosed without a clear elucidation of pathophysiologic mechanisms. In addition to this massive disorder burden, the CDC now estimates that a large increase in the prevalence of ME/CFS after COVID-19 is expected to affect more than 150 million people by 2050 worldwide, a challenge still unresolved by global healthcare system [3].

To date, there are no definitive diagnostic case criteria, no accurate diagnostic tests, and no FDA-approved pharmacological treatments for PVFS. Because the exact aetiology of this disorder is not fully understood, together with the unpredictable nature of symptoms, the diagnosis and management of the disease can be challenging. The onset of disease is multifactorial (e.g., a combination of immunogenetic and environmental factors); can occur suddenly or develop gradually over time; and is typically associated with triggering events, which, in addition to viral infections, may include physical and emotional trauma [4]. PVFS is often triggered by common viral infections such as the Epstein–Barr virus (EBV), human herpesvirus (HHVs), cytomegalovirus (CMV), SARS-CoV-2 (COVID-19), amongst others [5,6].

ME/CFS, FM, and long COVID are debilitating multisystem conditions that affect most body systems and are characterised by overwhelming fatigue and widespread musculoskeletal pain that is not alleviated by rest and cannot be explained by any underlying medical condition. In addition to fatigue and chronic pain as the "prime" symptoms, individuals may experience an array of symptoms such as post-exertional malaise, unrefreshing sleep, cognitive impairments commonly known as "brain fog", orthostatic intolerance, and gastrointestinal complaints [7–9].

These conditions affect millions of people of any age, gender (although predominantly women), and socio-economic burden worldwide, and the widely varying impact on individuals' daily functioning and quality of life can be significant [10,11]. The severity of the disease can fluctuate in frequency and intensity over time among patients, ranging from mild to moderate symptoms, while others can be severely affected, with around 25% housebound or bedridden [12,13]. The above conditions are established disorders, and their background will not be described further. Long COVID is a more recently recognised disorder, and it is further described below.

Post-acute sequelae of SARS-CoV-2 infection (PASC), also known as post-COVID-19 condition or long COVID, is an emerging umbrella condition, defined as a constellation of ongoing, relapsing, or new symptoms experienced by people following an acute COVID-19 infection that continue for months and even years [14,15]. While most individuals recover from a COVID-19 infection within a few weeks, some of them continue to experience prolonged symptoms that can significantly impact their daily functioning and quality of life. People who experience long COVID sometimes refer to themselves as "long-haulers" [16]. The term "long COVID" will be used throughout this review.

A significant portion of convalescent COVID-19 patients, estimated at 10–30% (over 30 million people in the U.S., 20 million in Europe, and up to 180 million worldwide) may experience long COVID [17]. The wide variation in the estimated prevalence of long COVID within and between countries may result from a number of determinants, including the age and sex of subjects, comorbid health conditions, the timing of assessment, sociodemographic factors, self-reported questionnaire variabilities, etc. [18]. There is emerging evidence suggesting that some individuals with long COVID exhibit symptoms common to patients with ME/CFS and FM, indicating potential overlapping biological pathomechanisms, although this is still unclear [1].

The precise pathomechanism underlying long COVID is unknown and is the subject of ongoing research. Risk factors for long COVID include increasing age, obesity, pre-existing respiratory disorders, and sociodemographic factors [18]. However, it is not yet clear why some individuals develop long COVID, while others recover fully after an acute COVID-19 infection. Long COVID can affect individuals varying in the severity of initial infection, including asymptomatic children/adolescents [19]. Long-term longitudinal clinical and -omics studies are needed to determine if long COVID can lead to distinct subgroups using cluster analysis in some individuals with ME/CFS and FM [20,21].

ME/CFS, FM, and long COVID can occur independently or an coexist in some individuals with other comorbid health conditions, such as irritable bowel syndrome (IBS), and mood disorders, such as anxiety/depression, which can further complicate the understanding and management of these conditions [22]. There is currently no cure for these disorders; a multidisciplinary approach that focuses on symptom relief, pacing activities, and improving overall well-being for affected people is often employed [23–26]. While the exact cause of these illnesses remains unknown, ongoing research is crucial to unravel the complexities of the connection between these conditions, and to develop a prominent hypothesis to deepen our understanding of the aetiology, underlying pathomechanisms, and risk factors; to develop more effective diagnostic tools; and to identify more effective treatment strategies.

This article aims to evaluate the evidence relating to mitochondrial dysfunction in the pathogenesis of PVFS; in particular, it aims to review issues relating to the efficacy of coenzyme Q10 (CoQ10) supplementation as a novel therapeutic strategy for the treatment of post-viral fatigue syndrome.

2. Evidence of Mitochondrial Dysfunction in Post-Viral Fatigue Syndrome

Mitochondria, the cellular powerhouses responsible for energy production, have recently garnered attention in the research into PVFS due to their crucial role in cellular energy metabolism. In addition to their role in energy production, mitochondria have key roles in many other aspects of cell metabolism, including free radical metabolism, calcium homeostasis, pyrimidine and lipid synthesis, and apoptosis [27–29]. The accumulating literature has identified a link between mitochondrial dysfunction (including oxidative stress, redox imbalance, altered mitochondrial membrane potential/permeability, disrupted calcium homeostasis, and impaired ATP production) and low-grade systemic inflammation in ME/CFS, FM, and long COVID patients [30,31].

Research has indicated that patients with ME/CFS, FM, and long COVID often exhibit abnormalities in mitochondrial function. Studies have shown that decreased ATP production, impaired mitochondrial respiration, abnormal mitochondrial DNA levels, immune dysregulation, increased oxidative stress, imbalance redox metabolism, and chronic systemic inflammation perpetuate symptoms in these patients [32–34]. Additionally, abnormalities in the mitochondrial structure and function have been also observed in muscle biopsies, indicating a systemic impact on energy production. These findings suggest that mitochondrial dysfunction could contribute to the energy depletion and fatigue experienced in these disorders [35–37]. In addition to fatigue, these diseases are frequently accompanied by a variety of overlapping symptoms, such as cognitive impairments, sleep disturbances, brain fog, concentration/memory impairments, and muscle pain. These symptoms can be attributed, at least partially, to mitochondrial dysfunction, which can have an impact on brain energy metabolism [38,39] (Figure 1).

Several studies have reported mitochondrial abnormalities in skeletal muscle cells of ME/CFS patients compared to healthy controls. Another study reported lower mitochondrial respiration rates and increased mitochondrial reactive oxygen species production in the immune cells of ME/CFS patients. These findings suggest that there are potential mitochondrial impairments in ME/CFS, contributing to energy production deficits and oxidative stress [40,41]. Similarly, in FM, some studies have observed evidence of mitochondrial dysfunction. Research has shown reduced mitochondrial ATP production, impaired oxidative phosphorylation, and increased oxidative stress biomarkers in the muscle cells of FM patients. However, more studies are needed to validate and expand upon these findings [34,42].

Regarding post-COVID-19 syndrome, emerging research has indicated potential evidence of mitochondrial dysfunction in the blood immune cells of COVID-19 patients. When the COVID-19 virus first enters the host respiratory tract, infection is initiated via the binding of the spike protein with angiotensin-converting enzyme 2 (ACE2) receptors, with the subsequent utilization of the transmembrane protease-serine 2 (TMPRSS2) to enter host cells; the virus then hijacks the host cellular machinery for viral RNA replication and protein production [43]. In a similar manner, there is evidence that the SARS-CoV-

2 is able also to hijack the host cells' mitochondria for viral advantage, for example, to evade host immune response [44]. It is of note that many other viral, bacterial, fungal, or parasitic pathogens also modulate the host cells' mitochondrial function to evade a host immune response and to promote infection [45]. The subject of mitochondrial hijacking in fatigue-related disorders is further described in a subsequent section of this article.

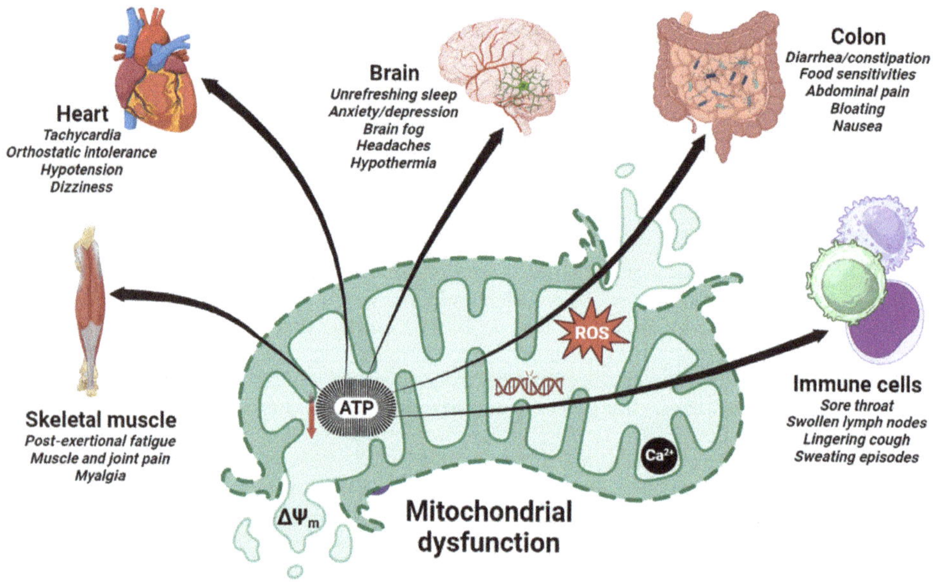

Figure 1. Schematic representation of mitochondrial dysfunction involved in the pathogenesis of post-viral fatigue syndrome. The most prevalent clinical features in these disorders affect the brain, the heart, skeletal muscle cells, immune cells, and the intestine (colon). Dysfunctions are commonly caused in multiple organ systems with a clinical spectrum that varies within and between patients. The resulting fall in ATP production due to a reduced mitochondrial membrane potential ($\Delta\Psi_m$) and an increased ROS generation has a deleterious effect on a number of major ATP-consuming organs in patients with PVFS causing the cardinal symptoms shown.

COVID-19 can cause systemic inflammation and oxidative stress, which may impact mitochondrial function. Preliminary studies have shown mitochondrial abnormalities in tissues and cells affected by COVID-19, including the lung epithelial cells and immune cells. However, more research is needed to understand the specific relationship between mitochondrial dysfunction and the post-COVID condition [46]. Several mechanisms may underlie mitochondrial dysfunction in PVFS. These include viral-induced mitochondrial damage, dysregulation of mitochondrial biogenesis and dynamics, immune-mediated mitochondrial dysfunction, and increased oxidative stress. Additionally, dysregulated mitochondrial calcium handling and impaired mitochondrial membrane potential may further contribute to the pathogenesis of PVFS [47–49].

One theory proposes that mitochondrial dysfunction in these diseases could be caused by a combination of genetic predisposition and environmental factors. Genetic variations in genes involved in mitochondrial function and energy metabolism, such as those related to the mitochondrial DNA, electron transport chain components, and oxidative stress response, may increase the susceptibility to mitochondrial dysfunction in individuals with PVFS. Moreover, various environmental triggers, including infectious agents, toxins, and physical or emotional stressors, have been proposed as potential triggers that can induce or exacerbate mitochondrial dysfunction in susceptible individuals. These triggers may lead to mitochondrial damage, oxidative stress, and inflammation, further impairing mitochondrial function and perpetuating the cycle of fatigue and other core symptoms in people with PVFS [50–55].

Understanding the connection between mitochondrial dysfunction and cardinal symptoms in PVFS has important clinical implications. Biomarkers of mitochondrial dysfunction, such as markers of oxidative stress and mitochondrial DNA damage, may aid in the diagnosis and subtyping of PVFS. Furthermore, targeting mitochondrial dysfunction through therapeutic interventions aimed at improving the mitochondrial function and reducing oxidative stress and imbalance redox holds promise for the management of PVFS. For example, supplementation with CoQ10 has shown promise in alleviating symptoms in some PVFS patients. However, further research is crucial to unravel the complexities of this connection, to develop targeted interventions to improve the quality of life for these individuals, and to explore the effectiveness and safety of such interventions [56–64]. The rationale for CoQ10 supplementation with regard to mitochondrial hijacking is considered in the following section.

3. Hijacking of Host Mitochondria in Post-Viral Fatigue Related Disorders

In addition to their role in cellular energy provision, mitochondria also have a key role in the host innate immune response in the first line defence against RNA viruses. Viral infection results in the activation of mitochondrial antiviral signalling proteins (MAVSs), which in turn results in the release of cytokines/chemokines and growth factors by the infected cell; this induces a further immune response which kills the infected host cell, facilitating clearance of the infecting virus [65,66]. Certain types of virus such as SARS-CoV-2 have adapted to promote viral survival and replication by suppressing the host immune response; by forming double-membrane vesicles (DMVs) around its RNA, thus shielding the latter from detection; and by inhibiting the MAVSs in the antiviral innate immune response [67]. While these DMVs are generally believed to be formed via viruses manipulating the endoplasmic reticulum (ER) membrane, the mechanism for importing and packaging proteins and RNA into these miniature organelles is not clearly understood [68]. One possible mechanism for importing viral RNA involves the virus exploiting the RNA localization mechanisms that the cell already possesses for endogenous double-membrane organelles, namely, the mitochondria.

In addition, the COVID-19 virus can directly impair the mitochondrial energy metabolism via targeted action on oxygen availability and utilization, and an effective host immune response will be impaired when the available mitochondrial energy is reduced [69]. COVID-19 viruses produce accessory proteins called open reading frames (ORFs), which interact with mitochondrial outer membrane receptors. One particular interaction involves an ORF-9 interaction with MAVSs in their role as mitochondrial import receptors and cytoplasmic viral recognition receptors [70]. Thus, ORFs have been shown to suppress the activity of MAVSs, thus limiting the initial host cell, innate immune, interferon, and antiviral responses. The interactions of the SARS-CoV-2 proteins such as ORFs and NSP with host cell mitochondrial proteins lead to the loss of membrane integrity and also cause dysfunction in the bioenergetics of the mitochondria.

The hijacking of the mitochondria by intracellular viral RNA and protein components also occurs during infections with the Ebola, Zika, and influenza A viruses [71]. It follows that drugs that help to prevent mitochondrial hijacking or restore mitochondrial function (of which CoQ10 would be an example) may provide novel therapeutic strategies to help prevent or treat the virus infection [72]. As noted in the section of this article on COVID-19 infections, to date variable outcomes have been reported from clinical studies supplementing CoQ10 in COVID-19 patients. Thus, an open study by Barletta et al. reported supplementation with 200 mg/day of CoQ10 and 200 mg/day of alpha lipoic acid for 2 months improved fatigue in chronic COVID-19 patients [73]. However, a randomised controlled trial supplementing CoQ10 (500 mg/day for 6 weeks) found no significant benefit on reducing the number or severity of symptoms in patients with the post-COVID-19 condition [74]. The development of novel therapies based on countering the effects of the viral hijacking of host mitochondria in post-infectious fatigue disorders therefore remains an area for more intensive future research.

4. Effects of Coenzyme Q10 Supplementation in Post-Viral Fatigue Related Conditions

All of the clinical studies described below supplemented the oxidised form of CoQ10 (ubiquinone) unless otherwise specified (Table 1).

Table 1. Summary of clinical trials conducted on mitochondria dysfunction-targeted CoQ10 supplementation in post-viral fatigue syndrome.

Population	Case Criteria	CoQ10 Daily Dose and Duration	Sample Size	Study Design	Outcomes	Refs.
FM	1990 ACR	300 mg for 40 days	20	RCT	Reduced chronic pain and fatigue, improved mitochondrial bioenergetic function, and reduced oxidative stress and inflammation	Cordero et al., 2013 [75]
FM	2010 ACR	300 mg for 40 days	20	RCT	Regulated serotonin levels in platelets and improved depression symptoms	Alcocer-Gómez et al., 2014 and 2017 [76,77]
FM	1990 ACR	300 mg for 40 days	20 cases 15 controls	Case-control study	Significant negative correlations between CoQ10 or catalase levels in PBMCs and headache parameters, restored biochemical parameters, and improved clinical symptoms	Cordero et al., 2012 [78]
FM	1990 ACR	2 × 200 mg for 6 months	22	Open-label crossover study	Significantly improved most pain-related outcomes by 24–37%, including fatigue (by ~22%) and sleep disturbance (by ~33%)	Di Pierro et al., 2017 [79]
FM	2010 ACR	Pregabalin with CoQ10 or pregabalin with placebo for 40 days	11	RCT crossover study	Reduced greater pain, anxiety, inflammation, and mitochondrial oxidative stress, along with increased GSH levels and superoxide dismutase levels	Sawaddiruk et al., 2019 [80]
FM	Not given	200 mg CoQ10 and 200 mg Ginkgo biloba extract for 84 days	25	Open-label pilot study	Improved quality of life and improved self-rating with 64% claiming to be better and only 9% claiming to feel worse	Lister et al., 2002 [81]
FM	2016 ACR	150 mg CoQ10 combined with vitamin D, alpha-lipoic acid, magnesium, and tryptophan or acupuncture treatment, both for 3 months	55	RCT	Reduced pain at 1 month after the start of therapy, strengthened after 3 months with the maintenance of treatment	Schweiger et al., 2020 [82]
Long COVID	eHRs from Israel Clalit Health Services provider	Not given	6953 cases 6530 controls	Retrospective case-control study	Case studies showing ubiquinone associated with significantly reduced odds for COVID-19 hospitalization (OR = 0.185, 95% CI (0.058–0.458), $p < 0.001$)	Israel et al., 2021 [83]
Long COVID	2015 IOM/NIH criteria for ME/CFS	100 mg CoQ10 and 100 mg alpha-lipoic acid (n = 116) or placebo (n = 58) for 60 days	174	Prospective observational study	Complete Fatigue Severity Scale response was reached more frequently in treatment group (53.5%) than in placebo (3.5%)	Barletta et al., 2023 [73]

Table 1. *Cont.*

Population	Case Criteria	CoQ10 Daily Dose and Duration	Sample Size	Study Design	Outcomes	Refs.
Long COVID	2021 WHO clinical case definition	500 mg or placebo for 6 weeks, with crossover treatment after a 4-week washout period	119	RCT crossover trial	No significant benefit on chronic COVID-19 symptoms	Hansen et al., 2023 [74]
ME/CFS	1994 CDC/Fukuda	200 mg CoQ10 and 20 mg of NADH (n = 104) or placebo (n = 103) for 12 weeks	207	RCT	Reduced cognitive fatigue perception and overall FIS-40 score and improved quality of life; improved sleep duration at 4 weeks and improved habitual sleep efficiency at 8 weeks	Castro-Marrero et al., 2021 [63]
ME/CFS	1994 CDC/Fukuda	400 mg CoQ10 and 200 mcg selenium for 8 weeks	27	Open-label exploratory study	Improved overall fatigue severity and global quality of life but no significant effect on sleep disturbances; increased total antioxidant capacity, reduced lipoperoxide levels, and decreased circulating cytokine levels	Castro-Marrero et al., 2022 [64]
ME/CFS	1994 CDC/Fukuda	150 mg ubiquinol or placebo for 3 months	20	RCT	Improved autonomic function and cognitive function	Fukuda et al., 2016 [84]

4.1. Coenzyme Q10 Supplementation in Fibromyalgia

With regard to interventions through nutritional supplementation in fibromyalgia, CoQ10 (alone or in nutrient combinations) has been shown to be effective in clinical studies for the symptomatic relief of this disorder. As noted in earlier sections of this article, fibromyalgia patients have depleted CoQ10 levels in tissues (typically 40–50% of the normal level), together with increased levels of mitochondrial dysfunction, oxidative stress, and inflammation, both in adults and in children/adolescents [85,86].

A randomised controlled clinical study by Cordero et al. [75] conducted in 20 FM patients found supplementation with CoQ10 (300 mg/day for 40 days) significantly reduced (by more than 50%) chronic pain and fatigue; there was a corresponding improvement in mitochondrial energy generation and reduced oxidative stress and inflammation. In this study, psychopathological symptoms (including anxiety/depression) were also significantly improved; this was linked to the effect of supplemental CoQ10 in reducing oxidative stress and inflammation, as well as increased levels of serotonin [76,77]. In addition, Cordero et al. [78] correlated headache symptoms with reduced CoQ10 levels and increased oxidative stress in the FM patients, with headache symptoms and oxidative stress levels significantly improved following CoQ10 supplementation (300 mg/day for 3 months). In adolescent FM patients (aged 8–17 years), Miyamae et al. [86] reported CoQ10 supplementation (100 mg/day for 3 months) significantly improved fatigue. In an open-label crossover study, supplementation with a water-soluble form of CoQ10 (400 mg/day for 6 months) resulted in significant reductions (by 20–40%) in chronic fatigue and pain [79].

A clinical study by Sawaddiruk et al. [80] described the role of supplementary CoQ10 in further reducing chronic pain in FM patients treated with pregabalin. In a double-blind randomised controlled study, the FM patients were treated either with pregabalin plus CoQ10 or pregabalin plus a placebo for 6 weeks. After a 2-week washout period, patients in the pregabalin plus CoQ10 group were switched to pregabalin plus a placebo, and vice-versa, for a further 6 weeks. Several parameters were monitored during the study, including the pain pressure threshold, pain score, and anxiety/depression level, as well as the biomarkers of antioxidant activity, inflammation, and mitochondrial dysfunction. While pregabalin alone reduced pain and anxiety/depression, there was no effect on inflammation and mitochondrial function. However, the treatment with pregabalin plus CoQ10 resulted in a significantly greater reduction in pain and anxiety/depression, together with a reduction in oxidative stress, inflammation, and mitochondrial dysfunction. The results from this study provide evidence that supplementary CoQ10 can provide further pain relief in FM patients treated with pregabalin, through reducing oxidative stress imbalance and inflammation and improving mitochondrial function.

With regard to nutrient combinations, an open uncontrolled study of 23 FM patients reported supplementation with 200 mg of CoQ10 and 200 mg of ginkgo biloba resulted in a significant improvement in health-related quality of life [81]. In a randomised controlled trial conducted in 21 FM patients supplemented with CoQ10, vitamin D, alpha-lipoic acid, magnesium, and tryptophan for 3 months, there was a significant reduction in pain [82].

4.2. Coenzyme Q10 Supplementation in Acute COVID-19 Infection

In a clinical study by Israel et al. [83], the intake of CoQ10 was associated with a significantly reduced risk of hospitalisation for COVID-19 patients. Fernandez-Ayala et al. [87] reviewed the evidence for mitochondrial dysfunction as a key factor determining the severity of a SARS-CoV-2 infection; in particular, the authors noted the increased susceptibility to a COVID-19 infection in individuals over 65 years of age, the same age by which endogenous CoQ10 levels have become substantially depleted. Similarly, Gvozdjakova et al. [72] consider one of the main consequences of a COVID-19 infection to be virus-induced oxidative stress-causing mutations in one or more of the genes responsible for CoQ10 biosynthesis, in turn resulting in mitochondrial dysfunction. Also of note is the computational study by Caruso et al. [88], in which the authors identified CoQ10 as a compound capable of inhibiting the SARS-CoV-2 virus, via binding to the active site of the main viral protease.

Clinical studies supplementing CoQ10 in COVID-19 patients (and also patients with long COVID) have reported mixed outcomes. In a prospective observational study, 116 patients with chronic COVID-19 were supplemented with 200 mg of CoQ10 and 200 mg of alpha-lipoic acid for 2 months versus 58 COVID-19 patients who received no treatment; the severity of fatigue was substantially reduced in the treated patients compared to the placebo group [73]. However, a randomised controlled intervention study comprising 121 chronic COVID-19 patients supplemented with 500 mg of CoQ10 per day for 6 weeks reported no significant benefit on chronic COVID-19 symptoms [74].

In patients severely affected by a COVID-19 infection, in addition to the "cytokine storm" and hyperinflammation status affecting the lung tissue, cardiac injury biomarkers may be elevated, characteristic of myocarditis and heart failure. While the precise mechanism underlying the damaging effect of COVID-19 infections on the heart function is not completely understood, attention has been focussed on the ACE-2 enzyme, which has roles both in cardiovascular function and the penetration of host cells by the SARS-CoV-2 infection.

It is well known that people with pre-existing medical conditions such as cardiovascular disease are at a greater risk of adverse outcomes following a COVID-19 infection. The acute effects of a COVID-19 infection in terms of cardiovascular function are well established, as noted above. What is less well known is the risk of longer-term cardiovascular dysfunction following a COVID-19 infection. Individuals who have been hospitalised because of a COVID-19 infection have a much higher risk of subsequently developing heart problems, including myocarditis, atrial fibrillation, myocardial infarction, heart failure, and stroke. However, it is not just people who have suffered more serious COVID-19 infections who are prone to developing heart problems; even people who were not hospitalised and seemed to have recovered from mild infection were subsequently found to be at risk of developing serious heart complications.

These conclusions were based on a number of clinical studies published in the medical literature, including studies led by Dr Ziad Al-Aly (Washington University Medical School, St. Louis, MO, USA), Dr Mouaz Al-Mallah (Debakey Heart Centre, Houston, TX, USA), and Prof. Colin Berry (Glasgow University). Dr Al-Aly's study comprising some 150,000 patients found both hospitalised and non-hospitalised individuals were at a substantially increased risk of developing a number of heart conditions, including myocarditis and heart failure [89]. The study by Dr Al-Mallah of 100 COVID-19 patients assessed via positron emission tomography/myocardial blood flow found that an infection doubled the risk of developing unhealthy endothelial cells lining the heart and blood vessels, increasing the likelihood of heart failure [90]. Additionally, Prof Berry's study, comprising more than 1000 patients, found that one in eight individuals who had been hospitalised due to COVID infection were later diagnosed with myocarditis [91]. The pathophysiological mechanisms by which SARS-CoV-2 infection causes longer term cardiovascular dysfunction is not completely understood. Possible contributory factors include direct cellular damage resulting from the viral invasion of cardiomyocytes and subsequent cell death, endothelial cell infection and endothelitis, persistent hyperactivation of the immune response, and persistence of the virus in tissues, possibly lying dormant for months or even years to be reactivated under conditions of stress/insults.

The above data provide a rationale for the use of supplemental CoQ10 to try and prevent the development of heart problems following COVID-19 infection; in addition, there is evidence that supplemental selenium may also be of benefit, as outlined below. There are several reasons why the nutritional supplements CoQ10 and selenium could be of benefit regarding COVID infection. Firstly, both CoQ10 and selenium have important roles in immune function and could help to prevent a COVID infection from taking place. Secondly, the combination of CoQ10 and selenium can reduce the excessive inflammation associated with virus infections, as well as inflammation in individuals without virus infections. Thirdly, CoQ10 and selenium have important roles in the normal function of the heart, and clinical trials supplementing CoQ10 and selenium have shown significant benefit in reducing the risk of developing heart disease in normal individuals as well as reducing mortality risk in heart failure patients [92–95]. It should be noted that the use of CoQ10 and selenium described above is a suggestion of the authors of this article and has not been explored in clinical trials to date, but an open-label exploratory study has been conducted to evaluate the efficacy of combined CoQ10 and selenium supplementation on clinical features and circulating biomarkers in ME/CFS patients [64]. Based on these findings, long-term supplementation with CoQ10 plus selenium suggests a potentially beneficial synergistic effect in patients with ME/CFS.

4.3. Coenzyme Q10 Supplementation in Myalgic Encephalomyelitis/Chronic Fatigue Syndrome

In a randomised controlled trial comprising 207 ME/CFS patients who were supplemented with 200 mg of CoQ10 and 20 mg of NADH per day for 3 months, or a placebo, there was a significant improvement in fatigue perception (assessed on the FIS-40 scale), health-related quality of life (36-item, short-form health survey) and sleep quality (assessed by a PSQI questionnaire) [63]. In an open-label study, 27 ME/CFS patients were supplemented with 400 mg of CoQ10 and 200 mcg of selenium per day for 8 weeks; there was a significant improvement in overall fatigue severity and global quality of life compared to the baseline among the participants [64]. Supplementation with CoQ10 for symptoms such as fatigue, pain, and cognitive dysfunction in ME/CFS has been suggested in an agreed report from the European Network on ME/CFS (EUROMENE consortium) [96]. In a randomised controlled trial, 43 ME/CFS patients were supplemented with the reduced CoQ10 form (ubiquinol) (150 mg/day for 3 months) or a placebo. Although there was no improvement in perceived fatigue (assessed by Chandler's fatigue scale), supplementation improved several other illness symptoms such as night-time awakenings [84].

A potential issue regarding the success or otherwise of clinical trials is the quality and bioavailability of the CoQ10 supplement used, and this is addressed in the following section.

5. Importance of CoQ10 Supplement Quality and Bioavailability

All prescription-type drugs require a marketing authorisation. To obtain a marketing authorisation, manufacturers must submit to the relevant regulatory authorities an extensive dossier of data relating to product manufacturing quality, together with proof of efficacy and safety [97]. Once marketing authorisation has been approved, products must be subject to a continual process of pharmacovigilance [98]. By contrast, products classed as food supplements are not subject to the same regulatory standards; there is no mandatory requirement relating to product quality or proof of efficacy and safety. As an example, surveys of Ginkgo biloba supplements available on the European and the US markets have reported issues with formulation discrepancies and adulteration problems. There is similarly no regulatory requirement for the manufacturers of most CoQ10 supplements to guarantee the quality, efficacy, and safety of their products [99–101].

To date, there is only one CoQ10 product produced to pharmaceutical standards for the adjunctive treatment of heart failure. Marketing authorisation approval acts as a guarantee relating to the accuracy of the stated dosage, the absence of adulterants, and their bioavailability. Products manufactured according to food supplement standards do not have this guarantee, which in turn may have adverse effects on the outcome of clinical studies utilising such products. In this regard, a recent review by Mantle & Hargreaves identified 38 clinical studies in which supplemental CoQ10 had been used to treat patients with primary CoQ10 deficiency. Only two of these studies provided information about the manufacturer of the supplement used. Based on this limited information, it becomes difficult to evaluate the outcomes of such studies in which poor-quality supplements may have been used [102].

The other key issue relevant to the success or otherwise of clinical studies is that of bioavailability. Bioavailability is defined as the proportion of an ingested substance that reaches the bloodstream. CoQ10 is a lipid-type substance and as such is absorbed from the digestive tract in the same general manner as other lipid substances. The process by which this takes place has been described in detail in the review by Mantle & Dybring [103] from which the following information has been summarised. Because of the particular chemical structure of CoQ10 (one of the most hydrophobic naturally occurring substances), the bioavailability of supplemental CoQ10 is low, estimated to be around 5% at most. One of the most effective methods to date for optimising the bioavailability of CoQ10 is based on a patented CoQ10 crystal modification process used in the manufacture of ubiquinone-form CoQ10 supplements [103].

Coenzyme Q10 is produced via a yeast fermentation process in the form of polymorphic crystals, which cannot be absorbed from the digestive tract. CoQ10 can be absorbed only as individual molecules, as noted above. To be effective as a supplement, the CoQ10 crystals must therefore be dissociated first into individual CoQ10 molecules prior to absorption. The above process involves changing the shape of the CoQ10 crystals in such a way as to increase the ratio of the crystals' surface area to the volume, thus making it easier for the crystals to dissolve into single molecules at body temperature. This modification to the CoQ10 crystalline form should remain in place throughout the shelf life of the CoQ10 preparation.

Supplement manufacturers may make extravagant claims about the bioavailability of their respective CoQ10 supplements, but the only definitive measure of bioavailability is that determined in human subjects, based on clinical studies published in the peer-reviewed medical literature. A good example in this regard is the bioavailability study by Lopez-Lluch et al. [104]. In this randomised controlled clinical trial, seven CoQ10 supplements differing in formulation (the CoQ10 crystal modification status, the type of carrier oil, the composition of other excipients, and the CoQ10 oxidation state) were administered in a single 100 mg dose to the same series of 14 healthy individuals, using a crossover/washout protocol. The bioavailability of the different formulations was quantified as the area under the curve at 48 h. The supplement that had been subject to the crystal modification process (Myoqinon) had the highest level of bioavailability, whilst the bioavailability of the same CoQ10 material that had not been subject to this process was reduced by 75%. It is of note that the Myoqinon formulation received a marketing authorisation within the E.U., as noted above, demonstrating the importance of utilising a CoQ10 product manufactured to pharmaceutical standards, rather than to food supplement standards.

Several studies have been carried out with the objective of improving the bioavailability of CoQ10 using a variety of agents; examples include polyethylene glycol, phosphorylated tocopherols, poloxamer/polyvinyl pyrrolidine, and hydrolysed proteins. However, again, the bioavailability of most of these formulations has not been directly compared with ubiquinone that has undergone crystal modification, the importance of which is demonstrated in the above Lopez-Lluch et al. study [104]. In addition, none of the modified forms of CoQ10 described above have been subject to an extensive evaluation of their efficacy and safety in randomised controlled trials. In comparison, the efficacy and the safety of the crystal-modified form of CoQ10 have been confirmed in a number of such clinical studies, an example being the Q-SYMBIO study in which supplemental CoQ10 was shown to substantially reduce the mortality risk in heart failure patients [95].

Notwithstanding the issues outlined above, it should be noted that there are other factors that may influence the success of clinical studies involving CoQ10 supplementation, as reviewed by Mantle et al. [105]. Examples include the problem that some individuals appear to have an inherently low capacity to absorb supplemental CoQ10 into the bloodstream, even with high bioavailability formulations—the reason for which is currently unknown. Additionally, the question of whether supplemental CoQ10 can effectively cross the blood–brain barrier in human subjects remains unclear.

6. Conclusions, Unresolved Issues, and Future Perspectives

Disorders constituting PVFS, namely, ME/CFS, FM, and long COVID, currently have no effective treatments. As part of a strategy to identify new treatment methods, we have identified considerable evidence for the involvement of mitochondrial dysfunction in the pathogenesis of these disorders. This, in turn, suggests a possible role for CoQ10 supplementation in the treatment of the above disorders, given the key role of CoQ10 in the normal mitochondrial function. Within mitochondria, CoQ10 has a key role as an electron carrier (from complexes I and II to complex III) in the mitochondrial electron transport chain during oxidative phosphorylation to generate ATP. In addition, CoQ10 serves as an important lipid-soluble antioxidant protecting the mitochondria from oxidative stress-induced damage resulting from reactive oxygen/nitrogen free radical species generated during oxidative phosphorylation. CoQ10 is also involved in the metabolism of pyrimidines, fatty acids, and mitochondrial uncoupling proteins, as well as in the regulation of the mitochondrial permeability transition pore [106]. Therefore, CoQ10 supplementation may ameliorate mitochondrial dysfunction and alleviate fatigue associated with PVFS through its ability to restore electron flow in the mitochondrial respiratory chain (MRC), which will enhance ATP generation by oxidative phosphorylation. Furthermore, exogenous CoQ10 will also enhance mitochondrial antioxidant capacity, which will protect the enzymes of the MRC from reactive oxygen species-induced impairment [107]. Interestingly, several clinical studies have demonstrated an association between decreased endogenous CoQ10 levels and an increased susceptibility to COVID-19 infection, and, consequently, some patients experiencing post-viral fatigue may have an underlying CoQ10 deficiency, which CoQ10 supplementation may restore [108].

Randomised controlled clinical trials have reported significant symptomatic benefits in the treatment of these disorders, particularly for FM; further randomised controlled trials are required to confirm the efficacy of CoQ10 supplementation in patients with ME/CFS and long COVID. It is of note that no serious adverse effects have been reported from clinical studies supplementing CoQ10 in patients with PVFS, or in a wide range of other chronic disorders. Other potential therapeutic agents for the treatment of PVFS have been suggested (reviewed by Chen et al. [109]); these include generalised antioxidants which can restore mitochondrial function, such as N-acetylcysteine; glutathione and catalase; IL-6R and IL-1 receptor blockers, such as the antibody tocilizumab, to reduce levels of pro-inflammatory cytokines; and mitochondrial calcium uniporter (MCU) inhibitors, such as ruthenium-265, mitoxantrone, and doxycycline, which can help restore mitochondrial function. However, in contrast to the use of CoQ10, none of the above agents have to date been investigated in randomised controlled trials for PVFS.

There are several unresolved issues relating to the CoQ10 intervention studies and mitochondrial dysfunction in PVFS that require further investigation; these include whether the bioavailability of CoQ10 could be improved through the use of alternative administration routes (e.g., intravenous, intraperitoneal, intramuscular, etc.), whether supplemental CoQ10 is able to cross the blood–brain barrier, and how CoQ10 is transported into and within cells, among others. With regard to future work, the question arises whether additional symptomatic benefits may be obtained through co-supplementation with other substances that have important roles in the mitochondrial function, as suggested by Castro-Marrero et al. and Mantle and Hargreaves [63,110]. The possibility of designing dietary interventions based on CoQ10 co-supplementation targeted specifically at boosting mitochondrial function to improve neuroimmune and inflammatory health outcomes in ME/CFS, FM, and long COVID appears well within reach within the next half decade. Mitochondria-dependent pathways may thereby represent an attractive therapeutic target for the amelioration of PVFS.

Author Contributions: Conceptualization and design, D.M., J.C.D. and J.C.-M.; formal analysis and investigation, D.M., I.P.H. and J.C.-M.; writing—original draft preparation, D.M., J.C.D. and J.C.-M.; writing—review and editing, D.M., J.C.D. and J.C.-M.; visualization, D.M. and J.C.-M. All authors have read and agreed to the published version of the manuscript.

Funding: This research received no external funding.

Institutional Review Board Statement: Not applicable.

Informed Consent Statement: Not applicable.

Data Availability Statement: Not applicable.

Conflicts of Interest: The authors declare no conflict of interest. Dr Mantle is medical adviser to Pharma Nord (UK) Ltd.

References

1. Komaroff, A.L.; Lipkin, W.I. ME/CFS and Long COVID share similar symptoms and biological abnormalities: Road map to the literature. *Front. Med.* **2023**, *10*, 1187163. [CrossRef] [PubMed]
2. Komaroff, A.L. Chronic "post-infectious" fatigue syndrome. *Trans. Am. Acad. Insur. Med.* **1993**, *76*, 82–95. [PubMed]
3. Poenaru, S.; Abdallah, S.J.; Corrales-Medina, V.; Cowan, J. COVID-19 and post-infectious myalgic encephalomyelitis/chronic fatigue syndrome: A narrative review. *Ther. Adv. Infect. Dis.* **2021**, *8*, 20499361211009385. [CrossRef] [PubMed]
4. Mahroum, N.; Shoenfeld, Y. Autoimmune Autonomic Dysfunction Syndromes: Potential Involvement and Pathophysiology Related to Complex Regional Pain Syndrome, Fibromyalgia, Chronic Fatigue Syndrome, Silicone Breast Implant-Related Symptoms and Post-COVID Syndrome. *Pathophysiology* **2022**, *29*, 414–425. [CrossRef] [PubMed]
5. Hamilton, W.T.; Gallagher, A.M.; Thomas, J.M.; White, P.D. The prognosis of different fatigue diagnostic labels: A longitudinal survey. *Fam. Pract.* **2005**, *22*, 383–388. [CrossRef] [PubMed]
6. Behan, P.O.; Behan, W.M.; Gow, J.W.; Cavanagh, H.; Gillespie, S. Enteroviruses and postviral fatigue syndrome. *Ciba Found. Symp.* **1993**, *173*, 146–154, discussion 154–159. [CrossRef] [PubMed]
7. Murga, I.; Aranburu, L.; Gargiulo, P.A.; Gomez Esteban, J.C.; Lafuente, J.V. Clinical Heterogeneity in ME/CFS. A Way to Understand Long-COVID19 Fatigue. *Front. Psychiatry* **2021**, *12*, 735784. [CrossRef] [PubMed]
8. Castro-Marrero, J.; Saez-Francas, N.; Santillo, D.; Alegre, J. Treatment and management of chronic fatigue syndrome/myalgic encephalomyelitis: All roads lead to Rome. *Br. J. Pharmacol.* **2017**, *174*, 345–369. [CrossRef]
9. Marshall-Gradisnik, S.; Eaton-Fitch, N. Understanding myalgic encephalomyelitis. *Science* **2022**, *377*, 1150–1151. [CrossRef]
10. Mazurkiewicz, I.; Chatys-Bogacka, Z.; Slowik, J.; Klich-Raczka, A.; Fedyk-Lukasik, M.; Slowik, A.; Wnuk, M.; Drabik, L. Fatigue after COVID-19 in non-hospitalized patients according to sex. *Brain Behav.* **2023**, *13*, e2849. [CrossRef]
11. Faro, M.; Saez-Francas, N.; Castro-Marrero, J.; Aliste, L.; Fernandez de Sevilla, T.; Alegre, J. Gender differences in chronic fatigue syndrome. *Reumatol. Clin.* **2016**, *12*, 72–77. [CrossRef] [PubMed]
12. Bonilla, H.; Quach, T.C.; Tiwari, A.; Bonilla, A.E.; Miglis, M.; Yang, P.C.; Eggert, L.E.; Sharifi, H.; Horomanski, A.; Subramanian, A.; et al. Myalgic Encephalomyelitis/Chronic Fatigue Syndrome is common in post-acute sequelae of SARS-CoV-2 infection (PASC): Results from a post-COVID-19 multidisciplinary clinic. *Front. Neurol.* **2023**, *14*, 1090747. [CrossRef] [PubMed]

13. Calabrese, C.; Kirchner, E.; Calabrese, L.H. Long COVID and rheumatology: Clinical, diagnostic, and therapeutic implications. *Best. Pract. Res. Clin. Rheumatol.* **2022**, *36*, 101794. [CrossRef] [PubMed]
14. Najafi, M.B.; Javanmard, S.H. Post-COVID-19 Syndrome Mechanisms, Prevention and Management. *Int. J. Prev. Med.* **2023**, *14*, 59. [CrossRef]
15. Natarajan, A.; Shetty, A.; Delanerolle, G.; Zeng, Y.; Zhang, Y.; Raymont, V.; Rathod, S.; Halabi, S.; Elliot, K.; Shi, J.Q.; et al. A systematic review and meta-analysis of long COVID symptoms. *Syst. Rev.* **2023**, *12*, 88. [CrossRef]
16. Haslam, A.; Olivier, T.; Prasad, V. The definition of long COVID used in interventional studies. *Eur. J. Clin. Investig.* **2023**, *53*, e13989. [CrossRef]
17. Arabi, M.; Al-Najjar, Y.; Sharma, O.; Kamal, I.; Javed, A.; Gohil, H.S.; Paul, P.; Al-Khalifa, A.M.; Laws, S.; Zakaria, D. Role of previous infection with SARS-CoV-2 in protecting against omicron reinfections and severe complications of COVID-19 compared to pre-omicron variants: A systematic review. *BMC Infect. Dis.* **2023**, *23*, 432. [CrossRef]
18. Raman, B.; Bluemke, D.A.; Luscher, T.F.; Neubauer, S. Long COVID: Post-acute sequelae of COVID-19 with a cardiovascular focus. *Eur. Heart J.* **2022**, *43*, 1157–1172. [CrossRef]
19. Ludvigsson, J.F. Case report and systematic review suggest that children may experience similar long-term effects to adults after clinical COVID-19. *Acta Paediatr.* **2021**, *110*, 914–921. [CrossRef]
20. Tate, W.P.; Walker, M.O.M.; Peppercorn, K.; Blair, A.L.H.; Edgar, C.D. Towards a Better Understanding of the Complexities of Myalgic Encephalomyelitis/Chronic Fatigue Syndrome and Long COVID. *Int. J. Mol. Sci.* **2023**, *24*, 5124. [CrossRef]
21. Yong, S.J.; Liu, S. Proposed subtypes of post-COVID-19 syndrome (or long-COVID) and their respective potential therapies. *Rev. Med. Virol.* **2022**, *32*, e2315. [CrossRef] [PubMed]
22. Barhorst, E.E.; Boruch, A.E.; Cook, D.B.; Lindheimer, J.B. Pain-Related Post-Exertional Malaise in Myalgic Encephalomyelitis/Chronic Fatigue Syndrome (ME/CFS) and Fibromyalgia: A Systematic Review and Three-Level Meta-Analysis. *Pain. Med.* **2022**, *23*, 1144–1157. [CrossRef]
23. Cardinali, D.P.; Brown, G.M.; Pandi-Perumal, S.R. Possible Application of Melatonin in Long COVID. *Biomolecules* **2022**, *12*, 1646. [CrossRef] [PubMed]
24. Porter, N.S.; Jason, L.A.; Boulton, A.; Bothne, N.; Coleman, B. Alternative medical interventions used in the treatment and management of myalgic encephalomyelitis/chronic fatigue syndrome and fibromyalgia. *J. Altern. Complement. Med.* **2010**, *16*, 235–249. [CrossRef] [PubMed]
25. Skilbeck, L. Patient-led integrated cognitive behavioural therapy for management of long COVID with comorbid depression and anxiety in primary care—A case study. *Chronic Illn.* **2022**, *18*, 691–701. [CrossRef] [PubMed]
26. Parker, M.; Sawant, H.B.; Flannery, T.; Tarrant, R.; Shardha, J.; Bannister, R.; Ross, D.; Halpin, S.; Greenwood, D.C.; Sivan, M. Effect of using a structured pacing protocol on post-exertional symptom exacerbation and health status in a longitudinal cohort with the post-COVID-19 syndrome. *J. Med. Virol.* **2023**, *95*, e28373. [CrossRef] [PubMed]
27. Annesley, S.J.; Fisher, P.R. Mitochondria in Health and Disease. *Cells* **2019**, *8*, 680. [CrossRef] [PubMed]
28. San-Millan, I. The Key Role of Mitochondrial Function in Health and Disease. *Antioxidants* **2023**, *12*, 782. [CrossRef]
29. Wallace, D.C. A mitochondrial bioenergetic etiology of disease. *J. Clin. Investig.* **2013**, *123*, 1405–1412. [CrossRef]
30. Komaroff, A.L.; Bateman, L. Will COVID-19 Lead to Myalgic Encephalomyelitis/Chronic Fatigue Syndrome? *Front. Med.* **2020**, *7*, 606824. [CrossRef]
31. Komaroff, A.L.; Lipkin, W.I. Insights from myalgic encephalomyelitis/chronic fatigue syndrome may help unravel the pathogenesis of postacute COVID-19 syndrome. *Trends Mol. Med.* **2021**, *27*, 895–906. [CrossRef] [PubMed]
32. Holden, S.; Maksoud, R.; Eaton-Fitch, N.; Cabanas, H.; Staines, D.; Marshall-Gradisnik, S. A systematic review of mitochondrial abnormalities in myalgic encephalomyelitis/chronic fatigue syndrome/systemic exertion intolerance disease. *J. Transl. Med.* **2020**, *18*, 290. [CrossRef] [PubMed]
33. Myhill, S.; Booth, N.E.; McLaren-Howard, J. Chronic fatigue syndrome and mitochondrial dysfunction. *Int. J. Clin. Exp. Med.* **2009**, *2*, 1–16. [PubMed]
34. Castro-Marrero, J.; Cordero, M.D.; Saez-Francas, N.; Jimenez-Gutierrez, C.; Aguilar-Montilla, F.J.; Aliste, L.; Alegre-Martin, J. Could mitochondrial dysfunction be a differentiating marker between chronic fatigue syndrome and fibromyalgia? *Antioxid. Redox Signal.* **2013**, *19*, 1855–1860. [CrossRef] [PubMed]
35. Tomas, C.; Brown, A.E.; Newton, J.L.; Elson, J.L. Mitochondrial complex activity in permeabilised cells of chronic fatigue syndrome patients using two cell types. *PeerJ* **2019**, *7*, e6500. [CrossRef] [PubMed]
36. Arnold, D.L.; Bore, P.J.; Radda, G.K.; Styles, P.; Taylor, D.J. Excessive intracellular acidosis of skeletal muscle on exercise in a patient with a post-viral exhaustion/fatigue syndrome. A 31P nuclear magnetic resonance study. *Lancet* **1984**, *1*, 1367–1369. [CrossRef]
37. Plioplys, A.V.; Plioplys, S. Electron-microscopic investigation of muscle mitochondria in chronic fatigue syndrome. *Neuropsychobiology* **1995**, *32*, 175–181. [CrossRef]
38. Pintos-Pascual, I.; Moreno-Torres, V.; Ibanez-Estellez, F.; Corrales-Rodriguez, P.; Trevino, A.; Corpas, M.; Corral, O.; Soriano, V.; de Mendoza, C. Is SARS-CoV-2 the only cause of long-COVID? *AIDS Rev.* **2022**, *24*, 183–196. [CrossRef]
39. Thapaliya, K.; Marshall-Gradisnik, S.; Barth, M.; Eaton-Fitch, N.; Barnden, L. Brainstem volume changes in myalgic encephalomyelitis/chronic fatigue syndrome and long COVID patients. *Front. Neurosci.* **2023**, *17*, 1125208. [CrossRef]

40. Tomas, C.; Brown, A.; Strassheim, V.; Elson, J.L.; Newton, J.; Manning, P. Cellular bioenergetics is impaired in patients with chronic fatigue syndrome. *PLoS ONE* **2017**, *12*, e0186802. [CrossRef]
41. Smits, B.; van den Heuvel, L.; Knoop, H.; Kusters, B.; Janssen, A.; Borm, G.; Bleijenberg, G.; Rodenburg, R.; van Engelen, B. Mitochondrial enzymes discriminate between mitochondrial disorders and chronic fatigue syndrome. *Mitochondrion* **2011**, *11*, 735–738. [CrossRef] [PubMed]
42. Cordero, M.D.; de Miguel, M.; Carmona-Lopez, I.; Bonal, P.; Campa, F.; Moreno-Fernandez, A.M. Oxidative stress and mitochondrial dysfunction in fibromyalgia. *Neuro Endocrinol. Lett.* **2010**, *31*, 169–173. [PubMed]
43. Bourgonje, A.R.; Abdulle, A.E.; Timens, W.; Hillebrands, J.L.; Navis, G.J.; Gordijn, S.J.; Bolling, M.C.; Dijkstra, G.; Voors, A.A.; Osterhaus, A.D.; et al. Angiotensin-converting enzyme 2 (ACE2), SARS-CoV-2 and the pathophysiology of coronavirus disease 2019 (COVID-19). *J. Pathol.* **2020**, *251*, 228–248. [CrossRef] [PubMed]
44. Singh, K.K.; Chaubey, G.; Chen, J.Y.; Suravajhala, P. Decoding SARS-CoV-2 hijacking of host mitochondria in COVID-19 pathogenesis. *Am. J. Physiol. Cell Physiol.* **2020**, *319*, C258–C267. [CrossRef] [PubMed]
45. Tiku, V.; Tan, M.W.; Dikic, I. Mitochondrial Functions in Infection and Immunity. *Trends Cell Biol.* **2020**, *30*, 263–275. [CrossRef] [PubMed]
46. Bojkova, D.; Klann, K.; Koch, B.; Widera, M.; Krause, D.; Ciesek, S.; Cinatl, J.; Munch, C. Proteomics of SARS-CoV-2-infected host cells reveals therapy targets. *Nature* **2020**, *583*, 469–472. [CrossRef] [PubMed]
47. Cabanas, H.; Muraki, K.; Eaton, N.; Balinas, C.; Staines, D.; Marshall-Gradisnik, S. Loss of Transient Receptor Potential Melastatin 3 ion channel function in natural killer cells from Chronic Fatigue Syndrome/Myalgic Encephalomyelitis patients. *Mol. Med.* **2018**, *24*, 44. [CrossRef]
48. Cabanas, H.; Muraki, K.; Balinas, C.; Eaton-Fitch, N.; Staines, D.; Marshall-Gradisnik, S. Validation of impaired Transient Receptor Potential Melastatin 3 ion channel activity in natural killer cells from Chronic Fatigue Syndrome/ Myalgic Encephalomyelitis patients. *Mol. Med.* **2019**, *25*, 14. [CrossRef]
49. Cabanas, H.; Muraki, K.; Eaton-Fitch, N.; Staines, D.R.; Marshall-Gradisnik, S. Potential Therapeutic Benefit of Low Dose Naltrexone in Myalgic Encephalomyelitis/Chronic Fatigue Syndrome: Role of Transient Receptor Potential Melastatin 3 Ion Channels in Pathophysiology and Treatment. *Front. Immunol.* **2021**, *12*, 687806. [CrossRef]
50. Cabanas, H.; Muraki, K.; Staines, D.; Marshall-Gradisnik, S. Naltrexone Restores Impaired Transient Receptor Potential Melastatin 3 Ion Channel Function in Natural Killer Cells from Myalgic Encephalomyelitis/Chronic Fatigue Syndrome Patients. *Front. Immunol.* **2019**, *10*, 2545. [CrossRef]
51. Missailidis, D.; Annesley, S.J.; Fisher, P.R. Pathological Mechanisms Underlying Myalgic Encephalomyelitis/Chronic Fatigue Syndrome. *Diagnostics* **2019**, *9*, 80. [CrossRef] [PubMed]
52. Morris, G.; Berk, M.; Galecki, P.; Maes, M. The emerging role of autoimmunity in myalgic encephalomyelitis/chronic fatigue syndrome (ME/cfs). *Mol. Neurobiol.* **2014**, *49*, 741–756. [CrossRef] [PubMed]
53. van Tilburg, M.A.L.; Parisien, M.; Boles, R.G.; Drury, G.L.; Smith-Voudouris, J.; Verma, V.; Khoury, S.; Chabot-Dore, A.J.; Nackley, A.G.; Smith, S.B.; et al. A genetic polymorphism that is associated with mitochondrial energy metabolism increases risk of fibromyalgia. *Pain* **2020**, *161*, 2860–2871. [CrossRef] [PubMed]
54. Ovrom, E.A.; Mostert, K.A.; Khakhkhar, S.; McKee, D.P.; Yang, P.; Her, Y.F. A Comprehensive Review of the Genetic and Epigenetic Contributions to the Development of Fibromyalgia. *Biomedicines* **2023**, *11*, 1119. [CrossRef] [PubMed]
55. Das, S.; Taylor, K.; Kozubek, J.; Sardell, J.; Gardner, S. Genetic risk factors for ME/CFS identified using combinatorial analysis. *J. Transl. Med.* **2022**, *20*, 598. [CrossRef]
56. Campisi, L.; La Motta, C. The Use of the Coenzyme Q10 as a Food Supplement in the Management of Fibromyalgia: A Critical Review. *Antioxidants* **2022**, *11*, 1969. [CrossRef] [PubMed]
57. Fernandez-Araque, A.; Verde, Z.; Torres-Ortega, C.; Sainz-Gil, M.; Velasco-Gonzalez, V.; Gonzalez-Bernal, J.J.; Mielgo-Ayuso, J. Effects of Antioxidants on Pain Perception in Patients with Fibromyalgia—A Systematic Review. *J. Clin. Med.* **2022**, *11*, 2462. [CrossRef] [PubMed]
58. Hargreaves, I.P.; Mantle, D. Targeted Treatment of Age-Related Fibromyalgia with Supplemental Coenzyme Q10. *Adv. Exp. Med. Biol.* **2021**, *1286*, 77–85. [CrossRef]
59. Lowry, E.; Marley, J.; McVeigh, J.G.; McSorley, E.; Allsopp, P.; Kerr, D. Dietary Interventions in the Management of Fibromyalgia: A Systematic Review and Best-Evidence Synthesis. *Nutrients* **2020**, *12*, 2664. [CrossRef]
60. Mehrabani, S.; Askari, G.; Miraghajani, M.; Tavakoly, R.; Arab, A. Effect of coenzyme Q10 supplementation on fatigue: A systematic review of interventional studies. *Complement. Ther. Med.* **2019**, *43*, 181–187. [CrossRef]
61. Castro-Marrero, J.; Cordero, M.D.; Segundo, M.J.; Saez-Francas, N.; Calvo, N.; Roman-Malo, L.; Aliste, L.; Fernandez de Sevilla, T.; Alegre, J. Does oral coenzyme Q10 plus NADH supplementation improve fatigue and biochemical parameters in chronic fatigue syndrome? *Antioxid. Redox Signal.* **2015**, *22*, 679–685. [CrossRef]
62. Castro-Marrero, J.; Saez-Francas, N.; Segundo, M.J.; Calvo, N.; Faro, M.; Aliste, L.; Fernandez de Sevilla, T.; Alegre, J. Effect of coenzyme Q10 plus nicotinamide adenine dinucleotide supplementation on maximum heart rate after exercise testing in chronic fatigue syndrome: A randomized, controlled, double-blind trial. *Clin. Nutr.* **2016**, *35*, 826–834. [CrossRef] [PubMed]
63. Castro-Marrero, J.; Segundo, M.J.; Lacasa, M.; Martinez-Martinez, A.; Sentanes, R.S.; Alegre-Martin, J. Effect of Dietary Coenzyme Q10 Plus NADH Supplementation on Fatigue Perception and Health-Related Quality of Life in Individuals with Myalgic

Encephalomyelitis/Chronic Fatigue Syndrome: A Prospective, Randomized, Double-Blind, Placebo-Controlled Trial. *Nutrients* **2021**, *13*, 2658. [CrossRef] [PubMed]
64. Castro-Marrero, J.; Domingo, J.C.; Cordobilla, B.; Ferrer, R.; Giralt, M.; Sanmartin-Sentanes, R.; Alegre-Martin, J. Does Coenzyme Q10 Plus Selenium Supplementation Ameliorate Clinical Outcomes by Modulating Oxidative Stress and Inflammation in Individuals with Myalgic Encephalomyelitis/Chronic Fatigue Syndrome? *Antioxid. Redox Signal.* **2022**, *36*, 729–739. [CrossRef] [PubMed]
65. Banoth, B.; Cassel, S.L. Mitochondria in innate immune signaling. *Transl. Res.* **2018**, *202*, 52–68. [CrossRef]
66. Vazquez, C.; Horner, S.M. MAVS Coordination of Antiviral Innate Immunity. *J. Virol.* **2015**, *89*, 6974–6977. [CrossRef]
67. Roingeard, P.; Eymieux, S.; Burlaud-Gaillard, J.; Hourioux, C.; Patient, R.; Blanchard, E. The double-membrane vesicle (DMV): A virus-induced organelle dedicated to the replication of SARS-CoV-2 and other positive-sense single-stranded RNA viruses. *Cell. Mol. Life Sci.* **2022**, *79*, 425. [CrossRef]
68. Wolff, G.; Melia, C.E.; Snijder, E.J.; Barcena, M. Double-Membrane Vesicles as Platforms for Viral Replication. *Trends Microbiol.* **2020**, *28*, 1022–1033. [CrossRef]
69. Singh, S.P.; Amar, S.; Gehlot, P.; Patra, S.K.; Kanwar, N.; Kanwal, A. Mitochondrial Modulations, Autophagy Pathways Shifts in Viral Infections: Consequences of COVID-19. *Int. J. Mol. Sci.* **2021**, *22*, 8180. [CrossRef]
70. Li, X.; Hou, P.; Ma, W.; Wang, X.; Wang, H.; Yu, Z.; Chang, H.; Wang, T.; Jin, S.; Wang, X.; et al. SARS-CoV-2 ORF10 suppresses the antiviral innate immune response by degrading MAVS through mitophagy. *Cell. Mol. Immunol.* **2022**, *19*, 67–78. [CrossRef]
71. Dutta, S.; Das, N.; Mukherjee, P. Picking up a Fight: Fine Tuning Mitochondrial Innate Immune Defenses Against RNA Viruses. *Front. Microbiol.* **2020**, *11*, 1990. [CrossRef] [PubMed]
72. Gvozdjakova, A.; Kucharska, J.; Sumbalova, Z.; Rausova, Z.; Chladekova, A.; Komlosi, M.; Szamosova, M.; Mojto, V. The importance of coenzyme Q10 and its ratio to cholesterol in the progress of chronic kidney diseases linked to non-communicable diseases. *Bratisl. Med. J.* **2020**, *121*, 693–699. [CrossRef] [PubMed]
73. Barletta, M.A.; Marino, G.; Spagnolo, B.; Bianchi, F.P.; Falappone, P.C.F.; Spagnolo, L.; Gatti, P. Coenzyme Q10 + alpha lipoic acid for chronic COVID syndrome. *Clin. Exp. Med.* **2023**, *23*, 667–678. [CrossRef] [PubMed]
74. Hansen, K.S.; Mogensen, T.H.; Agergaard, J.; Schiottz-Christensen, B.; Ostergaard, L.; Vibholm, L.K.; Leth, S. High-dose coenzyme Q10 therapy versus placebo in patients with post COVID-19 condition: A randomized, phase 2, crossover trial. *Lancet Reg. Health Eur.* **2023**, *24*, 100539. [CrossRef] [PubMed]
75. Cordero, M.D.; Alcocer-Gomez, E.; de Miguel, M.; Culic, O.; Carrion, A.M.; Alvarez-Suarez, J.M.; Bullon, P.; Battino, M.; Fernandez-Rodriguez, A.; Sanchez-Alcazar, J.A. Can coenzyme q10 improve clinical and molecular parameters in fibromyalgia? *Antioxid. Redox Signal.* **2013**, *19*, 1356–1361. [CrossRef]
76. Alcocer-Gomez, E.; Sanchez-Alcazar, J.A.; Cordero, M.D. Coenzyme q10 regulates serotonin levels and depressive symptoms in fibromyalgia patients: Results of a small clinical trial. *J. Clin. Psychopharmacol.* **2014**, *34*, 277–278. [CrossRef]
77. Alcocer-Gomez, E.; Culic, O.; Navarro-Pando, J.M.; Sanchez-Alcazar, J.A.; Bullon, P. Effect of Coenzyme Q(10) on Psychopathological Symptoms in Fibromyalgia Patients. *CNS Neurosci. Ther.* **2017**, *23*, 188–189. [CrossRef]
78. Cordero, M.D.; Cano-Garcia, F.J.; Alcocer-Gomez, E.; De Miguel, M.; Sanchez-Alcazar, J.A. Oxidative stress correlates with headache symptoms in fibromyalgia: Coenzyme Q10 effect on clinical improvement. *PLoS ONE* **2012**, *7*, e35677. [CrossRef]
79. Di Pierro, F.; Rossi, A.; Consensi, A.; Giacomelli, C.; Bazzichi, L. Role for a water-soluble form of CoQ10 in female subjects affected by fibromyalgia. A preliminary study. *Clin. Exp. Rheumatol.* **2017**, *35* (Suppl. S105), 20–27.
80. Sawaddiruk, P.; Apaijai, N.; Paiboonworachat, S.; Kaewchur, T.; Kasitanon, N.; Jaiwongkam, T.; Kerdphoo, S.; Chattipakorn, N.; Chattipakorn, S.C. Coenzyme Q10 supplementation alleviates pain in pregabalin-treated fibromyalgia patients via reducing brain activity and mitochondrial dysfunction. *Free Radic. Res.* **2019**, *53*, 901–909. [CrossRef]
81. Lister, R.E. An open, pilot study to evaluate the potential benefits of coenzyme Q10 combined with Ginkgo biloba extract in fibromyalgia syndrome. *J. Int. Med. Res.* **2002**, *30*, 195–199. [CrossRef] [PubMed]
82. Schweiger, V.; Secchettin, E.; Castellani, C.; Martini, A.; Mazzocchi, E.; Picelli, A.; Polati, E.; Donadello, K.; Valenti, M.T.; Dalle Carbonare, L. Comparison between Acupuncture and Nutraceutical Treatment with Migratens((R)) in Patients with Fibromyalgia Syndrome: A Prospective Randomized Clinical Trial. *Nutrients* **2020**, *12*, 821. [CrossRef] [PubMed]
83. Israel, A.; Schaffer, A.A.; Cicurel, A.; Feldhamer, I.; Tal, A.; Cheng, K.; Sinha, S.; Schiff, E.; Lavie, G.; Ruppin, E. Identification of drugs associated with reduced severity of COVID-19: A case-control study in a large population. *medRxiv* **2021**. [CrossRef]
84. Fukuda, S.; Nojima, J.; Kajimoto, O.; Yamaguti, K.; Nakatomi, Y.; Kuratsune, H.; Watanabe, Y. Ubiquinol-10 supplementation improves autonomic nervous function and cognitive function in chronic fatigue syndrome. *Biofactors* **2016**, *42*, 431–440. [CrossRef]
85. Cordero, M.D.; Diaz-Parrado, E.; Carrion, A.M.; Alfonsi, S.; Sanchez-Alcazar, J.A.; Bullon, P.; Battino, M.; de Miguel, M. Is inflammation a mitochondrial dysfunction-dependent event in fibromyalgia? *Antioxid. Redox Signal.* **2013**, *18*, 800–807. [CrossRef]
86. Miyamae, T.; Seki, M.; Naga, T.; Uchino, S.; Asazuma, H.; Yoshida, T.; Iizuka, Y.; Kikuchi, M.; Imagawa, T.; Natsumeda, Y.; et al. Increased oxidative stress and coenzyme Q10 deficiency in juvenile fibromyalgia: Amelioration of hypercholesterolemia and fatigue by ubiquinol-10 supplementation. *Redox Rep.* **2013**, *18*, 12–19. [CrossRef]
87. Moreno Fernandez-Ayala, D.J.; Navas, P.; Lopez-Lluch, G. Age-related mitochondrial dysfunction as a key factor in COVID-19 disease. *Exp. Gerontol.* **2020**, *142*, 111147. [CrossRef]

88. Caruso, F.; Rossi, M.; Pedersen, J.Z.; Incerpi, S. Computational studies reveal mechanism by which quinone derivatives can inhibit SARS-CoV-2. Study of embelin and two therapeutic compounds of interest, methyl prednisolone and dexamethasone. *J. Infect. Public. Health* **2020**, *13*, 1868–1877. [CrossRef]
89. Xie, Y.; Xu, E.; Bowe, B.; Al-Aly, Z. Long-term cardiovascular outcomes of COVID-19. *Nat. Med.* **2022**, *28*, 583–590. [CrossRef]
90. Ahmed, A.I.; Saad, J.M.; Han, Y.; Alahdab, F.; Malahfji, M.; Nabi, F.; Mahmarian, J.J.; Cooke, J.P.; Zoghbi, W.A.; Al-Mallah, M.H. Coronary Microvascular Health in Patients With Prior COVID-19 Infection. *JACC Cardiovasc. Imaging* **2022**, *15*, 2153–2155. [CrossRef]
91. Morrow, A.J.; Sykes, R.; McIntosh, A.; Kamdar, A.; Bagot, C.; Bayes, H.K.; Blyth, K.G.; Briscoe, M.; Bulluck, H.; Carrick, D.; et al. A multisystem, cardio-renal investigation of post-COVID-19 illness. *Nat. Med.* **2022**, *28*, 1303–1313. [CrossRef] [PubMed]
92. Mantle, D.; Heaton, R.A.; Hargreaves, I.P. Coenzyme Q10 and Immune Function: An Overview. *Antioxidants* **2021**, *10*, 759. [CrossRef] [PubMed]
93. Hargreaves, I.R.; Mantle, D. COVID-19, Coenzyme Q10 and Selenium. *Adv. Exp. Med. Biol.* **2021**, *1327*, 161–168. [CrossRef] [PubMed]
94. Alehagen, U.; Johansson, P.; Bjornstedt, M.; Rosen, A.; Dahlstrom, U. Cardiovascular mortality and N-terminal-proBNP reduced after combined selenium and coenzyme Q10 supplementation: A 5-year prospective randomized double-blind placebo-controlled trial among elderly Swedish citizens. *Int. J. Cardiol.* **2013**, *167*, 1860–1866. [CrossRef] [PubMed]
95. Mortensen, S.A.; Rosenfeldt, F.; Kumar, A.; Dolliner, P.; Filipiak, K.J.; Pella, D.; Alehagen, U.; Steurer, G.; Littarru, G.P.; Investigators, Q.S.S. The effect of coenzyme Q10 on morbidity and mortality in chronic heart failure: Results from Q-SYMBIO: A randomized double-blind trial. *JACC Heart Fail.* **2014**, *2*, 641–649. [CrossRef]
96. Nacul, L.; Authier, F.J.; Scheibenbogen, C.; Lorusso, L.; Helland, I.B.; Martin, J.A.; Sirbu, C.A.; Mengshoel, A.M.; Polo, O.; Behrends, U.; et al. European Network on Myalgic Encephalomyelitis/Chronic Fatigue Syndrome (EUROMENE): Expert Consensus on the Diagnosis, Service Provision, and Care of People with ME/CFS in Europe. *Medicina* **2021**, *57*, 510. [CrossRef]
97. Todic, M. Dossier for marketing authorization in the European Union. *Bosn. J. Basic Med. Sci.* **2003**, *3*, 56–60. [CrossRef]
98. Sardella, M.; Belcher, G.; Lungu, C.; Ignoni, T.; Camisa, M.; Stenver, D.I.; Porcelli, P.; D'Antuono, M.; Castiglione, N.G.; Adams, A.; et al. Monitoring the manufacturing and quality of medicines: A fundamental task of pharmacovigilance. *Ther. Adv. Drug Saf.* **2021**, *12*, 20420986211038436. [CrossRef]
99. Kressmann, S.; Muller, W.E.; Blume, H.H. Pharmaceutical quality of different Ginkgo biloba brands. *J. Pharm. Pharmacol.* **2002**, *54*, 661–669. [CrossRef]
100. Czigle, S.; Toth, J.; Jedlinszki, N.; Haznagy-Radnai, E.; Csupor, D.; Tekelova, D. Ginkgo biloba Food Supplements on the European Market—Adulteration Patterns Revealed by Quality Control of Selected Samples. *Planta Med.* **2018**, *84*, 475–482. [CrossRef]
101. Walkowiak, A.; Wnuk, K.; Cyrankiewicz, M.; Kupcewicz, B. Discrimination of Adulterated Ginkgo Biloba Products Based on 2T2D Correlation Spectroscopy in UV-Vis Range. *Molecules* **2022**, *27*, 433. [CrossRef]
102. Mantle, D.; Millichap, L.; Castro-Marrero, J.; Hargreaves, I.P. Primary Coenzyme Q10 Deficiency: An Update. *Antioxidants* **2023**, *12*, 1652. [CrossRef]
103. Mantle, D.; Dybring, A. Bioavailability of Coenzyme Q10: An Overview of the Absorption Process and Subsequent Metabolism. *Antioxidants* **2020**, *9*, 386. [CrossRef]
104. Lopez-Lluch, G.; Del Pozo-Cruz, J.; Sanchez-Cuesta, A.; Cortes-Rodriguez, A.B.; Navas, P. Bioavailability of coenzyme Q10 supplements depends on carrier lipids and solubilization. *Nutrition* **2019**, *57*, 133–140. [CrossRef]
105. Mantle, D.; Lopez-Lluch, G.; Hargreaves, I.P. Coenzyme Q10 Metabolism: A Review of Unresolved Issues. *Int. J. Mol. Sci.* **2023**, *24*, 2585. [CrossRef]
106. Crane, F.L. Biochemical functions of coenzyme Q10. *J. Am. Coll. Nutr.* **2001**, *20*, 591–598. [CrossRef]
107. Hargreaves, I.P. Coenzyme Q10 as a therapy for mitochondrial disease. *Int. J. Biochem. Cell Biol.* **2014**, *49*, 105–111. [CrossRef]
108. Polymeropoulos, V.M. A Potential Role of Coenzyme Q10 Deficiency in Severe SARS-CoV-2 Infection. *OBM Integr. Complement. Med.* **2020**, *5*, 042. [CrossRef]
109. Chen, T.H.; Chang, C.J.; Hung, P.H. Possible Pathogenesis and Prevention of Long COVID: SARS-CoV-2-Induced Mitochondrial Disorder. *Int. J. Mol. Sci.* **2023**, *24*, 8034. [CrossRef]
110. Mantle, D.; Hargreaves, I.P. Mitochondrial Dysfunction and Neurodegenerative Disorders: Role of Nutritional Supplementation. *Int. J. Mol. Sci.* **2022**, *23*, 12603. [CrossRef]

International Journal of
Molecular Sciences

MDPI

Article

Uridine as a Regulator of Functional and Ultrastructural Changes in the Brain of Rats in a Model of 6-OHDA-Induced Parkinson's Disease

Nina I. Uspalenko [1,2], Alexei A. Mosentsov [1], Natalia V. Khmil [1], Lyubov L. Pavlik [1], Natalia V. Belosludtseva [1,2], Natalia V. Khunderyakova [1,2], Maria I. Shigaeva [1], Vasilisa P. Medvedeva [1,2], Anton E. Malkov [1], Valentina F. Kitchigina [1] and Galina D. Mironova [1,2,*]

1 Institute of Theoretical and Experimental Biophysics, Russian Academy of Sciences, Pushchino 142290, Russia; nina_uspalenko@mail.ru (N.I.U.); makcvel.95@mail.ru (A.A.M.); nat-niig@yandex.ru (N.V.K.); pavlikl@mail.ru (L.L.P.); nata.imagination@gmail.com (N.V.B.); nkhunderyakova@gmail.com (N.V.K.); shigaeva-marija@rambler.ru (M.I.S.); vasilisa.medv@mail.ru (V.P.M.); malkovae@gmail.com (A.E.M.); vkitchigina@gmail.com (V.F.K.)

2 Pushchino State Natural Science Institute, Pushchino 142290, Russia

* Correspondence: mironova40@mail.ru or mironovagd@iteb.pushchino.ru

Abstract: Using a model of Parkinson's disease (PD) induced by the bilateral injection of neurotoxin 6-hydroxydopamine (6-OHDA) into rat brain substantia nigra (SN), we showed uridine to exert a protective effect associated with activation of the mitochondrial ATP-dependent potassium (mitoK-ATP) channel. Injection of 4 µg neurotoxin evoked a 70% decrease in the time the experimental animal spent on the rod in the RotaRod test, an increase in the amount of lipid peroxides in blood serum and cerebral-cortex mitochondria and the rate of reactive oxygen species formation, and a decrease in Ca^{2+} retention in mitochondria. Herewith, lymphocytes featured an increase in the activity of lactate dehydrogenase, a cytosolic enzyme of glycolysis, without changes in succinate-dehydrogenase activity. Structural changes occurring in the SN and striatum manifested themselves in the destruction of mitochondria, degeneration of neurons and synapses, and stratification of myelin sheaths in them. Subcutaneous injections of 30 µg/kg uridine for 22 days restored the neurotoxin-induced changes in these parameters to levels close to the control. 5-Hydroxydecanoate (5 mg/kg), a specific mitoK-ATP channel inhibitor, eliminated the beneficial effect of uridine for almost all characteristics tested, indicating the involvement of the mitoK-ATP channel in the protective effect of uridine. The mechanism of the protective effect of uridine and its therapeutic applications for the prevention and treatment of PD are discussed.

Keywords: Parkinson's disease; 6-hydroxydopamine; uridine; mitochondria; mitochondrial ATP-dependent potassium channel; oxidative stress; structure; neurons; synapses

1. Introduction

Parkinson's disease (PD) is a neurodegenerative disorder the probability of the development of which significantly increases with age. It is expected that, as a result of overall aging of the world population, the number of patients with PD will significantly increase [1]. Elucidation of the mechanisms of its occurrence and search for new approaches to its prevention and treatment are an urgent problem. The most common method of PD treatment to date has been the dopaminergic replacement therapy with levodopa, which only temporarily mitigates the symptoms of motor deficits [2].

One of the main processes underlying neurodegenerative disorders, in particular, PD, is mitochondrial dysfunction. Taking into account the high energy needs of the body, especially of the brain, this condition may have devastating consequences for the survival of neurons [3].

The mitochondrial dysfunction in brain tissues is commonly caused by an excessive production of reactive oxygen species (ROS), whose level increases with age [4]. At the same time, an increase in the ROS content in the substantia nigra (SN) and striatum induces the oxidation of dopamine accompanied by the death of dopaminergic neurons, which is a cause of PD development [5]. The lack of a radical therapy encourages the development of new approaches to the prevention and treatment of PD using currently available experimental models.

Since PD patients are found to feature an inhibition of respiratory chain complex I in mitochondria [5], one of the methods of modeling PD is the use of 6-hydroxydopamine (6-OHDA), which inhibits this complex [5,6]. This neurotoxin is unable to cross the hematoencephalic barrier and is therefore administered directly into the SN or striatum. Entering the dopaminergic neurons with the help of a dopamine transporter, 6-OHDA initiates an increase in the amount of ROS in them [6]. This can damage the protein structures of the brain tissue, affect the function of neurons, and lead to motor impairments [4]. An increase in the level of ROS also results in the oxidation of dopamine followed by its degradation and, as a consequence, severe mitochondrial dysfunction [7].

We have previously found that the injection of uridine to animals leads to an increase in the concentration of uridine diphosphate (UDP), a natural activator of the mitochondrial ATP-dependent potassium (mitoK-ATP) channel, which normalizes oxidative exchange and eliminates mitochondrial dysfunction [8–11].

In this work, we studied the therapeutic action of uridine in a model of neurotoxin-induced PD in rats and the degree of the involvement of the mitoK-ATP channel in the development of Parkinson's syndrome.

2. Results

2.1. *Effect of Uridine on the Behavior of Animals in a Model of PD Created by the Bilateral Injection of 6-OHDA into the Substantia Nigra*

In a model of PD created by the bilateral injection of 6-OHDA into the rat brain SN, we observed a disturbance of the dopaminergic nigrostriatal pathway and an impairment of the motor function. Nissl staining used to quantitatively assess the fate of dopaminergic neurons in the substantia nigra pars compacta after administration of the neurotoxin revealed that 70% of the neurons died. Upon creation of the model, the rats were in a calm environment with free access to water and food; in the postoperative period, they were under daily control. Additionally, the animals were administered Ringer's solution (5 mL per day). Motor impairments were assessed using the RotaRod behavioral test on the 22nd day after the injection of the neurotoxin (Figure 1A).

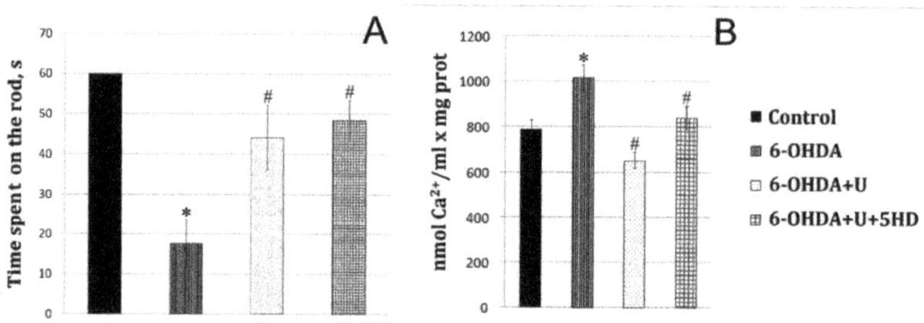

Figure 1. Effect of uridine on the motor function and ion exchange in rat brain mitochondria after the bilateral injection of 6-OHDA into the substantia nigra. (**A**) Estimation of the motor function on the 22nd day after the injection. *y*-axis: the time the animals move at a speed of 8 cm/s before falling from the RotaRod device. (**B**) Calcium retention capacity of rat brain mitochondria in the normal state and in a PD model. The results are presented as the mean ± SEM. * $p < 0.05$, relative to the control, # $p < 0.05$, relative to the 6-OHDA group.

Administration of the neurotoxin decreased by 70% the time spent by the animal on the rotating rod compared to the control group (Figure 1A). To correct 6-OHDA-induced impairments, uridine was injected intraperitoneally at a concentration of 30 mg/kg of body weight. After the injection of the neurotoxin together with uridine, the time spent on the rod increased to approach that of the control values. 5-Hydroxydecanoate (5-HD), a specific inhibitor of the mitoK-ATP channel, did not eliminate the protective effect of uridine within the time the animal was on the rotating rod.

2.2. *Effect of Uridine on the Calcium Exchange in Rat Brain Mitochondria after the Bilateral Administration of 6-OHDA into the Substantia Nigra*

Disturbance of calcium homeostasis observed in PD is known to lead to cell death. The cell death is, presumably, associated with the overload of mitochondria with calcium, which promotes the development of oxidative stress in them and changes the permeability of the mitochondrial membrane followed by the opening of a nonspecific pore and the death of dopaminergic neurons [12,13].

The results of the present study showed that the administration of the neurotoxin to model PD decreased the calcium retention capacity of mitochondria by 63% relative to the control. Injection of uridine at a concentration of 30 mg/kg of body weight together with 6-OHDA increased the calcium retention capacity of mitochondria to the control level. Application of 5-HD completely eliminated the beneficial action of uridine (Figure 1B).

2.3. *Effect of Uridine on the Oxidative Exchange in Rat Brain Mitochondria after the Bilateral Injection of 6-OHDA into the Substantia Nigra*

The rate of hydrogen peroxide formation in the experiments was determined in a system with Amplex Red and horseradish peroxidase. It was found that the neurotoxin increased the rate of hydrogen peroxide formation in rat brain mitochondria in the experimental group by 23% compared to the control groups. The injection of uridine together with the neurotoxin decreased the characteristic to values even below the control, and the injection of 5-HD in combination with uridine eliminated the protective effect of uridine, increasing the rate of hydrogen peroxide formation (Figure 2A).

When diffusing through biological membranes, hydrogen peroxide can react with unsaturated fatty acids of lipids, which leads to the destruction of membranes. One of the products of these reactions is malondialdehyde (MDA). In this work, we determined the content of lipid peroxidation products in brain mitochondria (Figure 2B). In rats injected with the neurotoxin, the content of MDA was, by 18%, higher than in the control group. The injection of uridine decreased the MDA content in brain mitochondria to a level significantly lower than in the control (Figure 2B), which is consistent with our data indicating a decrease in the rate of hydrogen peroxide formation in the brain (Figure 2A).

The measurements showed that the MDA content in the blood serum of rats with PD increased by 37%, and the treatment with uridine lowered this characteristic to the control level (Figure 2C). At the same time, the injection of 5-HD to animals receiving uridine treatment eliminated the effect of uridine in the blood serum and increased the MDA level by 45% relative to the MDA content in the group of animals treated with uridine.

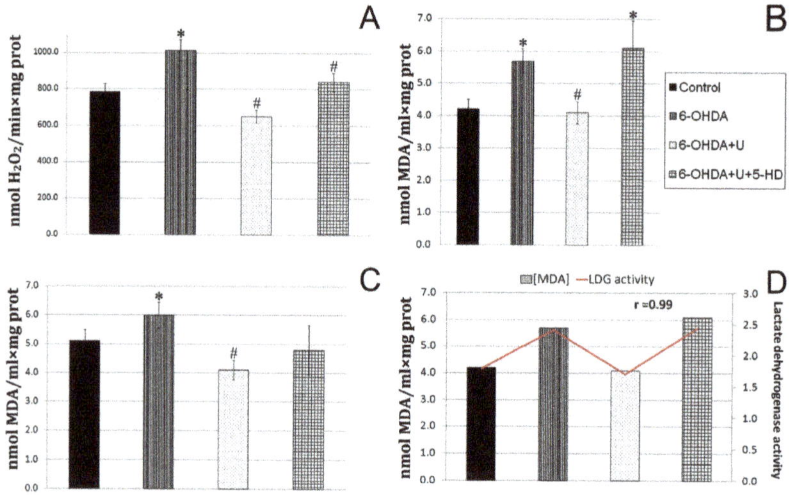

Figure 2. Effect of uridine on the rate of hydrogen peroxide formation and MDA production in rat brain mitochondria and blood serum after the bilateral injection of 6-OHDA into the substantia nigra. (**A**) The rate of hydrogen peroxide formation by rat brain mitochondria on the 22nd day after the administration of 6-OHDA. (**B**) Concentration of lipid peroxidation products in rat brain mitochondria on the 22nd day after the injection of 6-OHDA. (**C**) Concentration of lipid peroxidation products in blood serum of rats on the 22nd day after the injection of 6-OHDA. (**D**) A correlation between the content of TBA-active products in the blood serum and the LDG activity in lymphocytes. The results are presented as the mean ± SEM. * $p < 0.05$, relative to the control, # $p < 0.05$, relative to the 6-OHDA group.

2.4. *Effect of Uridine on Succinate Dehydrogenase and Lactate Dehydrogenase Activities in Blood Lymphocytes in a PD Model*

A cytobiochemical determination of the activity of the key mitochondrial enzyme, succinate dehydrogenase (SDH), in immobilized blood lymphocytes in a blood smear from PD rats did not reveal any significant differences from the control. After the injection of uridine to sick animals, the activity of SDH increased by 80% compared to the control. The application of 5-HD reduced the beneficial effect of uridine. Measurements of the activity of the glycolysis enzyme, lactate dehydrogenase (LDH), in blood lymphocytes in a smear from PD rats showed that it increased by 35% compared to the control, and the treatment with uridine decreased the activation to that of the control value. The administration of the 5-HD inhibitor abolished the effect of uridine, increasing the LDH level by 37% to the level in the group of sick rats. Thus, in the mitochondria of blood lymphocytes from rats with PD, glycolysis dominated over oxidative phosphorylation; the administration of uridine enhanced mitochondrial respiration by 80% and reduced glycolysis. The injection of 5-HD completely abolished the effect of uridine (Table 1).

Table 1. Succinate dehydrogenase and lactate dehydrogenase activities in lymphocytes in experimental parkinsonism.

Group	SDH Activity, Relative Units	LDH Activity, Relative Units
Control	1.14	1.78
6-OHDA	1.37	2.41 *
6-OHDA+U	1.82 *	1.70
6-OHDA+U + 5-HD	1.00	2.44 *

* $p < 0.05$, relative to the control.

The characteristics of glycolysis (activity of LDH) in lymphocytes and oxidative stress (MDA level) in serum were revealed to have a direct positive correlation with coefficient $r = 0.99$. In animals with Parkinson's syndrome, the LDH activity increased by 37%, and the MDA content rose by 35%. Treatment with uridine decreased both characteristics to the values for the control group, and 5-HD completely abolished the effect of uridine in lymphocytes and serum. The reduction in SDH activity and the increase in LDH indicate the disturbance of energetic processes in lymphocytes in PD, which shows up in the retardation of aerobic oxidation and enhancement of glycolysis; this is in line with the literature data [14].

2.5. Ultrastructures of Substantia Nigra and Striatum Neurons after the Bilateral Administration of 6-OHDA and the Protective Effect of Uridine on These Structures

Images of the ultrastructure of the dopaminergic neuron in the SN were obtained 22 days after the induction of Parkinson's syndrome in rats by the bilateral injection of 6-OHDA into the SN (Figure 3).

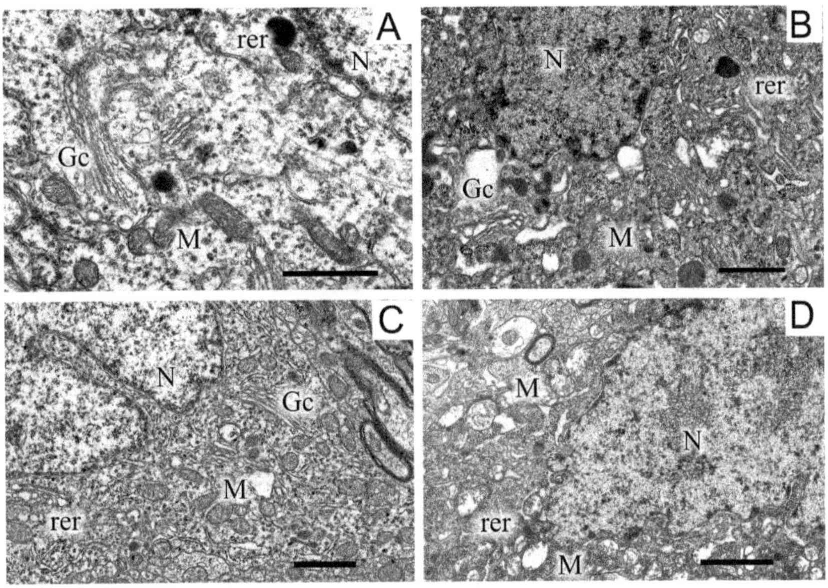

Figure 3. A region of a dopaminergic neuron from the substantia nigra in the control (**A**), in a model of parkinsonism (**B**), in the presence of uridine (**C**), and in the presence of uridine and 5-HD (**D**). N, nucleus; Gc, Golgi complex; M, mitochondrion; rer, endoplasmic reticulum. Scale bar = 1 μm.

Exposure to the neurotoxin resulted in the appearance of a large number of dark neurons (Figure 3B). As compared with the control (Figure 3A), where the neurons of the SN had a light cytoplasm and a light nucleus, the neurons from experimental animals had a high electron density of the cytoplasm, a dense nucleus with a convoluted sheath, enlarged cisterns of both the endoplasmic reticulum and the Golgi complex, as well as a disordered structure of mitochondria in which vacuoles appeared. The cytoplasm of a neuron contained a large number of lysosomes and lipofuscin granules. The number of mitochondria significantly (by almost 1.5 times) increased as compared with the control (2.22 ± 0.18 in the experiment, 1.13 ± 0.09 in the control). Administration of uridine prevented the structure of neurons from becoming damaged; as a result, they had a morphology similar to that of neurons in the control group (Figure 3C). They had a light cytoplasm and a light nucleus with flattened cisternae of the reticulum. The structure of their mitochondria was not damaged. Administration of the mitoK-ATP channel inhibitor,

5-HD, together with uridine abolished the beneficial effect of uridine: neurons with a dense cytoplasm and with mitochondria having abnormalities in the vicinity of cristae appeared, vacuoles emerged, and the lysis of the stroma occurred (Figure 3D). Uridine also decreased the number of mitochondria in presynaptic endings to that of the control value (1.2 ± 0.08), and 5-HD eliminated the effect of uridine, decreasing their number to the level recorded in pathology (2.3 ± 0.2).

In the neuropil of SN neurons, we observed significant structural damage to the myelin sheaths of axons (Figure 4B,D).

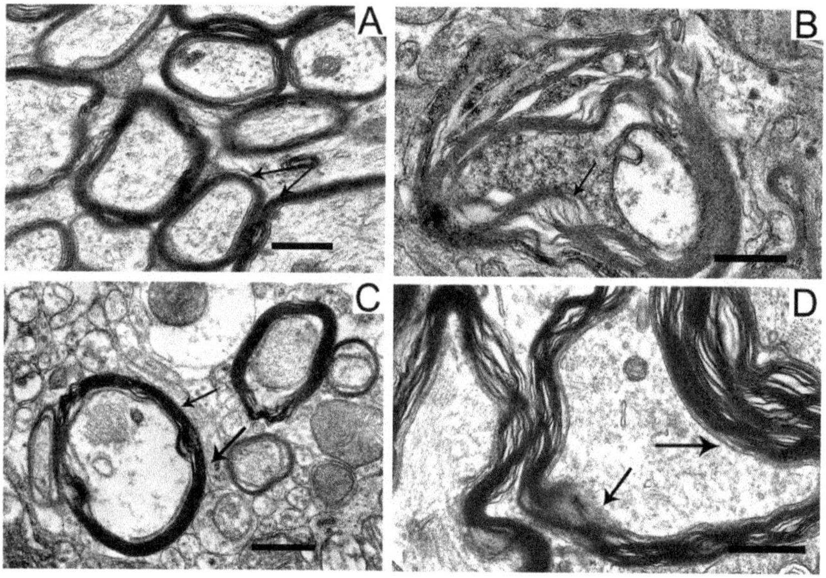

Figure 4. Myelin sheaths of axons in the neuropil of substantia nigra neurons in the control (**A**), in a model of parkinsonism (**B**), in the presence of uridine (**C**), and in the presence of uridine and 5-HD (**D**). Myelin sheaths are shown by arrows. Scale bar = 0.5 μm.

Compared with the control (Figure 4A), in neurons damaged by the neurotoxin, we noted a pronounced stratification of membrane layers of the myelin sheath and the protrusion of its part toward the cytoplasm (Figure 4B). After the administration of uridine, the myelin structure remained similar to that in the control (Figure 4C). Administration of 5-HD together with uridine abolished the protective effect of uridine; in this case, the myelin sheaths of axons remained untwisted (Figure 4D).

Along with disruptions in the SN structure, we observed changes in the striatum. They were in many respects similar to those found in the SN and consisted in the appearance of dark neurons with a dark cytoplasm and a dark nucleus, which had an untwisted sheath (Figure 5).

The cisternae of the reticulum and the Golgi complex in the cytoplasm were dilated (Figure 5B) as compared with the light cytoplasm and the light nucleus in the control (Figure 5A). After treatment with uridine, the structure of a neuron became close to that of the intact neuron, with a light cytoplasm and a light nucleus and flattened cisternae of the Golgi complex and the reticulum (Figure 5B). 5-HD abolished the protective effect of uridine (cf. Figure 5B,D). In the 6-OHDA group of animals, in the neurons of the striatum, we observed an increase in the number of mitochondria in presynaptic endings by 1.5 times compared with the control (2.7 ± 0.2). After the administration of uridine, their number remained at the control level (1.7 ± 0.1), and in the group of animals treated with uridine in combination with 5-HD, it did not differ from the value for experimental animals (2.2 ± 0.2).

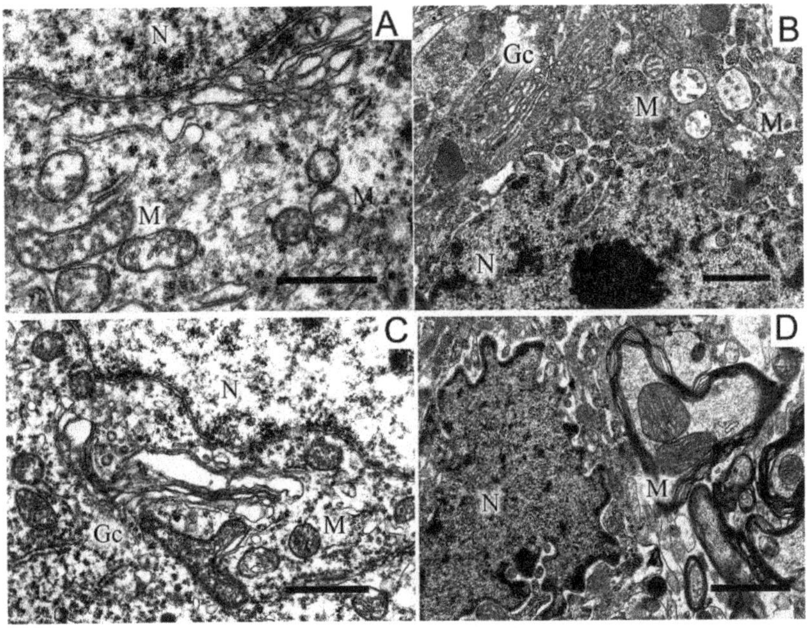

Figure 5. A region of a neuron from the striatum in the control (**A**), in a model of parkinsonism (**B**), in the presence of uridine (**C**), in the presence of uridine and 5-HD (**D**). N, nucleus; Gc, Golgi complex; M, mitochondrion; rer, endoplasmic reticulum. Scale bar = 1 μm.

The termini of axons of dopaminergic neurons of the SN commonly form axo-dendritic synapses in the striatum. Analysis of the state of axons in the striatum in control (Figure 6A) and experimental (Figure 6B,C) animals showed that the modeling of parkinsonism induced a significant restructuring of axo-dendritic synapses in this area.

In experimental rats, dilated axo-dendritic synaptic endings with significant accumulation of synaptic vesicles were found (Figure 6C). Synaptic vesicles in these synapses were packed very densely to form a continuous conglomerate. Along with these changes, the degeneration of axons by the "dark type" was observed in some places in the striatum of experimental animals (Figure 6B). As seen in Figure 6B, degenerating axons had a high electron density and swollen mitochondria. In the striatum of experimental animals, synaptic endings with perforated multiple postsynaptic indurations were found (Figure 6B). It should be noted that, in control animals, only single postsynaptic indurations were encountered in postsynaptic endings (Figure 6A). Uridine prevented the dilatation of axo-dendritic synaptic endings and the accumulation of synaptic vesicles in them, the degradation of axons, the swelling of mitochondria localized therein, and the appearance of multiple perforated postsynaptic indurations (Figure 6C).

The structure of myelin sheaths in the neuropil of striatal neurons was also disordered in the rat PD model (Figure 7).

Sheaths with stratified lamellae and membrane protrusions appeared (Figure 7B). After the administration of uridine (Figure 7C), the structure of myelin remained resistant to damage and retained a close-to-intact appearance (for Figure 7A). The injection of 5-HD eliminated the protective effect of uridine (Figure 7D), and stratified myelin lamellae were seen.

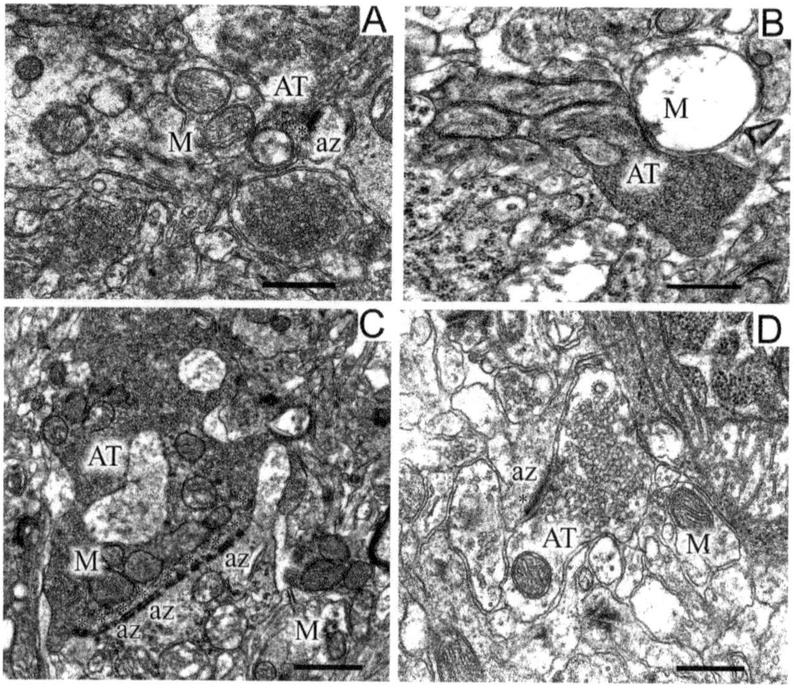

Figure 6. Regions of the neuropil of striatum neurons in the control (**A**), in a model of parkinsonism (**B**,**C**), and after the injection of uridine (**D**). Panel (**B**) shows a destroyed, swollen mitochondria and a large dark axon terminus, panel (**C**) shows synaptic endings with perforated multiple postsynaptic densities. AT, axon terminus; M, mitochondrion; az, active zone (asterisks). Scale bar = 1 μm.

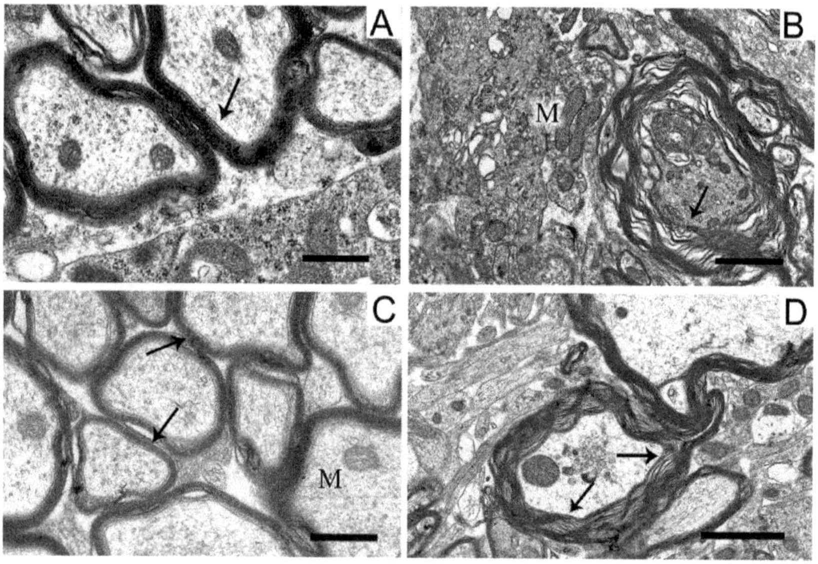

Figure 7. Myelin sheaths of axons in the neuropil of the striatum in the control (**A**), in a model of parkinsonism (**B**), in the presence of uridine (**C**), and in the presence of uridine and 5-HD (**D**). Myelin sheaths are shown by arrows. M, mitochondrion. Scale bar = 0.5 μm.

3. Discussion

The work proposes a new approach to the prevention and treatment of PD. The approach is based on the activation of the mitoK-ATP channel by its natural activator, which leads to an enhancement of energy metabolism, normalization of oxidative metabolism in brain tissues, and, as a consequence, a decrease in mitochondrial dysfunction developing in this disease.

A characteristic sign of PD is the progressive degeneration of dopaminergic neurons in the compact part of the SN and striatum, which leads to a decline in the motor activity of animals [4,7]. Uridine administered after the injection of neurotoxin 6-OHDA was found to increase the motor activity of rats more than threefold as compared with that for the 6-OHDA group (Figure 1A). This may presumably be due to the known ability of uridine to increase the synthesis of coenzyme A (CoA) and thereby to activate the functioning of the Krebs cycle, i.e., to enhance the energy metabolism in the rat body [15]. It also follows from the data obtained that the calcium metabolism in brain mitochondria of experimental animals is disturbed, which may contribute to the opening of cyclosporin-sensitive pores in them. In turn, the opening of the pore leads to cell death by necrosis or apoptosis [12].

PD is also characterized by an oxidative metabolism disturbance in brain tissues expressed in the accumulation of ROS, as well as by an increase in the rate of hydrogen peroxide production. This is probably due to the fact that, being structurally similar to dopamine, 6-OHDA enters the cell by means of dopamine and norepinephrine transporters, where it increases the concentration of ROS both enzymatically (using mitochondrial monoamine oxidase B) and nonenzymatically [4]. Furthermore, as rotenone, it is capable of inhibiting the function of the respiratory chain complex I, which also leads to the accumulation of peroxide radicals. An increase in the amount of ROS in tissues causes the oxidation of intracellular-compartment structures of dopaminergic neurons, as well as the oxidation of dopamine, which is manifested in the appearance of cognitive and motor impairments typical of PD [1,4,16].

We used uridine to correct biochemical impairments caused by the administration of 6-OHDA. At the concentrations applied, this nucleoside prevents the development of hypoxia in tissues, as shown in our previous research [11]. Administration of uridine to rats with Parkinson's syndrome completely prevented ion exchange disorders in these organelles, as well as a neurotoxin-induced increase in the formation rate and number of peroxide compounds in mitochondria and blood serum. At the same time, the energy metabolism in lymphocytes was also normalized.

Modeling of PD in rats revealed significant changes in the structures of rat brain SN and striatum. Each of these regions is of critical significance for the development of PD. Their structures are part of the extrapyramidal motor system, which is responsible for the regulation of motor function and muscle tone and is involved in many vegetative functions, such as respiration, cardiac activity, and blood vessel tone [17].

Morphological changes are observed in neurons, presynaptic endings, and in the myelin sheath of the SN and striatum. These changes may be a cause of a decrease in energy efficiency and ATP level in brain tissues, which leads to progressive degeneration of dopaminergic neurons in the compact region of the SN and striatum [18]. An increase in the number of mitochondria in synaptic endings may be an indicator of an enhancement of their activity aimed at maintaining the mechanisms of plasticity. It is assumed that the dysfunction of mitochondria and an increase in their number followed by the induction of apoptosis markers may be associated with the accumulation of mitochondrial DNA mutations due to the impact of ROS [19].

It is considered that neurodegeneration begins in synaptic junctions, as they are the first to be damaged in PD [20]. An increase in the number of perforated synapses in the PD model found in this work is usually considered to be a compensation for the degeneration of dopaminergic cells, which leads to a delay in or prevention of the development of the disease [21]. Similar plastic changes in synaptic endings of the striatum have been previously observed in a model of induced autoimmune synucleinopathy [22].

Upon administration of the neurotoxin, we observed a disruption of myelin sheaths known to be required for the separation of nerves from one another and the enhancement of nerve pulse transmission. At these structural disorders, signals become mixed, and the normal movements of the animal become impossible [23]. The above-described disorders in SN and striatum neurons, as well as in myelin sheaths, have been also found in our earlier work on a model of PD induced by rotenone, an inhibitor of the respiratory chain complex I [10], which indirectly indicates the identity of the pathology created in these models.

The study using the inhibitory analysis shows that the mechanism by which uridine affects the biochemical parameters and structure of experimental animals' brains is associated to a greater extent with the activation of the mitoK-ATP channel, because 5-HD, the channel inhibitor, abolishes the positive effect of uridine almost completely. We explain this by an increase in the concentration of UDP, an activator of this channel, in tissues at the administration of uridine [24]. It is known that UDP does not enter the cell but forms in tissues from uridine, which penetrates through the hematoencephalic barrier [8,9]. Activation of the channel is known to enhance the cyclization of potassium in mitochondria, which lowers their membrane potential ($\Delta\Psi_m$) [25,26]. It has been shown earlier that a 10% decrease in $\Delta\Psi_m$ diminishes the rate of peroxide formation in mitochondria sevenfold [27].

As the effect of uridine on brain tissues is almost completely eliminated by 5-HD, a selective inhibitor of the mitoK-ATP channel, we suggest that this channel is involved in maintaining metabolic processes and integrity of the brain structure in PD and, probably, in the development of the disease. The assumption about the role of the channel in the development of PD is consistent with our earlier data on a significant (3–5-fold) decrease in the activity of this channel with age [28]. The fact that the incidence of PD is generally recognized to rise with age [1,29] confirms the existence of a correlation between the disturbance of the mitoK-ATP channel function and the development of PD. Thus, the data obtained in the present research are indicative of the involvement of mitochondria and the mitoK-ATP channel in the development of PD.

Still, as 5-HD did not always completely abolish the effect of uridine, other metabolic pathways of this nucleoside can be also assumed to be involved in protecting the rat body from the neurotoxin. One of such pathways, as we noted above, can be the synthesis of acetyl-CoA from uridine, which is important for the recovery of the Krebs cycle energy equivalents, NADH and $FADN_2$, known to be depleted during the development of oxidative stress in toxic models of PD [15]. In this regard, the administration of uridine can significantly enhance the energy and ion metabolism in mitochondria, which prevents motor dysfunction in sick animals. The mechanism of the protective action of uridine in PD can also be related to the formation of UDP glucose involved in glycogen synthesis [30,31]. As for the effect of uridine on the prevention of structural changes in myelin in our PD model, this can be associated with an increased formation of cytidine triphosphate (CTP) from UTP, the concentration of which increases after the administration of uridine [8,9]. An increase in CTP in tissues stimulates the synthesis of brain phospholipids, which, probably, does prevent the breakdown of the myelin sheath [32].

Since the mitoK-ATP channel inhibitor eliminated the beneficial effect of uridine in almost all cases, we assume that the main mechanism of action of this metabolite is through the activation of the channel. The activation of the channel leads to an acceleration of potassium cyclization in mitochondria, which lowers their membrane potential to induce a "mild uncoupling". Herewith, the rate of peroxide formation in mitochondria decreases, oxidative metabolism normalizes, and both the calcium overload of cells and the neurotoxin-induced structural changes in the brain tissue are prevented.

4. Materials and Methods

Wistar male rats (N = 23) weighing 190–220 g were used. The animals were housed in a vivarium at the Institute of Theoretical and Experimental Biophysics, Russian Academy of Sciences. All manipulations with animals were carried out in compliance with the Council Directive 2010/63 EU of the European Parliament and the Regulations of the

European Convention for the Protection of Vertebrate Animals Used for Scientific Purposes (Strasbourg, France).

4.1. Stereotaxic Intervention and Groups of Animals

In this series of experiments, animals were divided into four groups: (1) the control group; to the SN of both brain hemispheres, 4 μL of a 0.2% L-ascorbic acid solution was injected (N = 5); (2) the 6-OHDA group; 4 μg of neurotoxin 6-OHDA dissolved in 6 μL of a 0.2% L-ascorbic acid solution was injected (N = 6); (3) the 6-OHDA + U group; after the injection of 6-OHDA, the mitoK-ATP channel activator, uridine (U), was daily administered intraperitoneally for 22 days at a dose of 30 mg/kg of body weight (N = 6); (4) the 6-OHDA+U + 5-HD group; after the injection of 6-OHDA, uridine (U) was administered daily, and 15 min after the injection of uridine, the mitoK-ATP channel inhibitor, 5-HD, was subcutaneously injected at a dose of 5 mg/kg of body weight (N = 6).

For anesthesia, Xylozin (4 mg/kg of body weight) and Zoletil (60 mg/kg) were used. 6-OHDA (5 mg) was dissolved in 0.8 mL of 300 mM sodium chloride (a sterile saline infusion solution) with 0.1% ascorbic acid. Operations were carried out on a stereotaxic frame using a 10 mL micro syringe (Hamilton Co., Reno, NV, USA) by the method described by Torres and Dunnett [33]. The neurotoxin was injected bilaterally along the coordinates (anterior-posterior = −2.0 mm, lateral = −5.2 mm, ventral = −8.2 mm) [34].

4.2. Behavioral Testing

The endurance and motor coordination of animals were assessed on a RotaRod device (Neurobotics, Moscow, Zelenograd, Russia) on the 22nd day after surgery. The facility was a rotating horizontal rod with lateral vertical baffles. An experimenter placed a rat into the facility and controlled the running of the animal. The time during which the animal stayed on the rotating rod (speed 8 cm/s) was measured.

4.3. Isolation of Mitochondria

Rats were decapitated on the 22nd day after surgery. Brain tissue fragments were washed and homogenized by a manual homogenizer in an isolation medium (230 mM mannitol, 70 mM sucrose, 1.0 mM EDTA, and 10 mM HEPES-KOH, pH 7.4). Homogenates were centrifuged at 12,000× *g* for 10 min. The supernatant was poured into a new test tube and centrifuged again at 12,000× *g* for 10 min. Then, the supernatant was removed and the sediment was homogenized to a homogenous state in a washing medium (0.075 M sucrose, 0.225 M mannitol, 10 mM HEPES-KOH, pH 7.4) and centrifuged at 12,000× *g* for 10 min. The resulting sediment was collected and further homogenized with the washing medium. All procedures were carried out on ice in a cold room at +4 °C.

4.4. Calcium Retention Capacity

The Ca^{2+} retention capacity of mitochondria from the brain of rats in the norm and in experimental parkinsonism was determined using a Record-4 potentiometric system with a Ca^{2+}-selective electrode (NikoAnalit, Moscow, Russia). The incubation medium contained 150 mM KCl, 1 mM NaH_2PO_4, 10 μM EGTA, and 10 mM HEPES-KOH (pH 7.4). The concentration of the mitochondrial protein in a cuvette was 1 mg/mL. The substrates used were 5 mM malate and 5 mM potassium gluconate. $CaCl_2$ was added in fractions of 25 μM every 30 s. The calcium retention capacity was calculated as nmol Ca^{2+}/mL × mg protein.

4.5. Rate of H_2O_2 Formation in Brain Mitochondria

The generation of hydrogen peroxide by rat brain mitochondria was measured using a fluorimeter (Varian Medical Systems, Palo Alto, CA, USA) at an excitation of 570 nm and an emission of 585 nm. The reaction mixture contained 120 mM KCl, 5 mM KH_2PO_4, 10 mM HEPES-KOH, and 0.5 mM EGTA, pH 7.4. The hydrogen peroxide production was measured at 37 °C in the presence of 20 μM Amplex Red and 2 U/mL horseradish peroxidase. To avoid the impact of optical effects associated with mitochondrial swelling, the activity of mitochondria was measured using the two-wave mode of registration (572–600 nm) [35]. The concentration of mitochondria in the measurement medium was 0.2 mg/mL. The rate was expressed in nmol H_2O_2/min × mg protein.

4.6. Concentration of Lipid Peroxidation Products in Brain Mitochondria and Blood Serum

The concentration of lipid peroxidation products in rat brain mitochondria and blood serum was determined from the reaction of 250–275 µL of 5% SDS, 900 µL of 20% CH_3COONa, 300 µL of a 0.8% solution of thiobarbituric acid (TBA), and 50–25 µL serum or mitochondria. Eppendorf dishes with the reaction mixture were incubated for 1 h at 90 °C. Then, the liquid was centrifuged at 2000× *g* for 5 min. The product was a trimethine complex of characteristic pink color (λ_{max} = 532 nm). The measurement was performed on a spectrophotometer (Shimadzu Europa GmbH, Kyoto, Japan) at 532–650 nm. The results were expressed in nmol/min × mg protein.

4.7. Succinate Dehydrogenase and Lactate Dehydrogenase Activities in Lymphocytes

The activities of succinate dehydrogenase (SDH) in mitochondria in peripheral blood and lactate dehydrogenase (LDH) in the cytosol in lymphocytes in peripheral blood were determined by a biocytochemical method (license no. 2364868, Russia) from the reduction in nitro blue tetrazolium (NBT) to dark blue formazan [36]. Smears were prepared on a Blood Smear Preparation Device (Microscopy Vision, Dornbirn, Austria), dried for 30–60 min, fixed in a 60% solution of acetone buffered with 10 mM HEPES (Sigma, St. Louis, MO, USA) (pH 5.2–5.5) for 30 s, rinsed with distilled water, and dried. Then, smears were incubated at 37 °C for 1 h in a medium containing 125 mM KC1, 10 mM HEPES, and 1 mg/mL of NBT, pH 7.2 ± 0.05. The incubation medium was supplemented with 5 mM lactic acid, 5 mM malonic acid, and 0.5 mM NADH to determine the activity of LDH and with 5 mM succinic acid to determine the activity of SDH. Smears were washed with distilled water, dried, and stained in a 0.05% neutral red solution. Samples were examined at a magnification of 10 × 100. On each smear, 100 cells collected from the edge of the smear were examined. Samples were photographed using the program BioImages, which makes it possible to measure the mean area of a smear stained by diformazan (in μm^2) in a sample of 100 lymphocytes.

4.8. Transmission Electron Microscopy

After decapitation, pieces of the SN were taken from rats. The material was fixed immediately, by placing tissue samples in a 2.5% solution of glutaraldehyde in 0.1 M cacodylate buffer (pH 7.4). Postfixation was performed with 2% osmium tetroxide in 0.1 M cacodylate buffer (pH 7.4). Dehydration was carried out in alcohols of increasing concentration and acetone. Dehydrated samples were embedded in Epon 812 resin. Ultrathin sections 60–70 nm thick were made on an ultramicrotome (Leica EM UC7, Wetzlar, Germany). Sections were contrasted with 1% uranyl acetate and zinc citrate. Samples were scanned using a transmission electron microscope (JEOL JEM-100B, Tokyo, Japan). The total number of mitochondria (nMch) on microphotographs was calculated.

4.9. Statistical Analysis

All values are given as the means ± standard error of the means. Statistical analysis was performed by the paired *t*-test. Differences are significant at * $p < 0.05$ and ** $p < 0.01$. MS Excel, ImageJ (Java 1.6.0_12, RRID: SCR_003070, LOCI, University of Wisconsin, Madison, Wisconsin, USA), Origin 2016 (OriginLab, Northampton, MA, USA), and Prism GraphPad 7 (GraphPad Software, RRID: SCR_002798) softwares were used for data and statistical analysis.

5. Conclusions

Based on the data obtained, it was concluded that the natural metabolite uridine protects the rat body against impairments induced by the administration of neurotoxin 6-

OHDA and prevents negative consequences observed when modeling PD. The mechanism of the protective effect of uridine is mainly associated with the activation of the mitoK-ATP channel, which reduces the oxidative stress and the mitochondrial dysfunction in tissues. In this connection, uridine can be considered to be a metabolite that prevents the development of PD and can be used as a therapeutic means at its early stages.

Author Contributions: G.D.M. conceived the study and contributed to the discussion of the results and preparation of the manuscript; N.I.U., A.A.M., N.V.K. (Natalia V. Khmil), M.I.S., A.E.M. and V.F.K. were involved in conducting the experiments, in writing—original draft, and in performing statistical analysis. N.V.K. (Natalia V. Khunderyakova) and V.P.M. determined the mitochondrial enzymes of lymphocytes. N.V.B. determined the calcium retention capacity. L.L.P. performed the transmission electron microscopy. All authors have read and agreed to the published version of the manuscript.

Funding: The study was supported by the Russian Science Foundation (project no. 23-25-00441).

Institutional Review Board Statement: All procedures with animals were performed in accordance with experimental protocols approved by the Bioethics Committee of the Institute of Cell Biophysics. Experiments were carried out according to Act708n (23 August 2010) of the Russian Federation National Ministry of Public Health, which states the rules of laboratory practice for the care and use of laboratory animals, and the Council Directive 2010/63 EU of the European Parliament on the Protection of Animals Used for Scientific Purposes.

Informed Consent Statement: Not applicable.

Data Availability Statement: The data presented in this study are available on request from the corresponding author.

Conflicts of Interest: The authors declare no conflict of interest.

References

1. Balestrino, R.; Schapira, A.H.V. Parkinson disease. *Eur. J. Neurol.* **2020**, *27*, 27–42. [CrossRef] [PubMed]
2. Lee, T.K.; Yankee, E.L. A review on Parkinson's disease treatment. *Neuroimmunol. Neuroinflamm.* **2021**, *8*, 222–244. [CrossRef]
3. Rose, J.; Brian, C.; Woods, J.; Pappa, A.; Panayiotidis, M.I.; Powers, R.; Franco, R. Mitochondrial dysfunction in glial cells: Implications for neuronal homeostasis and survival. *Toxicology* **2017**, *391*, 109–115. [CrossRef] [PubMed]
4. Anik, M.I.; Mahmud, N.; Masud, A.A.; Khan, M.I.; Islam, M.N.; Uddin, S.; Hossain, M.K. Role of reactive oxygen species in aging and age-related diseases: A review. *ACS Appl. Bio Mater.* **2022**, *5*, 4028–4054. [CrossRef] [PubMed]
5. Gao, X.Y.; Yang, T.; Gu, Y.; Sun, X.H. Mitochondrial dysfunction in Parkinson's disease: From mechanistic insights to therapy. *Front. Aging Neurosci.* **2022**, *14*, 885500. [CrossRef]
6. Barata-Antunes, S.; Teixeira, F.G.; Mendes-Pinheiro, B.; Domingues, A.V.; Vilaça-Faria, H.; Marote, A.; Silva, D.; Sousa, R.A.; Salgado, A.J. Impact of aging on the 6-OHDA-induced rat model of Parkinson's disease. *Int. J. Mol. Sci.* **2020**, *21*, 3459. [CrossRef]
7. Burbulla, L.F.; Song, P.; Mazzulli, J.R.; Zampese, E.; Wong, Y.C.; Jeon, S.; Santos, D.P.; Blanz, J.; Obermaier, C.D.; Strojny, C.; et al. Dopamine oxidation mediates mitochondrial and lysosomal dysfunction in Parkinson's disease. *Science* **2017**, *357*, 1255–1261. [CrossRef]
8. Krylova, I.B.; Selina, E.N.; Bulion, V.V.; Rodionova, O.M.; Evdokimova, N.R.; Belosludtseva, N.V.; Shigaeva, M.I.; Mironova, G.D. Uridine treatment prevents myocardial injury in rat models of acute ischemia and ischemia/reperfusion by activating the mitochondrial ATP-dependent potassium channel. *Sci. Rep.* **2021**, *11*, 16999. [CrossRef]
9. Mironova, G.D.; Khrenov, M.O.; Talanov, E.Y.; Glushkova, O.V.; Parfenyuk, S.B.; Novoselova, T.V.; Lunin, S.M.; Belosludtseva, N.V.; Novoselova, E.G.; Lemasters, J.J. The role of mitochondrial KATP channel in anti-inflammatory effects of uridine in endotoxemic mice. *Arch. Biochem. Biophys.* **2018**, *654*, 70–76. [CrossRef]
10. Mosentsov, A.A.; Rozova, E.V.; Belosludtseva, N.V.; Mankovskaya, I.N.; Putiy, Y.V.; Karaban, I.N.; Mikheeva, I.B.; Mironova, G.D. Does the operation of mitochondrial ATP-dependent potassium channels affect the structural component of mitochondrial and endothelial dysfunctions in experimental parkinsonism? *Bull. Exp. Biol. Med.* **2021**, *170*, 431–435. [CrossRef]
11. Krylova, I.B.; Safonova, A.F.; Evdokimova, N.R. Correction of hypoxic state by metabolic precursors of endogenous activator of mitochondrial ATP-dependent K^+ channels. *Rev. Clin. Pharmacol. Drug Ther.* **2018**, *16*, 25–31. [CrossRef]
12. Belosludtsev, K.N.; Dubinin, M.V.; Belosludtseva, N.V.; Mironova, G.D. Mitochondrial Ca^{2+} transport: Mechanisms, molecular structures, and role in cells. *Biochem. (Mosc.)* **2019**, *84*, 593–607. [CrossRef] [PubMed]
13. Ludtmann, M.H.R.; Abramov, A.Y. Mitochondrial calcium imbalance in Parkinson's disease. *Neurosci. Lett.* **2018**, *663*, 86–90. [CrossRef] [PubMed]
14. Werner, C.; Doenst, T.; Schwarzer, M. Metabolic Pathways and Cycles. In *The Scientist's Guide to Cardiac Metabolism*, 1st ed.; Schwarzer, M., Doenst, T., Eds.; Elsevier Science: Amsterdam, The Netherlands, 2015; pp. 39–55. ISBN 978-012-802-394-5.

15. Zhu, D.; Wei, Y.; Yin, J.; Liu, D.; Ang, E.L.; Zhao, H.; Zhang, Y. A pathway for degradation of uracil to acetyl coenzyme A in *Bacillus megaterium*. *Appl. Environ. Microbiol.* **2020**, *86*, e02837-19. [CrossRef] [PubMed]
16. Silva, T.P.; Poli, A.; Hara, D.B.; Takahashi, R.N. Time course study of microglial and behavioral alterations induced by 6-hydroxydopamine in rats. *Neurosci. Lett.* **2016**, *622*, 83–87. [CrossRef] [PubMed]
17. Lu, Y.; Zhang, X.; Zhao, L.; Yang, C.; Pan, L.; Li, C.; Liu, K.; Bai, G.; Gao, H.; Yan, Z. Metabolic disturbances in the striatum and substantia nigra in the onset and progression of MPTP-induced parkinsonism model. *Front. Neurosci.* **2018**, *12*, 90. [CrossRef]
18. Guo, J.D.; Zhao, X.; Li, Y.; Li, G.R.; Liu, X.L. Damage to dopaminergic neurons by oxidative stress in Parkinson's disease (Review). *Int. J. Mol. Med.* **2018**, *41*, 1817–1825. [CrossRef]
19. Todorova, V.; Blokland, A. Mitochondria and synaptic plasticity in the mature and aging mervous system. *Curr. Neuropharmacol.* **2017**, *15*, 166–173. [CrossRef]
20. Soukup, S.F.; Vanhauwaert, R.; Verstreken, P. Parkinson's disease: Convergence on synaptic homeostasis. *EMBO J.* **2018**, *37*, e98960. [CrossRef] [PubMed]
21. Merino-Galán, L.; Jimenez-Urbieta, H.; Zamarbide, M.; Rodríguez-Chinchilla, T.; Belloso-Iguerategui, A.; Santamaria, E.; Fernández-Irigoyen, J.; Aiastui, A.; Doudnikoff, E.; Bézard, E.; et al. Striatal synaptic bioenergetic and autophagic decline in premotor experimental parkinsonism. *Brain* **2022**, *145*, 2092–2107. [CrossRef] [PubMed]
22. Sergeeva, T.N.; Sergeev, V.G.; Vezheeva, O.A. Electron-microscopy studies of rat brain neurodegenerative changes in the model of autoimmune synucleopathie. *Bull. Udmurt. Univ. Ser. Biology. Earth Sci.* **2011**, *4*, 113–118. (In Russian)
23. Papuć, E.; Rejdak, K. The role of myelin damage in Alzheimer's disease pathology. *Arch. Med. Sci.* **2020**, *16*, 345–351. [CrossRef] [PubMed]
24. Mironova, G.D.; Negoda, A.E.; Marinov, B.S.; Paucek, P.; Costa, A.D.; Grigoriev, S.M.; Skarga, Y.Y.; Garlid, K.D. Functional distinctions between the mitochondrial ATP-dependent K^+ channel (mitoKATP) and its inward rectifier subunit (mitoKIR). *J. Biol. Chem.* **2004**, *279*, 32562–32568. [CrossRef] [PubMed]
25. Schönfeld, P.; Gerke, S.; Bohnensack, R.; Wojtczak, L. Stimulation of potassium cycling in mitochondria by long-chain fatty acids. *Biochim. Biophys. Acta (BBA) Bioenerg.* **2003**, *1604*, 125–133. [CrossRef]
26. Garlid, K.D.; Paucek, P. Mitochondrial potassium transport: The K^+ cycle. *Biochim. Biophys. Acta (BBA) Bioenerg.* **2003**, *1606*, 23–41. [CrossRef]
27. Korshunov, S.S.; Skulachev, V.P.; Starkov, A.A. High protonic potential actuates a mechanism of production of reactive oxygen species in mitochondria. *FEBS Lett.* **1997**, *416*, 15–18. [CrossRef]
28. Shigaeva, M.; Gritsenko, E.; Murzaeva, S.; Gorbacheva, O.; Talanov, E.; Mironova, G. Age-related changes in the functioning of the mitochondrial potassium-transporting system. *Biofizika* **2010**, *55*, 1030–1037. [CrossRef]
29. Strickland, M.; Yacoubi-Loueslati, B.; Bouhaouala-Zahar, B.; Pender, S.L.F.; Larbi, A. Relationships between ion channels, mitochondrial functions and inflammation in human aging. *Front. Physiol.* **2019**, *10*, 158. [CrossRef]
30. Belosludtseva, N.V.; Starinets, V.S.; Mikheeva, I.B.; Belosludtsev, M.N.; Dubinin, M.V.; Mironova, G.D.; Belosludtsev, K.N. Effect of chronic treatment with uridine on cardiac mitochondrial dysfunction in the C57BL/6 mouse model of high-fat diet streptozotocin-induced diabetes. *Int. J. Mol. Sci.* **2022**, *23*, 10633. [CrossRef]
31. Skinner, O.S.; Blanco-Fernández, J.; Goodman, R.P.; Kawakami, A.; Shen, H.; Kemény, L.V.; Joesch-Cohen, L.; Rees, M.G.; Roth, J.A.; Fisher, D.E.; et al. Salvage of ribose from uridine or RNA supports glycolysis in nutrient-limited conditions. *Nat. Metab.* **2023**, *5*, 765–776. [CrossRef]
32. Tracey, T.J.; Steyn, F.J.; Wolvetang, E.J.; Ngo, S.T. Neuronal lipid metabolism: Multiple pathways driving functional outcomes in health and disease. *Front. Mol. Neurosci.* **2018**, *11*, 10. [CrossRef] [PubMed]
33. Torres, E.; Dunnett, S. 6-OHDA lesion models of Parkinson's disease in the rat. In *Animal Models of Movement Disorders*; Part of the Neuromethods Book Series; Humana Press: Totowa, NJ, USA, 2011; Volume 61, pp. 267–279. [CrossRef]
34. Paxinos, G.; Watson, C. *The Rat Brain in Stereotaxic Coordinates*, 6th ed.; Academic Press: Burlington, MA, USA, 2007; pp. 166–191, ISBN 978-008-047-515-8.
35. Ferranti, R.; da Silva, M.M.; Kowaltowski, A.J. Mitochondrial ATP-sensitive K^+ channel opening decreases reactive oxygen species generation. *FEBS Lett.* **2003**, *536*, 51–55. [CrossRef] [PubMed]
36. Kondrashova, M.; Zakharchenko, M.; Khunderyakova, N. Preservation of the in vivo state of mitochondrial network for ex vivo physiological study of mitochondria. *Int. J. Biochem. Cell Biol.* **2009**, *41*, 2036–2050. [CrossRef] [PubMed]

International Journal of *Molecular Sciences*

MDPI

Review

Mitochondrial Dysfunction as a Potential Mechanism Mediating Cardiac Comorbidities in Parkinson's Disease

Agustina Salis Torres [1,2], Ji-Eun Lee [1,3], Andrea Caporali [4], Robert K. Semple [4], Mathew H. Horrocks [2,5,†] and Vicky E. MacRae [1,*,†]

1 The Roslin Institute and R(D)SVS, University of Edinburgh, Easter Bush, Midlothian EH25 9RH, UK; asalist@ed.ac.uk (A.S.T.); jlee20@ed.ac.uk (J.-E.L.)
2 EaStCHEM School of Chemistry, University of Edinburgh, Edinburgh EH9 3FJ, UK; mathew.horrocks@ed.ac.uk
3 IRR Chemistry Hub, Institute for Regeneration and Repair, University of Edinburgh, Edinburgh EH16 4UU, UK
4 Centre for Cardiovascular Science, Queen's Medical Research Institute (QMRI), The University of Edinburgh, 47 Little France Crescent, Edinburgh EH16 4TJ, UK; acaporal@exseed.ed.ac.uk (A.C.); rsemple@exseed.ed.ac.uk (R.K.S.)
5 MRC Human Genetics Unit, Institute for Genetics and Molecular Medicine, The University of Edinburgh, Edinburgh EH4 2XU, UK
* Correspondence: vicky.macrae@roslin.ed.ac.uk
† These authors contributed equally to this work.

Abstract: Individuals diagnosed with Parkinson's disease (PD) often exhibit heightened susceptibility to cardiac dysfunction, reflecting a complex interaction between these conditions. The involvement of mitochondrial dysfunction in the development and progression of cardiac dysfunction and PD suggests a plausible commonality in some aspects of their molecular pathogenesis, potentially contributing to the prevalence of cardiac issues in PD. Mitochondria, crucial organelles responsible for energy production and cellular regulation, play important roles in tissues with high energetic demands, such as neurons and cardiac cells. Mitochondrial dysfunction can occur in different and non-mutually exclusive ways; however, some mechanisms include alterations in mitochondrial dynamics, compromised bioenergetics, biogenesis deficits, oxidative stress, impaired mitophagy, and disrupted calcium balance. It is plausible that these factors contribute to the increased prevalence of cardiac dysfunction in PD, suggesting mitochondrial health as a potential target for therapeutic intervention. This review provides an overview of the physiological mechanisms underlying mitochondrial quality control systems. It summarises the diverse roles of mitochondria in brain and heart function, highlighting shared pathways potentially exhibiting dysfunction and driving cardiac comorbidities in PD. By highlighting strategies to mitigate dysfunction associated with mitochondrial impairment in cardiac and neural tissues, our review aims to provide new perspectives on therapeutic approaches.

Keywords: mitochondria; mitochondrial dysfunction; Parkinson's disease (PD); cardiac dysfunction

1. Introduction

Parkinson's disease (PD) is the second most common neurodegenerative disorder, impacting 1% to 3% of individuals aged over 65. With longer life expectancies, both the prevalence and impact of PD are growing globally [1]. Advanced aging is also related with the increasing prevalence of cardiac dysfunction and, therefore, it is reasonable to explore potential connections between PD and cardiac issues [2]. Individuals with PD exhibit a heightened susceptibility to cardiac dysfunction, suggesting a complex interplay between the two conditions [1,3–7]. Cardiovascular disorders have been identified in approximately 80% of PD patients [8]. Several studies have highlighted the association between PD and increased risks of myocardial infarction, congestive failure and all-cause mortality in PD patients [1,9]. A case-control study with a three-year follow-up observed a significantly increased risk of acute myocardial infarction in PD patients [9]. Additionally, PD patients may develop cardiomyopathies, arrhythmias, or sudden cardiac death, though the incidence is debated [10]. The mechanisms mediating these associations, whether direct or indirect, remain unproven. However, aberrant protein aggregation, clearance disruption, oxidative stress, neuroinflammation, and mitochondrial damage have all been suggested as potential contributors [1]. Notably, mitochondrial dysfunction and shared oxidative mechanisms have been proposed as candidate factors mediating the heightened risk of cardiac dysfunction in PD [3].

Given the extensive evidence of mitochondrial dysfunction in the development and progression of both cardiac dysfunction and PD, it is plausible that these two conditions share common underlying pathophysiological mechanisms, thereby potentially mediating cardiac comorbidities in PD patients. Mitochondria serve as dynamic cellular powerhouses, centrally involved in adenosine triphosphate (ATP) generation through oxidative phosphorylation (OXPHOS) [11]. This functionality impacts essential cellular processes, such as metabolism, redox balance, calcium (Ca^{2+}) regulation, apoptosis and signal transduction, forming an interconnected network [12]. Compromised mitochondria lead to reduced energy production, altered cellular metabolism and disrupted regulation of reactive oxygen species (ROS). These changes collectively contribute to cellular damage and dysfunction, initiating a pathophysiological cascade associated with both cardiac dysfunction and PD [13–15]. Recognising this overlap suggests a promising avenue for integrated treatment strategies targeting the common underlying mechanisms of both conditions. By exploring these shared pathways, this review aims to address research gaps and propose integrated therapeutic strategies focusing on mitochondrial dysfunction to manage both cardiac comorbidities in PD patients as well as the management of PD itself, emphasising the need for future investigations.

1.1. *Parkinson's Disease*

Parkinson's disease (PD) is a prevalent neurodegenerative disorder affecting both motor and cognitive functions [16]. Clinical features of PD include bradykinesia, resting tremor, rigidity and later-stage postural instability [17]. Influenced by age, PD prevalence ranges from 0.5–1% in individuals aged 59–69 to 1–3% in those over 80. It is anticipated that by 2030, there will be an increase of over 30% in PD prevalence due to demographic aging [17]. The intricate interplay of genetic and environmental factors contributes to PD development, with 10–15% of cases exhibiting familial links and approximately 5% showing Mendelian inheritance patterns [18]. Polygenic risk factors contribute to the disorder, with 23 'PARK' genes identified [17]. Well-established PD genes linked to mitochondrial dysfunction include autosomal dominant forms (e.g., synuclein-alpha (SNCA) and leucine-rich repeat kinase 2 (LRRK2) mutations) and autosomal recessive forms (e.g., Parkin RBR E3 Ubiquitin Protein Ligase (PRKN), PTEN-induced kinase 1 (PINK1) and ATPase cation Transporting 13A2 (ATP13A2) mutations) [17–19]. Environmental factors thought to influence the development of PD include smoking, caffeine consumption and pesticide exposure [20–22]. PD's primary cause is the loss of dopaminergic (DA) neurons in the substantia nigra pars compacta (SNpc), leading to motor symptoms and reduced dopamine levels [23]. The complexity of PD arises from mechanisms including protein misfolding, aggregation, mitochondrial dysfunction, oxidative stress, energy depletion, excitotoxicity and neuroinflammation [24–27]. Among these, protein misfolding and accumulation within intracellular spaces stand out as prominent hypotheses in PD aetiology [28]. PD exhibits the presence of misfolded amyloid proteins within the intracellular spaces of SNpc neurons, forming structures known as Lewy bodies. These Lewy bodies encapsulate multiple misfolded amyloid proteins, including α-synuclein, phosphorylated tau (p-tau) and amyloid beta protein (Aβ) [28].

Mitochondria's dynamic properties are crucial in neurons due to their substantial energy demands [29]. Mitochondrial dysfunction significantly contributes to PD progression, resulting in heightened oxidative stress and influencing various cellular pathways

(Figure 1) [25]. In pathology, α-synuclein undergoes oligomerisation at mitochondrial membranes [30]. These α-synuclein oligomers disrupt the normal functioning of ATP synthase, leading to mitochondrial dysfunction characterised by impaired respiration and the opening of the permeability transition pore (PTP), ultimately leading to neuronal toxicity and cell death [31,32]. This dysfunction further impairs mitophagy, compromises trafficking, alters mitochondrial dynamics and disrupts calcium ion (Ca^{2+}) balance [33]. The interaction of α-synuclein oligomers with neuronal membranes disrupts calcium signalling through increased lipid permeability and induction of ion channel formation [34,35]. Therefore, addressing mitochondrial dysfunction in PD presents an attractive avenue for therapeutic interventions in PD management.

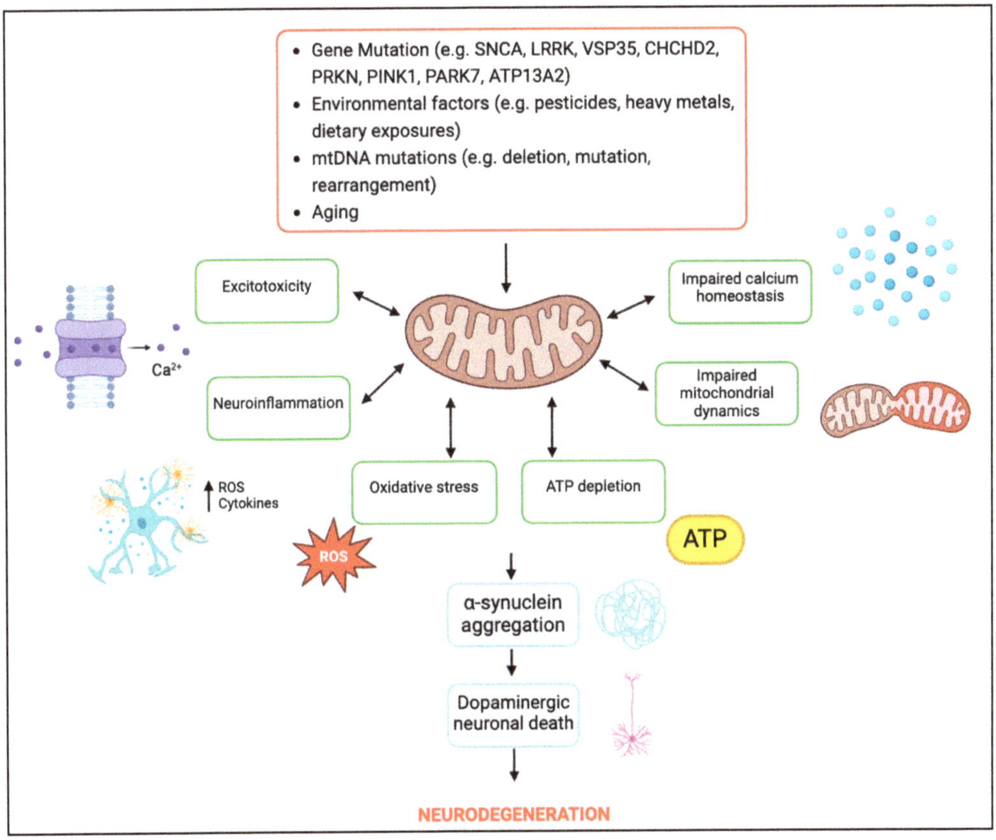

Figure 1. Mitochondrial Dysfunction in Parkinson's Disease (PD). Various factors, including genetic susceptibility, environmental influences, mtDNA mutations and aging, have been implicated in the onset of Parkinson's disease. Notably, abnormalities in mitochondrial metabolic function, morphology and homeostasis are observed, which contribute to the formation of α-synuclein aggregates and the subsequent death of dopaminergic (DA) neurons, thereby driving the progression of neurodegeneration. SNCA, Synuclein Alpha; LRRK, leucine-rich repeat kinase 2; VSP35, Vacuolar protein sorting ortholog 35; CHCHD2, Coiled-coil-helix-coiled-coil-helix domain containing 2; PINK1, PTEN-induced kinase 1; PARK7, Parkinson disease protein 7; PRKN, parkin RBR E3 ubiquitin protein ligase; ATP13A2, ATPase Cation Transporting 13A2; mtDNA, mitochondrial DNA; Ca^{2+}, calcium ions; ROS, Reactive Oxygen Species; ATP, Adenosine triphosphate.

1.2. Cardiac Dysfunction

Cardiac dysfunction is a major global health concern significantly contributing to morbidity and mortality, particularly in the context of advanced aging. Despite significant progress in the prevention and treatment of cardiovascular diseases (CVD), they remain the leading cause of death worldwide, accounting for approximately 17.9 million deaths in 2019 [36]. The global incidence of these diseases has nearly doubled between 1993 and 2019, with projections indicating a continued rise until 2024 [37]. A significant portion of cardiac dysfunction cases is attributed to coronary heart disease (CHD). CHD involves the narrowing or blockage of coronary arteries due to plaque accumulation, leading to reduced blood flow and contributing to conditions such as angina, myocardial infarction, and heart failure [38]. Myocardial infarction, or heart attack, occurs when blood flow to a part of the heart muscle is severely reduced or completely blocked, causing tissue damage or death due to lack of oxygen [39]. Heart failure is characterised by the heart's inability to pump blood efficiently, resulting in inadequate circulation to meet the body's needs [40]. Despite advancements in treatment and management strategies, these conditions continue to pose significant health challenges globally.

The role of mitochondria in cardiac function is gaining attention as a potential therapeutic avenue due to its involvement in several cardiac-related pathogenesis. Established risk factors such as hypertension, insulin resistance, diabetes and obesity have been associated with disruptions in cardiac mitochondrial dynamics, mitophagy irregularities and mitochondrial metabolic dysfunction [41–49]. These are also established risk factors in PD [50–53]. Studies highlight the involvement of cardiac myocardial mitochondrial imbalances in cardiac dysfunction [54,55]. Additionally, aberrant mitochondrial morphology and dysfunction are recognised as significant indicators of heart failure [56]. This highlights a potential role of mitochondria in cellular processes related to the progression of cardiac dysfunction and PD.

2. The Many Faces of Mitochondrial Function

Mitochondria are dynamic cellular structures with a central role in cellular function, primarily serving as the major generators of the chemical energy necessary to fuel the cell's biochemical reactions [57]. However, their functions extend beyond energy production, encompassing areas such as cellular metabolism, calcium ion (Ca^{2+}) regulation, redox signalling, cellular homeostasis and adaptation to stress (Figure 2) [58–60]. Their multifaceted functions make mitochondria indispensable components within tissues like the brain and heart, where they play essential roles in maintaining physiological integrity. Both organs, characterised by high metabolic demands, depend on a consistent supply of nutrients to support their functions. The heart maintains a continuous rhythmic beating, and a subset of neurons in the brain remains active at all times, preventing these tissues from entering a state of complete rest [61–63]. Additionally, they both undergo rapid shifts in function, as cardiac workload can vary significantly during physical exercise, and individual neurons undergo swift alterations in action potential during specific cognitive tasks [61,64,65]. As a result, mitochondrial dysfunction in these tissues can lead to significant consequences, contributing to the development of neurodegenerative and heart diseases. Here we explore the various roles mitochondria play in both the brain and heart.

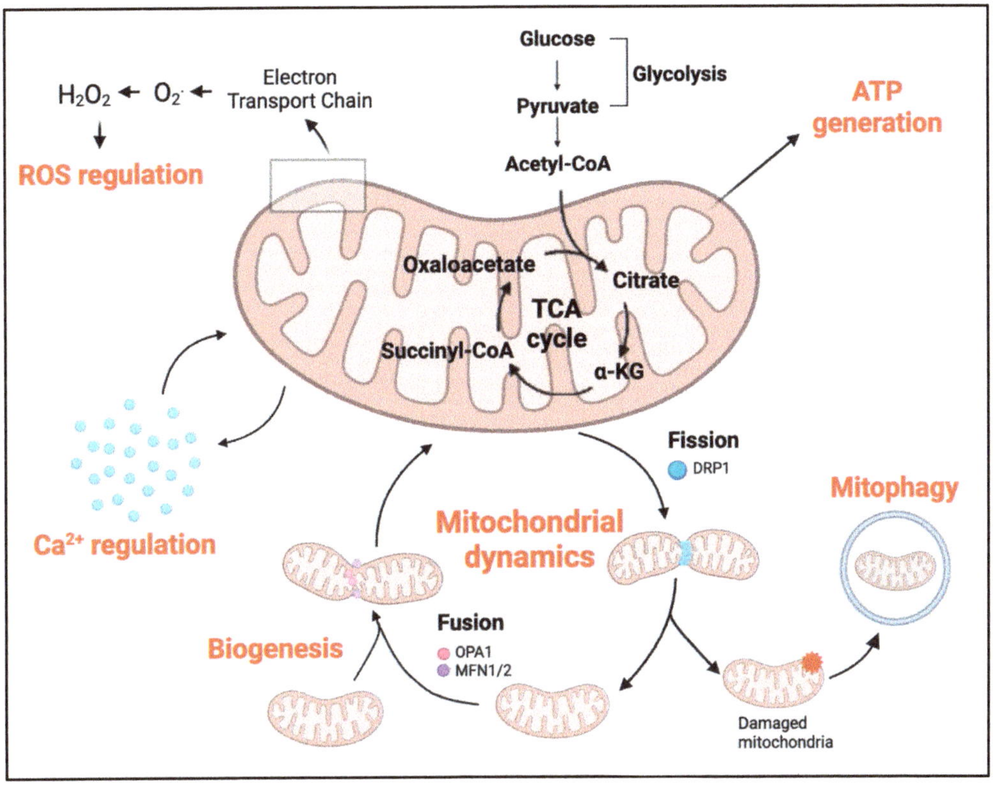

Figure 2. Mitochondrial function. Mitochondria are dynamic organelles crucial for energy generation, highlighted through oxidative phosphorylation. Their functionality is regulated by dynamic processes including fusion, enabling exchange of contents between mitochondria, and fission, facilitating organelle division and distribution. Mitochondrial biogenesis ensures the replenishment of these organelles, balancing turnover and maintenance. Mitophagy removes dysfunctional mitochondria, safeguarding cellular integrity. Regulation of ROS production within mitochondria is essential for redox homeostasis and physiological processes such as cell differentiation, senescence, signal transduction and adaptation to hypoxic conditions. Calcium homeostasis modulates signalling pathways and influences cellular functions. Ca^{2+}, calcium ion; ATP, Adenosine triphosphate; DRP1, Dynamin-related Protein 1; OPA1, optic Atrophy 1; MFN1/2, Mitofusin-1/2; H_2O_2, hydrogen peroxide; O_2, dioxygen; TCA, tricarboxylic acid; α-KG, alpha-ketoglutarate; CoA, coenzyme A.

2.1. The Role of Mitochondria in Brain Function

Despite constituting just 2% of the body's weight, the human brain exerts a substantial energy demand, accounting for 20% of the body's total energy consumption [66,67]. The heightened metabolic expenditure, essential for fundamental neural functions within the central nervous system, is primarily attributed to the intricate morphology of neurons, finely regulated ion gradients and ceaseless activity across billions of synapses [68]. Mitochondrial ATP production is essential for various synaptic processes, including the operation of ion channels, pumps, receptors and the release of neurotransmitters through Ca^{2+}-induced fusion of synaptic vesicles with the presynaptic membrane (exocytosis), as well as the subsequent recycling of neurotransmitters [69–71]. During an action potential, axonal terminals expend a significant amount of ATP—approximately 4.5×10^8 ATP molecules, compared to 3×10^6 ATP for resting potentials and basic cellular maintenance [72]. The majority of neuronal ATP is consumed by membrane pumps like the sodium-potassium pump (Na^+/K^+ ATPase) and Ca^{2+} ATPase, accounting for 55% of total production to maintain the resting potential [73]. Synaptic vesicle recycling also demands substantial energy, involving ATP for both glutamate vesicle events and restoring ionic gradient within neuronal terminals [67,74]. Most of the ATP in these cells is primarily generated through oxygen-dependent metabolism within the mitochondria, meeting the brain's energy demand through the oxidation of glucose via glycolysis and OXPHOS to produce ATP [61,70,71]. In cases of PD, a systemic deficiency in complex I of the ETC leads to ATP depletion, a characteristic observed in many patients with the disease [23]. This was first discovered in the early 1980s when individuals injected themselves with 1-methyl-4-phenyl-1,2,3,6-tetrahydropyridine (MPTP), leading to the accumulation of its toxic metabolite, 1-methyl-4-phenylpyridinium (MPP^+), in the mitochondria, ultimately causing DA neuronal death by reducing ATP synthesis and increasing ROS production [23,75].

Beyond ATP synthesis, mitochondria also play a critical role in ROS regulation and Ca^{2+} signalling, requiring their mutual interplay for fine-tuning modulation [76]. ROS play a crucial role in both the induction of long-term potentiation (LTP) through redox modifications of target proteins and the regulation of synaptic plasticity-related signalling molecules, receptors and channels [77,78]. For example, ROS bidirectionally modulates Ca^{2+} handling, including cytoplasmic influx, buffering and release from intracellular stores [79]. The precise regulation of ROS production is crucial for normal neuronal function, as conditions that induce oxidative/nitrosative stress can lead to excessive Ca^{2+} release, potentially triggering pathological responses and neuronal cell death, which has been shown to be a significant contributor to DA neuronal loss in PD [80]. In terms of Ca^{2+} regulation, neuronal mitochondria are essential for maintaining intracellular Ca^{2+} homeostasis, either by directly buffering Ca^{2+} or by providing the ATP necessary for the activity of the plasma membrane Ca^{2+} ATPase, effectively modulating cytosolic Ca^{2+} responses during neuronal excitation [69,81]. As a result, mitochondria possess a remarkable capacity to influence numerous Ca^{2+}-dependent functions within neurons [81]. In PD, DA neurons in the substantia nigra are susceptible to Ca^{2+}-overload via essential voltage-gated L-type channels that regulate their pace making activity [82]. This in turn leads to an increase in oxidative stress, further damaging DA neurons and contributing to the progression of PD [83]. Other factors, such as increased mitophagy, increased mitochondrial DNA (mtDNA) damage and defective mitochondrial biogenesis/dynamics, further contribute to the progression of PD [75].

2.2. The Role of Mitochondria in Cardiac Function

In the heart, mitochondria play a crucial role in meeting the high-energy demands of cardiomyocytes, the primary cell type found in the heart responsible for generating contractile force [84,85]. Mitochondria occupy roughly one-third of the volume within these cells [86]. Moreover, they are responsible for generating over 95% of the ATP in adult cardiomyocytes, which is crucial for facilitating muscle contraction and ion transport [87,88]. The continuous and rapid synthesis of ATP is crucial to sustain this heightened energy flux. In failing human myocardium and in the heart of animal models of severe heart failure, myocardial ATP levels are 30% lower than in healthy myocardium [89,90]. Remarkably, there is a significant correlation between the ATP content in myocardial tissue and in vivo contractile function in human biopsies of failing hearts [91]. Under normal conditions, mitochondria efficiently convert different substrates, including fatty acids, glucose and ketone bodies, into ATP (Figure 3) [92]. Fatty acids are the preferred substrate, accounting for 60–90% of the myocardium's energy supply [92]. They are metabolised through fatty acid β-oxidation (FAO) within the mitochondria, leading to the generation of acetyl-CoA, which enters the tricarboxylic acid (TCA) cycle, subsequently producing FADH2 and NADH [87]. These electron carriers are crucial for fuelling the electron transport chain (ETC), facilitating ATP synthesis and consuming oxygen [87]. Under conditions of reduced FAO, such as during stress, glucose becomes the primary energy source instead [93]. Glucose undergoes glycolysis in the cytosol, resulting in the production of pyruvate, which is then converted to acetyl-CoA, subsequently entering the TCA cycle and ETC [87]. In cases of heart failure, there is a shift in the utilisation of these mitochondrial energy substrates [94]. Research has shown that hypertrophied hearts have lower rates of fatty acid oxidation and higher rates of glycolysis compared to healthy hearts, indicating a gradual shift in substrate utilisation from fatty acid to glucose consumption [95].

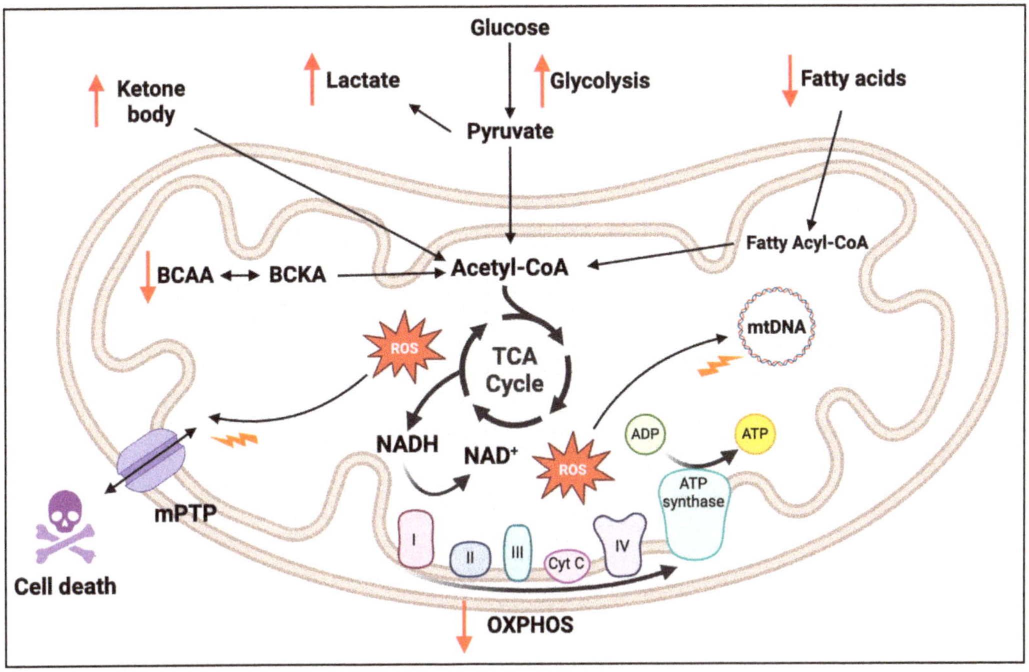

Figure 3. Cardiac metabolism in failing heart. In heart failure, metabolic shifts include decreased fatty acid oxidation, enhanced glycolysis, reduced glucose oxidation, increased lactate, increased ketone oxidation, decreased branched-chain amino acid oxidation and decreased oxidative phosphorylation. The abnormal substrate utilisation results in an increased production of radical oxygen species which can damage mitochondrial DNA and induce cell death by triggering the opening of the mitochondrial permeability transition pore. BCAA, branched-chain amino acids; BCKA, branched-chain keto acid; OXPHOS, oxidative phosphorylation; mPTP, mitochondrial permeability transition pore; NADH, nicotinamide adenine dinucleotide, NAD^+, Nicotinamide adenine dinucleotide; CoA, coenzyme A; ATP, Adenosine triphosphate; ADP, Adenosine diphosphate; Cyt C, Cytochrome C.

Beyond ATP production, mitochondria also play important roles in regulating Ca^{2+} homeostasis, redox status and lipid synthesis [87]. Particularly, mitochondrial Ca^{2+} plays a pivotal role in regulating cardiac excitation–contraction coupling (ECC) [96]. This regulatory function encompasses two primary aspects: firstly, mitochondrial Ca^{2+} is involved in shaping cytosolic Ca^{2+} signals by effectively absorbing and buffering Ca^{2+} ions, contributing to the fine-tuning of contractile activity within cardiac myocytes [96]. Secondly, mitochondrial Ca^{2+} uptake influences cellular metabolism and the necessary energy supply for muscle contractions, facilitated through a calcium-dependent mechanism extending to key enzymes within the TCA cycle, as well as various components of the ETC and the mitochondrial F1/F0 ATP synthase [96]. In cases of heart failure, energy deficiency becomes intertwined with dysregulated Ca^{2+} transport, resulting in excitation–contraction uncoupling and impaired cardiac function [94]. Redox signalling also holds substantial significance within cardiac ECC. The oxidative modification of specific proteins orchestrates various aspects of the cardiac ECC machinery, influencing processes such as sarcoplasmic reticulum (SR) Ca^{2+} release and uptake, ionic fluxes and contractile function [97]. Additionally, redox signalling extends its influence to other critical physiological processes, including cell differentiation and the maintenance of homeostatic and stress response pathways, such as adaptation to hypoxia/ischemia [98]. In pathological conditions, an excessive accumulation of mitochondrial reactive oxygen species (mROS) can lead to unfavourable cardiac remodelling and fibrosis [98]. Research suggests an excessive amount of mROS to promote sudden cardiac death and cause proteome remodelling [99]. Moreover, the generation of mROS during the early stages of reperfusion has been implicated in the promotion of myocardial ischemia/reperfusion (I/R) injury [94]. In essence, mitochondria hold a critical role in maintaining overall health, and any dysregulation in these cellular structures can significantly contribute to the development of heart failure.

3. Mitochondrial Dysfunction

3.1. Bioenergetic Deficits

Mitochondrial ATP production is the main energy source for intracellular metabolic pathways [100]. This process involves oxidative phosphorylation (OXPHOS), which comprises two closely interlinked components: (1) the electron transport chain (ETC), located within the inner mitochondrial membrane, and (2) chemiosmosis coupling, driven by an electrochemical gradient [101]. During OXPHOS, electrons derived from substrates like glucose and fatty acids traverse the ETC, simultaneously pumping protons across the mitochondrial membrane. Protons subsequently flow back through ATP synthase, converting adenosine diphosphate (ADP) and inorganic phosphate (Pi) into ATP [102].

Bioenergetic disruptions, primarily associated with mitochondrial dysfunction, are well-documented in cardiac pathophysiology and conditions like PD (Table 1) [62,103,104]. This imbalance in mitochondrial bioenergetics can result in impaired basic functions, affecting oxygen and substrate availability, thus altering metabolism and causing inefficient energy utilisation [103,105]. For instance, during ischemia, compromised OXPHOS and a shift to anaerobic glycolysis lead to reduced intracellular ATP levels, altered pH and lactic acid accumulation [106]. In hypertrophic and failing hearts, initial pressure overload induces a shift from fatty acid to glucose oxidation. This shift leads to a significant decrease in ATP concentration and alterations in substrate utilisation, contributing to a progressive myocardial degeneration [105,106].

Altered metabolism and energy utilisation is also a hallmark in PD. Evidence shows that neurons adopt glycolysis as a low-efficient compensatory mode of energy production in response to mitochondrial dysfunction [103]. A Drosophila PD model based on the inactivation of the DJ-1beta gene (ortholog of human PARK7), showed protein metabolism alterations and a shift from the TCA to glycolytic pathway to obtain ATP, together with an increase in the expression of some urea cycle enzymes [107]. Furthermore, during stress, astrocytes increase lactate production through glycolysis to support neurons. This bioenergetic shift between lactate and glucose levels can alter mitochondrial function and redox pairs that control bioenergetic-pathway feedback, potentially leading to further mitochondrial damage, glutamate toxicity and eventual neurodegeneration [108]. Studies also suggest that increased microglial activation, which display metabolic shifts from oxidative phosphorylation to glycolysis, contributes to amyloid deposition in PD [109,110].

Damage of mitochondrial electron transport chain (ETC) affecting complex I (NADH:ubiquinone oxidoreductase), and a reduction of maximal OXPHOS capacity have been widely reported in cardiac and PD pathogenesis [103,106]. This dysfunction in complex I translates into an increased ROS production and a decrease in energy supply, contributing to disease progression [106,111]. Reduced complex I activity has been identified in the SNpc of PD patients and human failing myocardium [106,112–114]. Recent research utilising a mouse knockout model demonstrated that complex I disruption can induce PD [108]. Similarly, defects in single subunits of mitochondrial complex I have been associated with cardiac hypertrophy, ischemia/reperfusion (I/R) injury, as well as diabetic complications and stroke in pre-clinical studies [115]. Mitochondrial bioenergetic deficiencies in the failing heart not only diminish ATP production but also impede high-energy phosphotransferase system activity, including creatine kinase and adenylate kinase [116,117]. This impedes the efficient transfer of ATP to myofibrils, compromising heart contractility. Additionally, reduced myofibrillar ATPase activity leads to decreased energy utilisation efficiency [116].

Antioxidants have become increasingly recognised as promising therapeutic avenues to counter bioenergetic deficits. Coenzyme Q10, an essential antioxidant and integral component of the ETC known to be depleted in PD, has shown promise in reversing complex I deficits observed in PD patient-derived cultures [106,118,119]. Additionally, in preclinical PD models, it demonstrated efficacy in mitigating the loss of dopamine neurons [120]. Similarly, in a canine model of isoproterenol-induced heart failure, coenzyme Q10 supplementation improves left ventricular function [121]. Alpha-lipoic acid (ALA) has also emerged as a powerful antioxidant and cofactor for mitochondrial enzymes involved in energy production. ALA alleviates motor deficits in PD models by regulating iron metabolism, reducing ROS accumulation and protecting mitochondria, ultimately preventing ferroptosis, a type of iron-driven cell death, through the silent information regulator 1/nuclear factor erythroid 2-related factor 2 (SIRT1/NRF2) signalling pathway [122]. Furthermore, ALA exhibits potent antioxidant properties and has potential protective effects against risk factors associated with cardiac dysfunction, including modulation of blood lipids, protection against low-density lipoprotein (LDL) oxidation and regulation of hypertension [123]. This convergence highlights potential mitochondrial-level interplay and suggests shared underlying mechanisms or vulnerabilities related to mitochondrial bioenergetic deficits in both conditions.

Table 1. Summary of mitochondrial pathways disrupted in cardiac dysfunction and Parkinson's disease, and potential common mechanisms.

Pathway	Cardiac Dysfunction	Parkinson's Disease	Common Mechanisms	References
Bioenergetic Pathways	• Impaired OXPHOS leads to reduced ATP production, affecting cardiac contractility. • Ischemia shifts metabolism from fatty acid oxidation to glucose metabolism, reducing ATP and increasing myocardial stress.	• Impaired OXPHOS forces reliance on less efficient glycolysis for energy, leading to energy deficits and neuronal dysfunction. • Increased lactate and metabolic stress contribute to neurodegeneration.	• Both exhibit a shift from OXPHOS to glycolysis under stress, reducing ATP production and energy efficiency	[103,106,124,125]
Electron Transport Chain (ETC)	• Dysfunction in complexes I-V reduces ATP, increases ROS, and impaired mitochondrial membrane potential, causing oxidative stress and affecting energy supply for cardiac function. • Contributes to heart failure, arrhythmias, and decreased cardiac output.	• Dysfunction, particularly in Complex I, impairs NADH oxidation, reducing ATP production, increasing ROS and causing oxidative damage. • Contributes to neuronal death and progressive loss of dopamine-producing neurons.	• ETC dysfunction reduces ATP production and increases ROS, causing oxidative stress and cellular damage in both conditions.	[106,126,127]
ROS Production	• Exacerbated by impaired ETC function and increased electron leakage. • Activation of NADPH oxidase and inflammatory pathways further contributes to the heightened ROS levels, promoting oxidative stress and cellular damage in the heart. • Oxidative damage to lipids, proteins, and DNA, as well as cellular apoptosis, necrosis and fibrosis.	• Increased ROS from mitochondrial dysfunction and dopamine dysregulation. • Inflammatory responses triggered by glial activation in response to neuronal damage contribute to ROS production, amplifying oxidative stress.	• Increased ROS production causes oxidative stress and cellular damage in both conditions.	[128,129]

Table 1. *Cont.*

Pathway	Cardiac Dysfunction	Parkinson's Disease	Common Mechanisms	References
Mitochondrial Dynamics	• Reduced MFN1/MFN2 and dysregulated DRP1 lead to mitochondrial fragmentation and dysfunction. • Reduced mitochondrial connectivity and compromised distribution of mitochondrial components. • Impaired mitochondrial quality control, reduced ATP production, increased oxidative stress, contributing to cardiac dysfunction and myocardial damage.	• Impaired MFN1/MFN2 and excessive DRP1 activity lead to fragmentation and neuronal death.	• Dysregulation in dynamics impairs energy production and increases oxidative stress in both.	[130,131]
Mitochondrial Biogenesis	• Decreased PGC-1α and TFAM expression reduce mitochondrial DNA replication and ATP production. • Leads to compromised cardiomyocyte energy supply. • Mutations or loss of function in PINK1/PRKN.	• Disrupted PGC-1α and PARIS signalling impair biogenesis and function. • Mutations or loss of function in PINK1/PRKN reduce mitochondrial number and function.	• Both involve dysregulation of PGC-1α and PINK1/PRKN, reducing biogenesis and increasing stress.	[132–134]
Mitochondrial Ca^{2+} Regulation	• Disrupted calcium uptake/efflux through the mitochondrial calcium uniporter (MCU) and sodium-calcium exchanger (NCLX), respectively. • Dysregulated ER-mitochondria transfer through voltage-dependent anion channel (VDAC). • Leads to opening of mPTP and loss of membrane potential, oxidative stress, impaired metabolism, and cell death.	• NCLX inhibition in familial forms of PD with PINK1 deficiency impairs calcium efflux, leading to calcium overload. This triggers the opening of the mPTP. • α-synuclein has been suggested to interact with mitochondrial calcium regulatory proteins, disrupting calcium homeostasis.	• Dysregulated calcium handling affects mitochondrial function and cell survival in both diseases.	[31,135]
Mitophagy	• Impaired PINK1/PRKN pathways reduce degradation of dysfunctional mitochondria. • Leads to oxidative stress and compromised cardiac function.	• Dysfunction in PINK1/PRKN impairs clearance, leading to neurodegeneration and inflammation. • Reduced lysosomal clearance of dysfunctional mitochondria exacerbates energy deficits and promotes accumulation of α-synuclein aggregates. • Increased vulnerability to toxins and oxidative stress, triggering neuroinflammation and glial activation.	• Dysfunctional mitophagy pathways cause accumulation of damaged mitochondria, increasing stress.	[136–139]
Lipid Peroxidation (LPO)	• Increased oxidative stress and LPO products, leading to impairment of mitochondrial respiration, cardiac ischaemia–reperfusion injury and diabetes.	• LPO products by oxidative stress induce the generation, accumulation, and modification of α-synuclein in dopaminergic neurons resulting in mitochondrial dysfunction.	• Increased oxidative stress and LPO products, especially related to promoting mitochondrial dysfunction.	[140,141]

OXPHOS, oxidative phosphorylation; ATP, Adenosine triphosphate; ROS, reactive oxygen species; NADH, nicotinamide adenine dinucleotide; ETC, electron transport chain; NADPH, nicotinamide adenine dinucleotide phosphate hydrogen; MFN1/2, Mitofusin-1/2; DRP1, Dynamin-related Protein; PGC-1α, Peroxisome proliferator-activated receptor-gamma coactivator; TFAM, mitochondrial transcription factor A; PINK1, PTEN-induced kinase 1; PRKN, parkin RBR E3 ubiquitin protein ligase; Ca^{2+}, calcium ions; mPTP, mitochondrial permeability transition pore; PD, Parkinson's disease; LPO, lipid peroxidation.

3.2. Mitochondrial DNA Defects

Mitochondria possess their own circular, double-stranded DNA, distinct from other cellular organelles [142]. The encoded components in mitochondrial DNA (mtDNA) are essential for cellular energy-generation, and defects in mtDNA can impair mitochondrial function [143]. The impact of mtDNA mutations on mitochondrial energy production deficiency is particularly pronounced in organs and tissues with inherent high energy demands, such as cardiac and neuronal tissues. Within these tissues, mtDNA mutations have the potential to induce myopathy, atrophy and progressive degeneration processes [13].

For instance, mtDNA defects play an important role in the development and progression of myocardial remodelling and failure after myocardial infarction (MI), at least in part, by inducing mitochondrial oxidative stress and damage to mtDNA, which leads to a decrease in mtDNA copy number, number of mitochondrial RNA (mtRNA) transcripts and oxidative capacity [144]. The pathways by which mtDNA mutations impact cardiac function involve a decrease in tRNAs and protein synthesis, including those vital for mitochondrial OXPHOS, leading to an increase in ROS production, subsequent mitochondrial oxidative stress and eventual apoptosis [145].

Similarly, studies have found brain region-specific accumulation of mtDNA damage in PD neuronal culture and animal models, as well as in human post-mortem brain tissue [146]. While mtDNA sequencing did not identify specific pathogenic mutations as a distinctive PD signature, an age-related rise in mtDNA deletions linked to respiratory chain dysfunction was observed in dopaminergic (DA) neurons of the substantial nigra [147]. These deletions were more prevalent in PD patients compared to age-matched controls, particularly in the substantia nigra, indicating a potential association with PD development [147].

Due to the proximity of mtDNA to the electron transport chain within mitochondria, it is more susceptible to damage from free radicals produced during oxidative phosphorylation [142]. The mutation rate of mtDNA is notably higher compared to nuclear DNA, and current knowledge attributes ROS damage as a major driver of mtDNA mutagenesis [145]. Additionally, research suggests that the mitochondrial DNA repair system may be less efficient than that of nuclear DNA, and mtDNA lacks the protective histone proteins, rendering it more susceptible to harmful agents [148]. If left unrepaired, mtDNA can disrupt the ETC, leading to increased ROS production thus initiating a vicious cycle that ultimately results in cellular energy depletion and apoptosis [149].

3.3. Genetic Susceptibility

Research on inherited forms of PD has identified several genes linked to mitochondrial dysfunction [29]. While the mitochondrial genetic factors associated with cardiac dysfunction are less extensively documented, the substantial overlap in mitochondrial dysfunction between cardiac pathology and PD suggests a potential shared genetic basis. Leading examples include Parkin RBR E3 Ubiquitin Protein Ligase (PRKN), PTEN-induced kinase 1 (PINK1) and Parkinson disease protein 7 (PARK7), with robust evidence linking them to the development of PD [150]. PRKN and PINK1 gene mutations are recognised as primary causes of autosomal recessive early-onset PD, with PRKN accounting for up to 42.2% of cases with an onset before the age of 20, and PINK1 representing 1–9% of all genetic PD [151,152]. In normal physiology, the shared pathway between PINK1, a protein kinase, and PRKN, an E3 ubiquitin ligase, serves to identify damaged mitochondria and activate a recruitment mechanism for the removal and replacement of dysfunctional components [136,153]. This PINK1/PRKN-mediated mitophagy critically governs cellular fate by eliminating impaired mitochondria, and components of this quality control pathway have already been found mutated in PD or linked to an elevated vulnerability to PD [136,153–156]. The loss of PRKN has been associated with dopaminergic neuronal loss and the accumulation of damaged mitochondria [157]. Interestingly, mutations in these genes also significantly contribute to the development of cardiac dysfunction [158]. PINK1 absence increases oxidative stress levels and disrupts mitochondrial function in cardiomyocytes, leading to cardiac dysfunction and hypertrophy [159]. PRKN deficiency exacerbates cardiac injury and reduces survival following myocardial infarction [158]. Therefore, targeting the modulation of PINK1/PRKN-mediated mitophagy could be considered a potential therapeutic approach to treat cardiac dysfunction [154].

An additional gene implicated in PD is PARK7, found within the mitochondria which serves as a protective factor against oxidative neuronal damage [142]. Its involvement in PD development has been well-documented [160,161]. Clinically, individuals with PARK7 mutations in PD exhibit an early onset of symptoms like dyskinesia, rigidity and tremors, amongst other PD-like symptoms [162]. In cardiac pathophysiology, PARK7 is associated with cardio-protection through the regulation of cardiac injury in models of I/R and acute myocardial infarctions [163–165]. Further investigation into the genetic underpinnings of both conditions will contribute valuable insights for targeted interventions and a more comprehensive understanding of their shared genetic susceptibility.

3.4. Mitochondrial Dynamics

Mitochondria exhibit a complex ability to adapt to varying physiological demands through dynamic processes known as fusion and fission. These intricate mechanisms play a role in shaping mitochondrial structure, function and cellular health [166]. Fusion involves the merging of two separate mitochondria into a singular organelle. This process is driven by large guanosine triphosphate (GTP)-hydrolysing enzymes of the dynamin superfamily—Mitofusin 1 (MFN1), MFN2 and Optic atrophy 1 (OPA1). MFN1 and MFN2, positioned on the outer membrane, orchestrate the fusion of outer membranes, while OPA1 is associated with the inner mitochondrial membrane [12]. Mitochondrial fission involves the division of a single mitochondrion into two organelles—a process primarily regulated by the dynamin-related protein 1 (DRP1). Upon activation, DRP1 translocates from the cytosol to the mitochondria. This translocation is facilitated by specific adaptor proteins, such as Fission protein 1 (FIS1), mitochondrial division protein 1 (MDV1) and mitochondrial fission factor (MFF), which are located on the outer mitochondrial membrane. Once at the outer membrane, DRP1 undergoes GTP-dependent oligomerisation, forming a spiral ring around the tubule, ultimately leading to its constriction and division. Dysregulation of fusion and fission processes can lead to distinct mitochondrial network morphologies. These morphological imbalances can influence cellular function and contribute to a range of physiological and pathophysiological conditions [166].

Maintaining proper mitochondrial dynamics is essential for the structural and functional integrity of the heart, both under normal conditions and during periods of stress. Imbalances in fusion or fission processes can result in either elongated or fragmented mitochondria, leading to compromised mitochondrial function (Table 1). In vitro studies suggest that increased mitochondrial fusion promotes cell senescence [167]. Animal models with inhibited mitochondrial fission exhibit adverse effects, exacerbating myocardial fibrosis and cardiomyocyte necrosis [168]. Reduced expression of DRP1 has been associated with heightened mitochondrial depolarisation in the heart, indicating its critical role in maintaining mitochondrial function [169]. In experimental models, mutations affecting DRP1 interactions have resulted in elongated mitochondrial networks, decreased mitochondrial enzyme complexes, ATP depletion and ultimately heart failure [170]. Interestingly, increased mitochondrial fission, predominantly mediated by upregulated DRP1, has been shown to play a significant role in I/R injury, contributing to mitochondrial dysfunction and decreased contractility [171]. Increased DRP1 also participates in opening the mitochondrial permeability transition pore (mPTP), exacerbating heart dysfunction in various pathological conditions such as I/R injury and chronic β-adrenergic receptor activation [172]. Evidence also suggests that DRP1-mediated mitochondrial fission contributes to cardiomyocyte death in conditions such as pressure overload and myocardial infarction [169]. Inhibiting DRP1, either genetically or pharmacologically, has shown promise in preventing mPTP opening, reducing infarct size and improving cardiovascular function in animal models of acute myocardial infarction [169]. Moreover, studies inducing heart failure in animal models and treating them with DRP1 inhibitors have demonstrated improvement in left ventricular function, accompanied by reduced expression of autophagy markers [170].

In PD, reduced DRP1 activity in mitochondria of PD mouse models with α-synucleinopathy lead to enlarged neuronal mitochondria and compromised neuronal integrity [173]. Deletion of DRP1 in mouse dopaminergic neurons prompts rapid degeneration of dopamine terminals and cell bodies in the midbrain by impairing mitochondrial dynamics in axons, resulting in reduced mitochondrial mass and disrupted mitochondrial movement coordination [174]. Interestingly, other studies suggest that neurotoxins associated with PD trigger DRP1-mediated fragmentation of mitochondria, indicating a predominant role for mitochondrial fission in pathology [175]. Exposure of cultured rat cortical neurons to acute rotenone induces rapid mitochondrial fragmentation and cell death, dependent on DRP1 [29]. The pharmacological inhibition of DRP1 by mitochondrial division inhibitor (Mdivi-1) in PD rats not only significantly alleviates behavioural deficits but also modulates mitochondrial function, enhances biogenesis and boosts the production of new-born dopaminergic neurons in the substantia nigra pars compacta [176].

The involvement of fusion proteins in mitochondrial dynamics in the heart has also been explored. Dysregulation of fusion proteins like MARF (analogous to human MFN) and OPA1 in Drosophila and mice models has been linked to cardiomyopathy and impaired heart function, whereas the overexpression of human MFN1/2 has shown promise in mitigating these effects [177]. In aging hearts, imbalanced mitochondrial dynamics contribute to cardiac dysfunction, characterised by reduced MFN1/2 and increased OPA1 and DRP1 expression [177]. Ischemic heart failure correlates with decreased OPA1 expression, exacerbating apoptosis and heart failure progression [178]. Studies involving specific deletion of MFN2 in cardiomyocytes demonstrate impaired mitochondrial fusion and cardiac hypertrophy, and altered expressions of MFN1/2 have been noted in ischemic and non-ischemic heart failure [179,180]. Inhibition of fission has shown efficacy in reducing I/R injury [181]. OPA1 mutant heart tissue displays increased ROS and compromised mitochondrial function, suggesting a potential role in heart disease progression [181].

In PD, deletion of MFN2 induces aberrant mitochondrial morphologies and impairs ETC activity, leading to a severe loss of nerve terminals in the striatum [130]. Additionally, mutations in the OPA1 gene have been associated with inherited forms of PD and other dementia, potentially through destabilisation of the cristae structure and activation of the apoptotic pathway [182]. MFN2 ablation also disrupts PRKN signalling initiating aberrant mitophagy [183]. Furthermore, overexpression of α-synuclein in transgenic mice results in reduced MFN1/2 protein levels, corresponding to diminished mitochondrial fusion and smaller mitochondria, while α-synuclein knockdown induces mitochondrial elongation [184].

The precise mechanisms governing fusion/fission protein modulation varies across different disease contexts, and further research is essential for developing effective interventions to mitigate disease progression. Promisingly, DRP1 inhibitors such as Mdivi-1, have shown potential in restoring the balance between fusion and fission dynamics [33,185]. Additionally, flavonoids have emerged as a therapeutic avenue for modulating mitochondrial fission. Administration in PD mouse models has demonstrated the restoration of mitochondrial dynamics by downregulating DRP1 expression and upregulating MFN1 expression in the hippocampus [186]. In cardiac pathology, interventions like 7,8-dihydroxyflavone (7,8-DHF) treatment in myocardial ischemic mice have shown promise in ameliorating cardiac dysfunction and cardiomyocyte abnormalities by suppressing mitochondrial fission [187]. The selective peptide inhibitor P110, targeting excessive mitochondrial fission, also emerges as a promising pharmacological intervention [188]. P110 has demonstrated cardioprotective effects by preserving cardiac mitochondria from I/R injury-induced damage, reducing myocardial infarct size and improving cardiac function in CVD models [170]. Similarly, in PD models, P110 shows neuroprotective properties by preserving mitochondrial function, mitigating neuronal death and potentially slowing neurodegeneration [189]. With its ability to safeguard mitochondria from damage and enhance mitochondrial function, these approaches hold promise for further investigation in clinical trials as therapeutic strategies for both cardiac dysfunction and PD.

3.5. Biogenesis Deficits

Mitochondrial biogenesis is a cellular response to heightened energy demands triggered by developmental signals and environmental stressors, involving the generation of new mitochondria from existing ones [190]. Mitochondria are descendants of an alpha-protobacteria endosymbiont and possess their own genetic material and capability for self-replication [191]. This process is vital for maintaining cellular balance, coordinating the equilibrium between generating new mitochondria through biogenesis and removing damaged ones via mitophagy [190]. Several growth factors are involved. Peroxisome proliferator-activated receptor-gamma coactivator (PGC-1α) serves as a central regulator, tiggering transcription factors like nuclear respiratory factors-1 (NRF1) and NRF2. These initiate the transcription of nuclear-encoded respiratory chain proteins expressed by the nuclear genome, ultimately leading in mitochondrial DNA replication [192,193]. Other transcription factors such as mitochondrial transcription factor A (TFAM) and dimethyladenosine transferase 2 (TFB2M) can then act in response to intracellular oxidative stress [192]. PGC-1α, regulated by AMP-activated protein kinase (AMPK), is often reduced in many diseases (Table 1) [193].

Mitochondrial biogenesis plays a crucial role in cardiac function [116]. In the heart, this association stems from diminished mitochondrial function in cardiac and skeletal muscles, characterised by changes in mitochondrial proteins and reduced levels of PGC-1α, along with its downstream transcription factors NRFs and TFAM [194]. This reduction in cardiac PGC-1α is consistently observed in various heart failure models [116,195–197]. Hearts with deletions in PGC-1α or PGC-1β are more susceptible to heart failure when exposed to pressure overload [196]. The chronic deactivation of the PGC-1α axis leads to decreased ATP production, impacting energy transfer and utilisation, ultimately resulting in decreased energy efficiency [116,194,195]. Research on PGC-1α knockout and transgenic mice have highlighted its influence on various pathways beyond mitochondrial biogenesis, underscoring the critical role of PGC-1α expression in determining energetic states [198]. Regarding mitochondrial biogenesis in PD, recent research involving PRKN-deficient human dopaminergic neurons found that the main driver of mitochondrial dysfunction was defective biogenesis [4,33]. This was attributed to increased levels of the PRKN substrates PARIS, leading to decreased PGC-1α expression [4,33]. Studies on PGC-1α knockout mice demonstrated a reduction in the expression of genes responsible for mitochondrial respiration, resulting in decreased enzymatic activities and lower ATP concentrations [199]. Additionally, diminished expression of a specific set of 425 PGC-1α responsible genes is closely correlated with PD pathology and subclinical Lewy body neuropathology. PGC-1α activation boosts expression of nuclear-encoded mitochondrial respiratory chain subunits, safeguarding dopaminergic neurons from damage by mutant α-synuclein or rotenone [199].

The reduction of the PGC-1α axis during cardiac dysfunction and PD, along with its ability to enhance energy production and reduce oxidative stress, highlights its potential as a target for preventing and treating these diseases [195,199]. One approach focuses on reducing acetylation of PGC-1α and PGC-1β proteins, negatively regulating their activity [195]. SIRT1, a deacetylase for PGC-1α/β, can be activated by compounds like resveratrol, leading to enhanced PGC-1 activity [200,201]. Resveratrol exhibits cardioprotective effects in various heart failure models through SIRT1 activation [202,203]. It also plays a neuroprotective role through the SIRT1/PGC-1α pathway in PD models [204,205].

Exercise has also emerged as a therapeutic strategy, promoting mitochondrial biogenesis and function via the SIRT1/PGC-1α pathway [33,198]. In a unilateral PD rat model, one week of intermittent moderate treadmill exercise prevented a decrease in PGC-1α and NRF1 expression [33]. Exercise training induced activation of the SIRT1 pathway, reducing cardiomyocyte apoptosis and oxidative damage [206]. Increased levels of SIRT and PGC-1α were found after moderate long-term exercise in rats and mice, suggesting that exercise can upregulate the SIRT1/PGC-1α pathway. This evidence supports the idea that exercise-induced SIRT1/PGC-1α activation promotes mitochondrial biogenesis and neuronal health [201,207]. This mechanism may contribute to the neuroprotective and cardioprotective benefits observes with exercise.

3.6. Calcium Dysregulation

Calcium ions (Ca^{2+}) serve as versatile signalling molecules in various physiological processes, encompassing muscle contraction, neuronal excitability, cell migration and cell growth [208]. Mitochondria play a pivotal role in regulating cellular Ca^{2+}. Beyond this role, mitochondrial Ca^{2+} has additional functions, such as influencing ATP production, cytosolic calcium levels and cell fate, including apoptosis control [208]. Extensive evidence underscores the critical role of mitochondrial Ca^{2+} in ATP production. In the context of the heart, the influx of Ca^{2+} into mitochondria assumes a critical stance in sustaining ATP production, thereby underpinning the contractile activity of cardiomyocytes [209]. Similarly, in neurons, mitochondrial Ca^{2+} buffering is essential for shaping Ca^{2+} signals and regulating various Ca^{2+}-dependent functions, such as neuronal excitability, synaptic transmission, gene expression and neuronal toxicity [81]. Any disruption in tightly regulated mitochondrial Ca^{2+} levels initiate a cascade of molecular malfunctions, resulting in mitochondrial dysfunction and abnormal Ca^{2+} signalling, leading to cellular degeneration.

Insufficient levels of Ca^{2+} within cardiac mitochondria can compromise their functionality, diminishing energy production and potentially inducing cellular damage or death (Table 1) [209]. Conversely, excessive Ca^{2+} accumulation can also severely disrupt cellular functions [210]. In heart failure, there is an imbalance between Ca^{2+} and ATP, leading to the oxidation of pyridine nucleotides within the mitochondrial matrix. This process may diminish ATP synthesis and cardiomyocyte contraction, while also triggering oxidative damage through NADPH oxidation, subsequently contributing to maladaptive cardiac remodelling [135]. Research findings indicate a substantial elevation in mitochondrial Ca^{2+} and ROS levels in a murine model of heart failure post-myocardial infarction [211]. Leaky ryanodine receptors (RyR2) channels on the sarcoplasmic reticulum (SR), which cause SR Ca^{2+} leakage, leads to mitochondrial Ca^{2+} overload and mitochondrial dysfunction. Mitigating RyR2 oxidative modification or phosphorylation has demonstrated a reduction in SR Ca^{2+} leak, leading to improved mitochondrial function and decreased severity of heart failure [211]. In instances of I/R injury, mitochondrial Ca^{2+} overload induces a sudden rise in mitochondrial membrane permeability, a significant driver of cell death [210]. Studies involving genetic deletion of the mitochondrial calcium uniporter (MCU) in adult mouse cardiomyocytes have shown protective effects against I/R injury. This intervention reduces mitochondrial Ca^{2+} overload, diminishes activation of the mitochondrial permeability transition pore, decreases infarct size and enhances cardiac function post-I/R [212]. Other studies, however, indicate that while MCU deletion leads to less mitochondrial Ca^{2+} accumulation during ischemia, it does not entirely prevent it, suggesting that mitochondrial Ca^{2+} overload during ischemia is not exclusively dependent on MCU [213]. Overall, the maintenance of a balanced level of mitochondrial Ca^{2+} is crucial for cardiomyocyte survival and function [209].

Chronic elevated Ca^{2+} levels, resulting from altered Ca^{2+} transient handling, are also a significant pathological hallmark of PD. This Ca^{2+} dysregulation affects cellular signalling and damages mitochondria, leading to cell death [31]. In PD neurons, mitochondrial Na^+/Ca^{2+} exchange (mNCX) mechanisms play a crucial role in neuronal Ca^{2+} homeostasis, acting as safeguards against cell death from excessive mitochondrial Ca^{2+} accumulation [214,215]. Recent findings suggest that the mitochondrial kinase PINK1 regulates calcium efflux from mitochondria through mNCX [214,216]. PINK1 deficiency leads to mitochondrial calcium overload, triggering increased ROS production, inhibiting glucose transport, reducing substrate delivery and compromising function [216]. Activating mNCX in PINK1 deficient models rescues pathogenic mitochondrial Ca^{2+} efflux, mitochondrial depolarisation and neuronal cell death through the protein kinase A (PKA) pathway [217]. In some cases, mitochondrial Ca^{2+} overload is linked to prolonged cytosolic Ca^{2+} levels [218]. The activation of plasma membrane L-type Cav1.3 Ca^{2+} channels induce independent, rhythmic pace making in dopaminergic neurons. Aging and stress factors associated with PD further intensify this neuronal activity [218]. Additionally, PD dopaminergic neurons exhibit a restricted Ca^{2+} buffering system. These elements collectively contribute to heightened mitochondrial Ca^{2+} uptake and activation of OXPHOS. While ensuring practical ATP synthesis, this process may result in mitochondrial hyperpolarisation, the generation of ROS, mitochondrial damage and the formation of defective organelles [218].

3.7. Mitophagy Impairment

Mitophagy is a highly coordinated cellular process involving the identification, capture and transport of damaged mitochondria to lysosomes for degradation [219]. This mechanism comprises three main phases: recognition of damaged mitochondria, formation of autophagic membranes around these targeted mitochondria and subsequent fusion of these autophagosomes with lysosomes [192]. This process is intricately linked with mitochondrial fusion, fission and biogenesis, ensuring the maintenance of appropriate mitochondria morphology, quantity, quality and turnover [220]. Regulation of mitophagy involves a network of proteins, including those associated with mitochondrial fusion (MFN1, MFN2, OPA1) and fission (DRP1, FIS1), as well as B-cell lymphoma 2 (BCL-2) family proteins and the PINK1/PRKN pathway [221]. Mitophagy plays a pivotal role in responding to various forms of stress, and dysregulation of this process contributes to the onset of several diseases (Table 1) [222,223].

In cardiac pathology, the functional significance of cardiac mitophagy has been revealed by loss-of-function mouse models of autophagy [224]. Mice with cardiac-specific autophagy related 5 (ATG5) or autophagy related 7 (ATG7) ablation, required for optimal autophagic responses, develop cardiac hypertrophy, left ventricular dilation, contractile dysfunction and premature death, along with mitochondrial misalignment and aggregation [225]. Biopsies from individuals with heart failure show downregulated autophagy-specific genes (beclin1 and LC3-II), indicating a potential association between mitophagy and heart failure development. Subsequent experiments on heart failure models have revealed that insufficient mitophagy aggravates heart injury [137]. The impact of PINK1 and PRKN is highly responsible for mitophagy impairment, and this impact extends to the cardiac system [226]. In Drosophila models, genetic deletion of either PINK1 or PRKN results in mitochondrial dysfunction and compromised cardiac contractibility [224]. Patients with end-stage heart failure exhibit reduced expression of PINK1, and its loss leads to mitochondrial dysfunction and excessive ROS accumulation [154]. Mutations leading to the reduced function of the PINK1/PRKN pathway have also been associated with the development of PD [152,227]. The expression of several mitophagy-related genes is altered in DA neurons derived from PRKN knockout isogenic induced pluripotent stem cells (iPSCs) [228]. Neurons differentiated from iPSCs carrying PRKN or PINK1 mutations demonstrate aberrant accumulation of phospho-ubiquitin and aggregated mitochondria [228]. Moreover, PINK1 and PRKN null Drosophila exhibit learning and memory abnormalities, weakened circadian rhythms, and underlying electrophysiological irregularities in clock neurons [136]. Overall, the evidence indicates mitophagy to play a role in the degeneration of dopaminergic neurons observed in PD progression [229].

The exploration of nutritional and pharmacological interventions to modulate autophagy/mitophagy as potential therapeutic strategies holds promise. Inhibitors of mTOR have demonstrated the ability to induce autophagy, offering protection against various cardiac pathologies and extending lifespan across different species [230]. Notably, the mTOR inhibitor rapamycin has been identified as contributing to the safeguarding of dopaminergic neurons and enhancing behavioural outcomes in mice with PD [230]. While no specific study has focused on the impact of mTOR inhibitors in targeting mitophagy for the treatment of cardiac dysfunction, research has shown the cardioprotective effects of rapamycin in pressure-overloaded and ischemic heart diseases [231]. AMPK activators have also emerged as potential therapeutic strategies. AMPK serves as a cellular energy sensor regulating metabolic pathways, including autophagy and mitophagy. Activation of AMPK promotes mitophagy and enhances mitochondrial function [232]. Pharmacological agents like metformin and resveratrol, known for activating AMPK, hold potential therapeutic benefits in cardiac function and PD [233,234]. Metformin, commonly used in type 2 diabetes (T2D) management, exerts neuroprotective effects through AMPK activation, reducing mitochondrial dysfunction, oxidative stress and α-synuclein aggregation [235,236]. Moreover, metformin has been shown to exert beneficial effects in myocardial ischemic injury, diabetic cardiomyopathy, cardiotoxicity and ventricular dysfunction [237]. Another therapeutic avenue is the use of nicotinamide adenine dinucleotide (NAD+) precursors. NAD+ plays a crucial role in cellular energy metabolism and mitochondrial function. Its levels decline with age and in various disease conditions, impairing mitochondrial health and contributing to disease progression. NAD+ precursors such as nicotinamide riboside (NR) and nicotinamide mononucleotide (NMN) have been shown to enhance mitophagy and improve mitochondrial function, offering potential therapeutic benefits for both cardiac dysfunction and PD [238,239]. For instance, NR was shown to prevent neuronal cell loss in patient-derived cell lines and Drosophila models of PD [240]. Supplementation with NAD+ precursors has been linked to significant reduction in systolic and diastolic blood pressure as well as C-reactive protein concentrations, indicating a decrease in inflammation and suggesting potential benefits for cardiovascular risk factors [241]. In heart failure, NMN administration mitigates mitochondrial dysfunction by reducing mitochondrial protein hyperacetylation, preserving mitochondrial ultrastructure, reducing ROS, preventing cell death and enhancing long-chain fatty acid oxidation [242]. These findings suggest a promising avenue for targeting mitochondrial health in the treatment of both cardiac comorbidities and PD.

3.8. Oxidative Stress and Lipid Peroxidation

Recently, growing evidence has highlighted oxidative stress and associated mitochondrial dysfunction to be critical players in the pathophysiologic processes involved in neurodegenerative conditions, suggesting a new paradigm for therapeutic treatments. Oxidative stress is characterized by an overproduction of ROS within cells. It results from perturbations in homeostatic mechanisms involved in pro- and antioxidant balance, whereby the balance of ROS and antioxidants observed under physiological conditions is disrupted due to the overproduction of free radicals. The most common ROS include singlet oxygen (O_2), superoxide anion radicals ($O_2^{\bullet -}$), hydroxyl radicals ($HO^{\bullet}$) and hydrogen peroxide (H_2O_2) [243]. These excess free radicals can lead to not only protein deposition and DNA damage, but also degradation of proteins and lipids [244].

The mitochondrion is the single most important cellular organelle involved in the generation of ROS [245], primarily as a consequence of aerobic respiratory processes, which are mediated by protein complexes within the inner mitochondrial membrane. Notably, the inner mitochondrial membrane is prone to lipid peroxidation (LPO) [246]. LPO is the formation of a free radical chain as a result of damage to the phospholipid layer of the cell through oxygen derived-free radicals [247]. Indeed, oxidative damage of lipids results in the formation of LPO products, which further attack lipids, resulting in the release of lipid peroxyl radicals, hydroperoxides, which subsequently target and induce the breakdown of proteins and DNA.

Lipids are major components of the structural and functional organization of the central nerve system (CNS), comprising almost 60% of the dry mass of human brain. Lipid properties and the effects in the CNS are directly determined by the proportion of specific fatty acids within their molecular structure and, in particular, by the content of long-chain polyunsaturated fatty acids (PUFAs) [248,249]. PUFAs can be classified as omega-3 (n-3) and omega-6 (n-6) fatty acids. Interestingly, within healthy dopaminergic neurons, LPO products induce the generation and accumulation of misfolded α-synuclein, resulting in insufficient dopamine production and the development of PD [140]. It has been recently demonstrated that reduced levels of glutathione, an antioxidant critical for protecting dopaminergic neurons in the SNpc from free radical damage, directly increases LPO levels [250]. Furthermore, clinical studies have reported significant upregulation of acrolein levels in the brain with PD [140,251]. Acrolein, which is an α, β-unsaturated aldehyde produced by the lipid peroxidation of PUFAs, promotes the initiation of LPO and further elevation of oxidative stress, as indicated by acrolein-induced increases in 4-hydroxy-2-alkenal (HNE) levels, formed by the peroxidation of omega-6 (n-6) PUFAs [252]. Additionally, acrolein acts on the modification of α-synuclein in dopaminergic neurons, leading to mitochondrial dysfunction and resulting in the ROS-mediated apoptosis of affected neurons [253]. Importantly, elevated levels of HNE and acrolein have both been reported in the CSF of living PD patients [253–255].

Numerous studies have also found that there are functional consequences in the heart following exposure to acrolein [256–258]. Due to the established role of LPO products in heart failure and cardiac ischaemia–reperfusion injury [259] and diabetes [260], they may play an underappreciated role in the pathophysiology of these disease processes in PD patients and warrant further investigation [257,261,262].

4. Future Perspectives

While there is a strong association between Parkinson's disease (PD) and cardiac complications, establishing a definitive cause-and-effect relationship remains challenging. Individuals with PD often exhibit a heightened susceptibility to cardiac dysfunction, including increased risk of myocardial infarction, heart failure and overall mortality. This review explores potential commonalities in the molecular mechanisms underlying cardiac comorbidities in PD. In this respect, it would be worthwhile to investigate whether this association is bidirectional—that is, whether there is also an increased risk of neurodegenerative diseases associated with cardiac conditions. The existing literature on this topic is sparse, indicating a valuable area for future research. Investigating these associations could provide important insights into the broader implications of the connection between neurodegenerative diseases and cardiac health. For instance, emerging evidence suggests that chronic cardiac dysfunction, such as heart failure, may raise the risk of developing neurodegenerative diseases like Alzheimer's disease (AD) and Parkinson's disease (PD) [263–265]. Age-related changes in cardiac haemodynamics, including alterations in cardiac output and arterial stiffness, could impair brain health and accelerate cognitive decline by affecting brain structure and function, potentially interacting with neurodegenerative processes in aging adults [266]. Cardiac dysfunction may also lead to reduced cerebral perfusion, which can impair cognitive function and accelerate neurodegeneration [265]. Additionally, cardiac issues may exacerbate existing neurodegenerative conditions by inducing systemic inflammation, further compromising brain health [267]. Interestingly, a recent study found that while myocardial infarction (MI) was associated with a higher risk of vascular dementia, particularly in patients who experienced a stroke post-MI, it was not linked to an increased risk of Alzheimer's disease or other dementias [268]. Furthermore, another study revealed that survivors of MI had a reduced risk of developing Parkinson's disease and secondary parkinsonism, indicating a possible inverse relationship between cardiovascular risk factors and these conditions [269]. These findings highlight the need for further research to clarify the pathogenetic and clinical connections between cardiovascular disease and Parkinson's disease. Such research could inform the development of new therapeutic strategies and improve our understanding of the complex interactions between these conditions.

Understanding the broader links between PD and cardiac comorbidities is crucial. Exploring specific key molecules in PD that may lead to cardiac insufficiency can yield valuable insights into these connections. Notably, few studies in PD patients have focused on identifying the molecular keys responsible for cardiac dysfunction. Several PD-associated genes, such as PRKN, PINK1, PARK7, LRRK2, and α-synuclein, are expressed in cardiac tissue. Although definitive clinical links between these genes and cardiac damage in PD are lacking, preclinical models, as discussed throughout the review, suggest that these genes may exert protective effects on the heart. PINK1 is crucial for heart function, regulating mitochondrial health during stress. Its deficiency leads to cardiac hypertrophy and increased susceptibility to ischemic injury in animal models [270]. PARK7 protects the heart against oxidative stress, with its absence heightening the risk of cardiac damage during ischemia [163]. Mutations in LRRK2 have also been associated with altered heart rate variability in PD patients [271]. Interestingly, aberrant α-synuclein aggregates have been found in the epicardial tissue of undiagnosed PD patients, suggesting a potential link to the disease's prodromal stage [8,272]. Furthermore, Lewy bodies have been identified in the myocardium of PD patients, particularly in the nerve fibres of arteries and atrial ganglia, while α-synuclein accumulation in myocardial tissue and coronary arteries suggests a possible connection to cardiac sympathetic dysfunction [8,273,274]. Given the elevated risk of heart disease in PD patients, assessing mutations in PD-related genes for potential links to cardiovascular disease is critical. However, despite these associations, direct evidence identifying specific molecular connections between PD and cardiac insufficiency remains limited. Given the overlap of mitochondrial dysfunction in both neurodegenerative and cardiovascular diseases, further research is essential to determine whether these identified molecules are key specific contributors to cardiac comorbidities in PD.

5. Conclusions

Mitochondria, crucial for both heart and brain function, are implicated in the development of cardiac dysfunction and PD. Mitochondrial dysfunction in these conditions can manifest through various mechanisms, such as bioenergetic deficits, mitochondrial DNA defects, genetic predispositions, disruptions in mitochondrial dynamics, biogenesis deficits, calcium dysregulation, impaired mitophagy and oxidative stress. Despite this observed association, the precise underlying mechanisms are not entirely clear. Hence, our review aims to explore the potential role of mitochondrial dysfunction as a mediator of cardiac comorbidities in PD. By uncovering common pathways and molecular targets relevant to both cardiac dysfunction and PD, there is potential for the elucidation of shared therapeutic targets. Exploring the role of mitochondrial dysfunction as a potential mechanism linking both conditions can provide new perspectives into their interconnectedness and highlight promising areas for future research.

Author Contributions: Conceptualization, V.E.M., A.S.T., J.-E.L. and M.H.H.; writing—original draft preparation, A.S.T. and J.-E.L.; writing—review and editing, V.E.M., M.H.H., R.K.S. and A.C.; visualization, A.S.T.; supervision, V.E.M., M.H.H., R.K.S. and A.C.; project administration, V.E.M. and M.H.H.; funding acquisition, V.E.M., M.H.H., R.K.S. and A.C. All authors have read and agreed to the published version of the manuscript.

Funding: This research was funded by (i) the British Heart Foundation (RE/18/5/3421) to V.E.M., M.H.H., A.C and R.K.S (ii) the Biotechnology and Biological Sciences Research Council (BBSRC) in the form of an Institute Strategic Programme Grant (BB/J004316/1, BBS/E/D/20221657 and BBS/E/RL/230001C) to V.E.M. and (iii) the Wellcome Trust (grant 210752) to R.K.S. The APC was funded by UK Research and Innovation (UKRI). For the purpose of open access, the author has applied a CC-BY public copyright license to any Author Accepted Manuscript version arising from this submission.

Acknowledgments: V.E.M is a member of the International Network on Ectopic Calcification (INTEC · itnintec.com).

Conflicts of Interest: The authors declare no conflicts of interest.

References

1. Park, J.-H.; Kim, D.-H.; Park, Y.-G.; Kwon, D.-Y.; Choi, M.; Jung, J.-H.; Han, K. Association of Parkinson Disease with Risk of Cardiovascular Disease and All-Cause Mortality: A Nationwide, Population-Based Cohort Study. *Circulation* **2020**, *141*, 1205–1207. [CrossRef] [PubMed]
2. Grosu, L.; Grosu, A.; Crisan, D.; Zlibut, A.; Perju-Dumbrava, L. Parkinson's Disease and Cardiovascular Involvement: Edifying Insights (Review). *Biomed. Rep.* **2023**, *18*, 25. [CrossRef] [PubMed]
3. Hong, C.T.; Hu, H.H.; Chan, L.; Bai, C.-H. Prevalent Cerebrovascular and Cardiovascular Disease in People with Parkinson’s Disease: A Meta-Analysis. *Clin. Epidemiol.* **2018**, *10*, 1147–1154. [CrossRef]
4. Jha, S.K.; Jha, N.K.; Kumar, D.; Ambasta, R.K.; Kumar, P. Linking Mitochondrial Dysfunction, Metabolic Syndrome and Stress Signaling in Neurodegeneration. *Biochim. Biophys. Acta BBA Mol. Basis Dis.* **2017**, *1863*, 1132–1146. [CrossRef]
5. Husnu, D.; Eftal Murat, B.; Hikmet, H. Cardiac Effects of Parkinson's Disease. *Open J. Park. Dis. Treat.* **2020**, *3*, 006–007. [CrossRef]
6. Potashkin, J.; Huang, X.; Becker, C.; Chen, H.; Foltynie, T.; Marras, C. Understanding the Links Between Cardiovascular Disease and Parkinson's Disease. *Mov. Disord.* **2020**, *35*, 55–74. [CrossRef]
7. Colín-Castelán, D.; Zaina, S. Associations between Atherosclerosis and Neurological Diseases, beyond Ischemia-Induced Cerebral Damage. *Rev. Endocr. Metab. Disord.* **2019**, *20*, 15–25. [CrossRef]

8. Cuenca-Bermejo, L.; Almela, P.; Navarro-Zaragoza, J.; Fernández Villalba, E.; González-Cuello, A.-M.; Laorden, M.-L.; Herrero, M.-T. Cardiac Changes in Parkinson's Disease: Lessons from Clinical and Experimental Evidence. *Int. J. Mol. Sci.* **2021**, *22*, 13488. [CrossRef] [PubMed]
9. Liang, H.-W.; Huang, Y.-P.; Pan, S.-L. Parkinson Disease and Risk of Acute Myocardial Infarction: A Population-Based, Propensity Score–Matched, Longitudinal Follow-up Study. *Am. Heart J.* **2015**, *169*, 508–514. [CrossRef]
10. Scorza, F.A.; Fiorini, A.C.; Scorza, C.A.; Finsterer, J. Cardiac Abnormalities in Parkinson's Disease and Parkinsonism. *J. Clin. Neurosci.* **2018**, *53*, 1–5. [CrossRef]
11. Brand, M.D.; Orr, A.L.; Perevoshchikova, I.V.; Quinlan, C.L. The Role of Mitochondrial Function and Cellular Bioenergetics in Ageing and Disease: Mitochondrial Function in Ageing and Disease. *Br. J. Dermatol.* **2013**, *169*, 1–8. [CrossRef]
12. Liu, Y.Z.; Li, Z.X.; Zhang, L.L.; Wang, D.; Liu, Y.P. Phenotypic Plasticity of Vascular Smooth Muscle Cells in Vascular Calcification: Role of Mitochondria. *Front. Cardiovasc. Med.* **2022**, *9*, 972836. [CrossRef] [PubMed]
13. Zhunina, O.A.; Yabbarov, N.G.; Grechko, A.V.; Starodubova, A.V.; Ivanova, E.; Nikiforov, N.G.; Orekhov, A.N. The Role of Mitochondrial Dysfunction in Vascular Disease, Tumorigenesis, and Diabetes. *Front. Mol. Biosci.* **2021**, *8*, 671908. [CrossRef]
14. Wang, Y.; Xu, E.; Musich, P.R.; Lin, F. Mitochondrial Dysfunction in Neurodegenerative Diseases and the Potential Countermeasure. *CNS Neurosci. Ther.* **2019**, *25*, 816–824. [CrossRef] [PubMed]
15. Siasos, G.; Tsigkou, V.; Kosmopoulos, M.; Theodosiadis, D.; Simantiris, S.; Tagkou, N.M.; Tsimpiktsioglou, A.; Stampouloglou, P.K.; Oikonomou, E.; Mourouzis, K.; et al. Mitochondria and Cardiovascular Diseases-from Pathophysiology to Treatment. *Ann. Transl. Med.* **2018**, *6*, 256. [CrossRef]
16. Fröhlich, F. Parkinson's Disease. In *Network Neuroscience*; Elsevier: Amsterdam, The Netherlands, 2016; pp. 291–296, ISBN 978-0-12-801560-5.
17. Kouli, A.; Torsney, K.M.; Kuan, W.-L. Parkinson's Disease: Etiology, Neuropathology, and Pathogenesis. In *Parkinson's Disease: Pathogenesis and Clinical Aspects*; Stoker, T.B., Greenland, J.C., Eds.; Codon Publications: Brisbane, Australia, 2018; ISBN 978-0-9944381-6-4.
18. Warner, T.T.; Schapira, A.H.V. Genetic and Environmental Factors in the Cause of Parkinson's Disease. *Ann. Neurol.* **2003**, *53*, S16–S25. [CrossRef] [PubMed]
19. Park, J.-S.; Davis, R.L.; Sue, C.M. Mitochondrial Dysfunction in Parkinson's Disease: New Mechanistic Insights and Therapeutic Perspectives. *Curr. Neurol. Neurosci. Rep.* **2018**, *18*, 21. [CrossRef] [PubMed]
20. Kieburtz, K.; Dorsey, E.R. Parkinson Disease Risks: Correctly Identifying Environmental Factors for a Chronic Disease. *J. Clin. Investig.* **2021**, *131*, e150252. [CrossRef]
21. Narayan, S.; Liew, Z.; Bronstein, J.M.; Ritz, B. Occupational Pesticide Use and Parkinson's Disease in the Parkinson Environment Gene (PEG) Study. *Environ. Int.* **2017**, *107*, 266–273. [CrossRef]
22. Hong, C.T.; Chan, L.; Bai, C.-H. The Effect of Caffeine on the Risk and Progression of Parkinson's Disease: A Meta-Analysis. *Nutrients* **2020**, *12*, 1860. [CrossRef]
23. Hauser, D.N.; Hastings, T.G. Mitochondrial Dysfunction and Oxidative Stress in Parkinson's Disease and Monogenic Parkinsonism. *Neurobiol. Dis.* **2013**, *51*, 35–42. [CrossRef] [PubMed]
24. Tan, J.M.M.; Wong, E.S.P.; Lim, K.-L. Protein Misfolding and Aggregation in Parkinson's Disease. *Antioxid. Redox Signal.* **2009**, *11*, 2119–2134. [CrossRef] [PubMed]
25. Moon, H.E.; Paek, S.H. Mitochondrial Dysfunction in Parkinson's Disease. *Exp. Neurobiol.* **2015**, *24*, 103–116. [CrossRef] [PubMed]
26. Wang, J.; Wang, F.; Mai, D.; Qu, S. Molecular Mechanisms of Glutamate Toxicity in Parkinson's Disease. *Front. Neurosci.* **2020**, *14*, 585584. [CrossRef] [PubMed]
27. Wang, Q.; Liu, Y.; Zhou, J. Neuroinflammation in Parkinson's Disease and Its Potential as Therapeutic Target. *Transl. Neurodegener.* **2015**, *4*, 19. [CrossRef]
28. Maiti, P.; Manna, J.; Dunbar, G.L. Current Understanding of the Molecular Mechanisms in Parkinson's Disease: Targets for Potential Treatments. *Transl. Neurodegener.* **2017**, *6*, 28. [CrossRef]
29. Van Laar, V.S.; Berman, S.B. Mitochondrial Dynamics in Parkinson's Disease. *Exp. Neurol.* **2009**, *218*, 247–256. [CrossRef]
30. Choi, M.L.; Chappard, A.; Singh, B.P.; Maclachlan, C.; Rodrigues, M.; Fedotova, E.I.; Berezhnov, A.V.; De, S.; Peddie, C.J.; Athauda, D.; et al. Pathological Structural Conversion of α-Synuclein at the Mitochondria Induces Neuronal Toxicity. *Nat. Neurosci.* **2022**, *25*, 1134–1148. [CrossRef]
31. Ludtmann, M.H.R.; Abramov, A.Y. Mitochondrial Calcium Imbalance in Parkinson's Disease. *Neurosci. Lett.* **2018**, *663*, 86–90. [CrossRef]
32. Reeve, A.K.; Ludtmann, M.H.; Angelova, P.R.; Simcox, E.M.; Horrocks, M.H.; Klenerman, D.; Gandhi, S.; Turnbull, D.M.; Abramov, A.Y. Aggregated α-Synuclein and Complex I Deficiency: Exploration of Their Relationship in Differentiated Neurons. *Cell Death Dis.* **2015**, *6*, e1820. [CrossRef]
33. Prasuhn, J.; Davis, R.L.; Kumar, K.R. Targeting Mitochondrial Impairment in Parkinson's Disease: Challenges and Opportunities. *Front. Cell Dev. Biol.* **2021**, *8*, 615461. [CrossRef] [PubMed]
34. Virdi, G.S.; Choi, M.L.; Evans, J.R.; Yao, Z.; Athauda, D.; Strohbuecker, S.; Nirujogi, R.S.; Wernick, A.I.; Pelegrina-Hidalgo, N.; Leighton, C.; et al. Protein Aggregation and Calcium Dysregulation Are Hallmarks of Familial Parkinson's Disease in Midbrain Dopaminergic Neurons. *npj Park. Dis.* **2022**, *8*, 162. [CrossRef] [PubMed]

35. Angelova, P.R.; Ludtmann, M.H.R.; Horrocks, M.H.; Negoda, A.; Cremades, N.; Klenerman, D.; Dobson, C.M.; Wood, N.W.; Pavlov, E.V.; Gandhi, S.; et al. Calcium Is a Key Factor in α-Synuclein Induced Neurotoxicity. *J. Cell Sci.* **2016**, *129*, 1792–1801. [CrossRef]
36. Global Burden of Disease Cancer Collaboration; Fitzmaurice, C.; Allen, C.; Barber, R.M.; Barregard, L.; Bhutta, Z.A.; Brenner, H.; Dicker, D.J.; Chimed-Orchir, O.; Dandona, R.; et al. Global, Regional, and National Cancer Incidence, Mortality, Years of Life Lost, Years Lived With Disability, and Disability-Adjusted Life-Years for 32 Cancer Groups, 1990 to 2015: A Systematic Analysis for the Global Burden of Disease Study. *JAMA Oncol.* **2017**, *3*, 524. [CrossRef]
37. Goldsborough, E.; Osuji, N.; Blaha, M.J. Assessment of Cardiovascular Disease Risk. *Endocrinol. Metab. Clin. North. Am.* **2022**, *51*, 483–509. [CrossRef] [PubMed]
38. Olvera Lopez, E.; Ballard, B.D.; Jan, A. Cardiovascular Disease. In *StatPearls*; StatPearls Publishing: Treasure Island, FL, USA, 2023.
39. Lu, L.; Liu, M.; Sun, R.; Zheng, Y.; Zhang, P. Myocardial Infarction: Symptoms and Treatments. *Cell Biochem. Biophys.* **2015**, *72*, 865–867. [CrossRef]
40. Gardner, R.S.; McDonagh, T.A.; Walker, N.L. *Heart Failure*; Oxford University Press: Oxford, UK, 2014; ISBN 978-0-19-967415-2.
41. Li, K.; Wan, B.; Li, S.; Chen, Z.; Jia, H.; Song, Y.; Zhang, J.; Ju, W.; Ma, H.; Wang, Y. Mitochondrial Dysfunction in Cardiovascular Disease: Towards Exercise Regulation of Mitochondrial Function. *Front. Physiol.* **2023**, *14*, 1063556. [CrossRef]
42. Eirin, A.; Lerman, A.; Lerman, L.O. Mitochondrial Injury and Dysfunction in Hypertension-Induced Cardiac Damage. *Eur. Heart J.* **2014**, *35*, 3258–3266. [CrossRef]
43. Eirin, A.; Lerman, A.; Lerman, L.O. Mitochondria: A Pathogenic Paradigm in Hypertensive Renal Disease. *Hypertension* **2015**, *65*, 264–270. [CrossRef]
44. Leem, J.; Koh, E.H. Interaction between Mitochondria and the Endoplasmic Reticulum: Implications for the Pathogenesis of Type 2 Diabetes Mellitus. *Exp. Diabetes Res.* **2012**, *2012*, 1–8. [CrossRef]
45. Ordog, K.; Horvath, O.; Eros, K.; Bruszt, K.; Toth, S.; Kovacs, D.; Kalman, N.; Radnai, B.; Deres, L.; Gallyas, F.; et al. Mitochondrial Protective Effects of PARP-Inhibition in Hypertension-Induced Myocardial Remodeling and in Stressed Cardiomyocytes. *Life Sci.* **2021**, *268*, 118936. [CrossRef] [PubMed]
46. Deng, Y.; Li, S.; Chen, Z.; Wang, W.; Geng, B.; Cai, J. Mdivi-1, a Mitochondrial Fission Inhibitor, Reduces Angiotensin-II- Induced Hypertension by Mediating VSMC Phenotypic Switch. *Biomed. Pharmacother.* **2021**, *140*, 111689. [CrossRef]
47. Anderson, E.J.; Kypson, A.P.; Rodriguez, E.; Anderson, C.A.; Lehr, E.J.; Neufer, P.D. Substrate-Specific Derangements in Mitochondrial Metabolism and Redox Balance in the Atrium of the Type 2 Diabetic Human Heart. *J. Am. Coll. Cardiol.* **2009**, *54*, 1891–1898. [CrossRef]
48. Ritov, V.B.; Menshikova, E.V.; He, J.; Ferrell, R.E.; Goodpaster, B.H.; Kelley, D.E. Deficiency of Subsarcolemmal Mitochondria in Obesity and Type 2 Diabetes. *Diabetes* **2005**, *54*, 8–14. [CrossRef]
49. Morino, K. Reduced Mitochondrial Density and Increased IRS-1 Serine Phosphorylation in Muscle of Insulin-Resistant Offspring of Type 2 Diabetic Parents. *J. Clin. Investig.* **2005**, *115*, 3587–3593. [CrossRef] [PubMed]
50. Chen, J.; Guan, Z.; Wang, L.; Song, G.; Ma, B.; Wang, Y. Meta-Analysis: Overweight, Obesity, and Parkinson's Disease. *Int. J. Endocrinol.* **2014**, *2014*, 1–7. [CrossRef]
51. Chen, J.; Zhang, C.; Wu, Y.; Zhang, D. Association between Hypertension and the Risk of Parkinson's Disease: A Meta-Analysis of Analytical Studies. *Neuroepidemiology* **2019**, *52*, 181–192. [CrossRef]
52. Ruiz-Pozo, V.A.; Tamayo-Trujillo, R.; Cadena-Ullauri, S.; Frias-Toral, E.; Guevara-Ramírez, P.; Paz-Cruz, E.; Chapela, S.; Montalván, M.; Morales-López, T.; Simancas-Racines, D.; et al. The Molecular Mechanisms of the Relationship between Insulin Resistance and Parkinson's Disease Pathogenesis. *Nutrients* **2023**, *15*, 3585. [CrossRef]
53. Xu, Q.; Park, Y.; Huang, X.; Hollenbeck, A.; Blair, A.; Schatzkin, A.; Chen, H. Diabetes and Risk of Parkinson's Disease. *Diabetes Care* **2011**, *34*, 910–915. [CrossRef]
54. Huang, C.-Y.; Lai, C.-H.; Kuo, C.-H.; Chiang, S.-F.; Pai, P.-Y.; Lin, J.-Y.; Chang, C.-F.; Viswanadha, V.P.; Kuo, W.-W.; Huang, C.-Y. Inhibition of ERK-Drp1 Signaling and Mitochondria Fragmentation Alleviates IGF-IIR-Induced Mitochondria Dysfunction during Heart Failure. *J. Mol. Cell. Cardiol.* **2018**, *122*, 58–68. [CrossRef]
55. Wang, B.; Nie, J.; Wu, L.; Hu, Y.; Wen, Z.; Dong, L.; Zou, M.-H.; Chen, C.; Wang, D.W. AMPKα2 Protects Against the Development of Heart Failure by Enhancing Mitophagy via PINK1 Phosphorylation. *Circ. Res.* **2018**, *122*, 712–729. [CrossRef] [PubMed]
56. Adaniya, S.M.; O-Uchi, J.; Cypress, M.W.; Kusakari, Y.; Jhun, B.S. Posttranslational Modifications of Mitochondrial Fission and Fusion Proteins in Cardiac Physiology and Pathophysiology. *Am. J. Physiol. Cell Physiol.* **2019**, *316*, C583–C604. [CrossRef] [PubMed]
57. Osellame, L.D.; Blacker, T.S.; Duchen, M.R. Cellular and Molecular Mechanisms of Mitochondrial Function. *Best. Pract. Res. Clin. Endocrinol. Metab.* **2012**, *26*, 711–723. [CrossRef] [PubMed]
58. Vakifahmetoglu-Norberg, H.; Ouchida, A.T.; Norberg, E. The Role of Mitochondria in Metabolism and Cell Death. *Biochem. Biophys. Res. Commun.* **2017**, *482*, 426–431. [CrossRef]
59. Collier, J.J.; Oláhová, M.; McWilliams, T.G.; Taylor, R.W. Mitochondrial Signalling and Homeostasis: From Cell Biology to Neurological Disease. *Trends Neurosci.* **2023**, *46*, 137–152. [CrossRef]
60. Granatiero, V.; De Stefani, D.; Rizzuto, R. Mitochondrial Calcium Handling in Physiology and Disease. In *Mitochondrial Dynamics in Cardiovascular Medicine*; Santulli, G., Ed.; Advances in Experimental Medicine and Biology; Springer International Publishing: Cham, Switzerland, 2017; Volume 982, pp. 25–47, ISBN 978-3-319-55329-0.

61. Ashrafi, G.; Ryan, T.A. Glucose Metabolism in Nerve Terminals. *Curr. Opin. Neurobiol.* **2017**, *45*, 156–161. [CrossRef]
62. Lopaschuk, G.D.; Karwi, Q.G.; Tian, R.; Wende, A.R.; Abel, E.D. Cardiac Energy Metabolism in Heart Failure. *Circ. Res.* **2021**, *128*, 1487–1513. [CrossRef]
63. Vergara, R.C.; Jaramillo-Riveri, S.; Luarte, A.; Moënne-Loccoz, C.; Fuentes, R.; Couve, A.; Maldonado, P.E. The Energy Homeostasis Principle: Neuronal Energy Regulation Drives Local Network Dynamics Generating Behavior. *Front. Comput. Neurosci.* **2019**, *13*, 49. [CrossRef] [PubMed]
64. Evans, D.L. Cardiovascular Adaptations to Exercise and Training. *Vet. Clin. North. Am. Equine Pract.* **1985**, *1*, 513–531. [CrossRef]
65. López-Doménech, G.; Kittler, J.T. Mitochondrial Regulation of Local Supply of Energy in Neurons. *Curr. Opin. Neurobiol.* **2023**, *81*, 102747. [CrossRef]
66. Ambekar, T.; Pawar, J.; Rathod, R.; Patel, M.; Fernandes, V.; Kumar, R.; Singh, S.B.; Khatri, D.K. Mitochondrial Quality Control: Epigenetic Signatures and Therapeutic Strategies. *Neurochem. Int.* **2021**, *148*, 105095. [CrossRef] [PubMed]
67. Shen, X.; Sun, P.; Zhang, H.; Yang, H. Mitochondrial Quality Control in the Brain: The Physiological and Pathological Roles. *Front. Neurosci.* **2022**, *16*, 1075141. [CrossRef] [PubMed]
68. Rangaraju, V.; Lewis, T.L.; Hirabayashi, Y.; Bergami, M.; Motori, E.; Cartoni, R.; Kwon, S.-K.; Courchet, J. Pleiotropic Mitochondria: The Influence of Mitochondria on Neuronal Development and Disease. *J. Neurosci.* **2019**, *39*, 8200–8208. [CrossRef] [PubMed]
69. Duarte, F.V.; Ciampi, D.; Duarte, C.B. Mitochondria as Central Hubs in Synaptic Modulation. *Cell. Mol. Life Sci.* **2023**, *80*, 173. [CrossRef] [PubMed]
70. Kann, O.; Kovács, R. Mitochondria and Neuronal Activity. *Am. J. Physiol. Cell Physiol.* **2007**, *292*, C641–C657. [CrossRef] [PubMed]
71. Zambrano, K.; Barba, D.; Castillo, K.; Noboa, L.; Argueta-Zamora, D.; Robayo, P.; Arizaga, E.; Caicedo, A.; Gavilanes, A.W.D. Fighting Parkinson's Disease: The Return of the Mitochondria. *Mitochondrion* **2022**, *64*, 34–44. [CrossRef]
72. Harris, J.J.; Jolivet, R.; Attwell, D. Synaptic Energy Use and Supply. *Neuron* **2012**, *75*, 762–777. [CrossRef]
73. Harris, J.J.; Attwell, D. The Energetics of CNS White Matter. *J. Neurosci.* **2012**, *32*, 356–371. [CrossRef] [PubMed]
74. Rangaraju, V.; Calloway, N.; Ryan, T.A. Activity-Driven Local ATP Synthesis Is Required for Synaptic Function. *Cell* **2014**, *156*, 825–835. [CrossRef]
75. Moradi Vastegani, S.; Nasrolahi, A.; Ghaderi, S.; Belali, R.; Rashno, M.; Farzaneh, M.; Khoshnam, S.E. Mitochondrial Dysfunction and Parkinson's Disease: Pathogenesis and Therapeutic Strategies. *Neurochem. Res.* **2023**, *48*, 2285–2308. [CrossRef]
76. Görlach, A.; Bertram, K.; Hudecova, S.; Krizanova, O. Calcium and ROS: A Mutual Interplay. *Redox Biol.* **2015**, *6*, 260–271. [CrossRef] [PubMed]
77. Massaad, C.A.; Klann, E. Reactive Oxygen Species in the Regulation of Synaptic Plasticity and Memory. *Antioxid. Redox Signal* **2011**, *14*, 2013–2054. [CrossRef] [PubMed]
78. Huddleston, A.T.; Tang, W.; Takeshima, H.; Hamilton, S.L.; Klann, E. Superoxide-Induced Potentiation in the Hippocampus Requires Activation of Ryanodine Receptor Type 3 and ERK. *J. Neurophysiol.* **2008**, *99*, 1565–1571. [CrossRef] [PubMed]
79. Doser, R.L.; Hoerndli, F.J. Regulation of Neuronal Excitability by Reactive Oxygen Species and Calcium Signaling: Insights into Brain Aging. *Curr. Res. Neurobiol.* **2021**, *2*, 100012. [CrossRef]
80. Zündorf, G.; Reiser, G. Calcium Dysregulation and Homeostasis of Neural Calcium in the Molecular Mechanisms of Neurodegenerative Diseases Provide Multiple Targets for Neuroprotection. *Antioxid. Redox Signal.* **2011**, *14*, 1275–1288. [CrossRef]
81. Walters, G.C.; Usachev, Y.M. Mitochondrial Calcium Cycling in Neuronal Function and Neurodegeneration. *Front. Cell Dev. Biol.* **2023**, *11*, 1094356. [CrossRef] [PubMed]
82. Surmeier, D.J. Calcium, Ageing, and Neuronal Vulnerability in Parkinson's Disease. *Lancet Neurol.* **2007**, *6*, 933–938. [CrossRef]
83. Guzman, J.N.; Sanchez-Padilla, J.; Wokosin, D.; Kondapalli, J.; Ilijic, E.; Schumacker, P.T.; Surmeier, D.J. Oxidant Stress Evoked by Pacemaking in Dopaminergic Neurons Is Attenuated by DJ-1. *Nature* **2010**, *468*, 696–700. [CrossRef]
84. Li, A.; Gao, M.; Liu, B.; Qin, Y.; Chen, L.; Liu, H.; Wu, H.; Gong, G. Mitochondrial Autophagy: Molecular Mechanisms and Implications for Cardiovascular Disease. *Cell Death Dis.* **2022**, *13*, 444. [CrossRef]
85. Woodcock, E.A.; Matkovich, S.J. Cardiomyocytes Structure, Function and Associated Pathologies. *Int. J. Biochem. Cell Biol.* **2005**, *37*, 1746–1751. [CrossRef]
86. Tian, R.; Colucci, W.S.; Arany, Z.; Bachschmid, M.M.; Ballinger, S.W.; Boudina, S.; Bruce, J.E.; Busija, D.W.; Dikalov, S.; Dorn, G.W.; et al. Unlocking the Secrets of Mitochondria in the Cardiovascular System: Path to a Cure in Heart Failure—A Report from the 2018 National Heart, Lung, and Blood Institute Workshop. *Circulation* **2019**, *140*, 1205–1216. [CrossRef] [PubMed]
87. Nguyen, B.Y.; Ruiz-Velasco, A.; Bui, T.; Collins, L.; Wang, X.; Liu, W. Mitochondrial Function in the Heart: The Insight into Mechanisms and Therapeutic Potentials. *Br. J. Pharmacol.* **2019**, *176*, 4302–4318. [CrossRef] [PubMed]
88. Zhao, Q.; Sun, Q.; Zhou, L.; Liu, K.; Jiao, K. Complex Regulation of Mitochondrial Function During Cardiac Development. *J. Am. Heart Assoc.* **2019**, *8*, e012731. [CrossRef]
89. Ingwall, J.S. Energy Metabolism in Heart Failure and Remodelling. *Cardiovasc. Res.* **2008**, *81*, 412–419. [CrossRef]
90. Neubauer, S. The Failing Heart—An Engine Out of Fuel. *N. Engl. J. Med.* **2007**, *356*, 1140–1151. [CrossRef] [PubMed]
91. Starling, R.C.; Hammer, D.F.; Altschuld, R.A. Human Myocardial ATP Content and in Vivo Contractile Function. *Mol. Cell. Biochem.* **1998**, *180*, 171–177. [CrossRef]
92. Murphy, E.; Ardehali, H.; Balaban, R.S.; DiLisa, F.; Dorn, G.W.; Kitsis, R.N.; Otsu, K.; Ping, P.; Rizzuto, R.; Sack, M.N.; et al. Mitochondrial Function, Biology, and Role in Disease: A Scientific Statement from the American Heart Association. *Circ. Res.* **2016**, *118*, 1960–1991. [CrossRef]

93. Tran, D.H.; Wang, Z.V. Glucose Metabolism in Cardiac Hypertrophy and Heart Failure. *J. Am. Heart Assoc.* **2019**, *8*, e012673. [CrossRef]
94. Liu, M.; Lv, J.; Pan, Z.; Wang, D.; Zhao, L.; Guo, X. Mitochondrial Dysfunction in Heart Failure and Its Therapeutic Implications. *Front. Cardiovasc. Med.* **2022**, *9*, 945142. [CrossRef] [PubMed]
95. Allard, M.F.; Schonekess, B.O.; Henning, S.L.; English, D.R.; Lopaschuk, G.D. Contribution of Oxidative Metabolism and Glycolysis to ATP Production in Hypertrophied Hearts. *Am. J. Physiol. Heart Circ. Physiol.* **1994**, *267*, H742–H750. [CrossRef]
96. Dedkova, E.N.; Blatter, L.A. Calcium Signaling in Cardiac Mitochondria. *J. Mol. Cell. Cardiol.* **2013**, *58*, 125–133. [CrossRef] [PubMed]
97. Santos, C.X.C.; Anilkumar, N.; Zhang, M.; Brewer, A.C.; Shah, A.M. Redox Signaling in Cardiac Myocytes. *Free Radic. Biol. Med.* **2011**, *50*, 777–793. [CrossRef] [PubMed]
98. Burgoyne, J.R.; Mongue-Din, H.; Eaton, P.; Shah, A.M. Redox Signaling in Cardiac Physiology and Pathology. *Circ. Res.* **2012**, *111*, 1091–1106. [CrossRef] [PubMed]
99. Dey, S.; DeMazumder, D.; Sidor, A.; Foster, D.B.; O'Rourke, B. Mitochondrial ROS Drive Sudden Cardiac Death and Chronic Proteome Remodeling in Heart Failure. *Circ. Res.* **2018**, *123*, 356–371. [CrossRef]
100. Jonckheere, A.I.; Smeitink, J.A.M.; Rodenburg, R.J.T. Mitochondrial ATP Synthase: Architecture, Function and Pathology. *J. Inherit. Metab. Dis.* **2012**, *35*, 211–225. [CrossRef]
101. Ahmad, M.; Wolberg, A.; Kahwaji, C.I. Biochemistry, Electron Transport Chain. In *StatPearls*; StatPearls Publishing: Treasure Island, FL, USA, 2023.
102. Juan, C.A.; Pérez de la Lastra, J.M.; Plou, F.J.; Pérez-Lebeña, E. The Chemistry of Reactive Oxygen Species (ROS) Revisited: Outlining Their Role in Biological Macromolecules (DNA, Lipids and Proteins) and Induced Pathologies. *Int. J. Mol. Sci.* **2021**, *22*, 4642. [CrossRef]
103. Requejo-Aguilar, R.; Bolaños, J.P. Mitochondrial Control of Cell Bioenergetics in Parkinson's Disease. *Free Radic. Biol. Med.* **2016**, *100*, 123–137. [CrossRef]
104. Zambon, F.; Cherubini, M.; Fernandes, H.J.R.; Lang, C.; Ryan, B.J.; Volpato, V.; Bengoa-Vergniory, N.; Vingill, S.; Attar, M.; Booth, H.D.E.; et al. Cellular α-Synuclein Pathology Is Associated with Bioenergetic Dysfunction in Parkinson's iPSC-Derived Dopamine Neurons. *Human. Mol. Genet.* **2019**, *28*, 2001–2013. [CrossRef]
105. Morciano, G.; Patergnani, S.; Bonora, M.; Pedriali, G.; Tarocco, A.; Bouhamida, E.; Marchi, S.; Ancora, G.; Anania, G.; Wieckowski, M.R.; et al. Mitophagy in Cardiovascular Diseases. *J. Clin. Med.* **2020**, *9*, 892. [CrossRef]
106. Hassanpour, S.H.; Dehghani, M.A.; Karami, S.Z. Study of Respiratory Chain Dysfunction in Heart Disease. *J. Cardiovasc. Thorac. Res.* **2018**, *10*, 1–13. [CrossRef]
107. Solana-Manrique, C.; Sanz, F.J.; Torregrosa, I.; Palomino-Schätzlein, M.; Hernández-Oliver, C.; Pineda-Lucena, A.; Paricio, N. Metabolic Alterations in a Drosophila Model of Parkinson's Disease Based on DJ-1 Deficiency. *Cells* **2022**, *11*, 331. [CrossRef] [PubMed]
108. Strope, T.A.; Birky, C.J.; Wilkins, H.M. The Role of Bioenergetics in Neurodegeneration. *Int. J. Mol. Sci.* **2022**, *23*, 9212. [CrossRef] [PubMed]
109. Cleland, N.R.W.; Al-Juboori, S.I.; Dobrinskikh, E.; Bruce, K.D. Altered Substrate Metabolism in Neurodegenerative Disease: New Insights from Metabolic Imaging. *J. Neuroinflammation* **2021**, *18*, 248. [CrossRef] [PubMed]
110. Zhao, Y.; Xu, H. Microglial Lactate Metabolism as a Potential Therapeutic Target for Alzheimer's Disease. *Mol. Neurodegener.* **2022**, *17*, 36. [CrossRef] [PubMed]
111. Marella, M.; Seo, B.B.; Yagi, T.; Matsuno-Yagi, A. Parkinson's Disease and Mitochondrial Complex I: A Perspective on the Ndi1 Therapy. *J. Bioenerg. Biomembr.* **2009**, *41*, 493–497. [CrossRef]
112. Onyango, I.; Bennett, J.; Stokin, G. Regulation of Neuronal Bioenergetics as a Therapeutic Strategy in Neurodegenerative Diseases. *Neural Regen. Res.* **2021**, *16*, 1467. [CrossRef]
113. Norat, P.; Soldozy, S.; Sokolowski, J.D.; Gorick, C.M.; Kumar, J.S.; Chae, Y.; Yağmurlu, K.; Prada, F.; Walker, M.; Levitt, M.R.; et al. Mitochondrial Dysfunction in Neurological Disorders: Exploring Mitochondrial Transplantation. *npj Regen. Med.* **2020**, *5*, 22. [CrossRef]
114. Scheubel, R.J.; Tostlebe, M.; Simm, A.; Rohrbach, S.; Prondzinsky, R.; Gellerich, F.N.; Silber, R.-E.; Holtz, J. Dysfunction of Mitochondrial Respiratory Chain Complex I in Human Failing Myocardium Is Not Due to Disturbed Mitochondrial Gene Expression. *J. Am. Coll. Cardiol.* **2002**, *40*, 2174–2181. [CrossRef]
115. Forte, M.; Palmerio, S.; Bianchi, F.; Volpe, M.; Rubattu, S. Mitochondrial Complex I Deficiency and Cardiovascular Diseases: Current Evidence and Future Directions. *J. Mol. Med.* **2019**, *97*, 579–591. [CrossRef]
116. Ventura-Clapier, R.; Garnier, A.; Veksler, V.; Joubert, F. Bioenergetics of the Failing Heart. *Biochim. Biophys. Acta BBA Mol. Cell Res.* **2011**, *1813*, 1360–1372. [CrossRef]
117. Walker, M.A.; Chavez, J.; Villet, O.; Tang, X.; Keller, A.; Bruce, J.E.; Tian, R. Acetylation of Muscle Creatine Kinase Negatively Impacts High-Energy Phosphotransfer in Heart Failure. *JCI Insight* **2021**, *6*, e144301. [CrossRef] [PubMed]
118. Mantle, D.; Heaton, R.A.; Hargreaves, I.P. Coenzyme Q10, Ageing and the Nervous System: An Overview. *Antioxidants* **2021**, *11*, 2. [CrossRef] [PubMed]

119. Grünewald, A.; Kumar, K.R.; Sue, C.M. New Insights into the Complex Role of Mitochondria in Parkinson's Disease. *Progress. Neurobiol.* **2019**, *177*, 73–93. [CrossRef] [PubMed]
120. The Parkinson Study Group QE3 Investigators; Beal, M.F.; Oakes, D.; Shoulson, I.; Henchcliffe, C.; Galpern, W.R.; Haas, R.; Juncos, J.L.; Nutt, J.G.; Voss, T.S.; et al. A Randomized Clinical Trial of High-Dosage Coenzyme Q10 in Early Parkinson Disease: No Evidence of Benefit. *JAMA Neurol.* **2014**, *71*, 543. [CrossRef] [PubMed]
121. Garjani, A.; Andalib, S.; Biabani, S.; Soraya, H.; Doustar, Y.; Garjani, A.; Maleki-Dizaji, N. Combined Atorvastatin and Coenzyme Q10 Improve the Left Ventricular Function in Isoproterenol-Induced Heart Failure in Rat. *Eur. J. Pharmacol.* **2011**, *666*, 135–141. [CrossRef]
122. Zheng, Q.; Ma, P.; Yang, P.; Zhai, S.; He, M.; Zhang, X.; Tu, Q.; Jiao, L.; Ye, L.; Feng, Z.; et al. Alpha Lipoic Acid Ameliorates Motor Deficits by Inhibiting Ferroptosis in Parkinson's Disease. *Neurosci. Lett.* **2023**, *810*, 137346. [CrossRef]
123. Wollin, S.D.; Jones, P.J.H. α-Lipoic Acid and Cardiovascular Disease. *J. Nutr.* **2003**, *133*, 3327–3330. [CrossRef]
124. Bhullar, S.K.; Dhalla, N.S. Status of Mitochondrial Oxidative Phosphorylation during the Development of Heart Failure. *Antioxidants* **2023**, *12*, 1941. [CrossRef]
125. Li, J.; Chen, L.; Qin, Q.; Wang, D.; Zhao, J.; Gao, H.; Yuan, X.; Zhang, J.; Zou, Y.; Mao, Z.; et al. Upregulated Hexokinase 2 Expression Induces the Apoptosis of Dopaminergic Neurons by Promoting Lactate Production in Parkinson's Disease. *Neurobiol. Dis.* **2022**, *163*, 105605. [CrossRef]
126. Deng, J.; Jiang, Y.; Chen, Z.B.; Rhee, J.-W.; Deng, Y.; Wang, Z.V. Mitochondrial Dysfunction in Cardiac Arrhythmias. *Cells* **2023**, *12*, 679. [CrossRef]
127. Li, J.-L.; Lin, T.-Y.; Chen, P.-L.; Guo, T.-N.; Huang, S.-Y.; Chen, C.-H.; Lin, C.-H.; Chan, C.-C. Mitochondrial Function and Parkinson's Disease: From the Perspective of the Electron Transport Chain. *Front. Mol. Neurosci.* **2021**, *14*, 797833. [CrossRef] [PubMed]
128. Moris, D.; Spartalis, M.; Spartalis, E.; Karachaliou, G.-S.; Karaolanis, G.I.; Tsourouflis, G.; Tsilimigras, D.I.; Tzatzaki, E.; Theocharis, S. The Role of Reactive Oxygen Species in the Pathophysiology of Cardiovascular Diseases and the Clinical Significance of Myocardial Redox. *Ann. Transl. Med.* **2017**, *5*, 326. [CrossRef] [PubMed]
129. Dias, V.; Junn, E.; Mouradian, M.M. The Role of Oxidative Stress in Parkinson's Disease. *J. Park. Dis.* **2013**, *3*, 461–491. [CrossRef] [PubMed]
130. Pozo Devoto, V.M.; Falzone, T.L. Mitochondrial Dynamics in Parkinson's Disease: A Role for α-Synuclein? *Dis. Models Mech.* **2017**, *10*, 1075–1087. [CrossRef] [PubMed]
131. Tokuyama, T.; Yanagi, S. Role of Mitochondrial Dynamics in Heart Diseases. *Genes* **2023**, *14*, 1876. [CrossRef] [PubMed]
132. Werbner, B.; Tavakoli-Rouzbehani, O.M.; Fatahian, A.N.; Boudina, S. The Dynamic Interplay between Cardiac Mitochondrial Health and Myocardial Structural Remodeling in Metabolic Heart Disease, Aging, and Heart Failure. *J. Cardiovasc. Aging* **2023**, *3*, 9. [CrossRef]
133. Asghar, M.; Odeh, A.; Fattahi, A.J.; Henriksson, A.E.; Miglar, A.; Khosousi, S.; Svenningsson, P. Mitochondrial Biogenesis, Telomere Length and Cellular Senescence in Parkinson's Disease and Lewy Body Dementia. *Sci. Rep.* **2022**, *12*, 17578. [CrossRef]
134. Castillo-Quan, J.I. Parkin' Control: Regulation of PGC-1α through PARIS in Parkinson's Disease. *Dis. Model. Mech.* **2011**, *4*, 427–429. [CrossRef]
135. Xu, H.; Cui, S.; Zhang, Y.; Ren, J. Mitochondrial Ca2+ Regulation in the Etiology of Heart Failure: Physiological and Pathophysiological Implications. *Acta Pharmacol. Sin.* **2020**, *41*, 1301–1309. [CrossRef]
136. Quinn, P.M.J.; Moreira, P.I.; Ambrósio, A.F.; Alves, C.H. PINK1/PARKIN Signalling in Neurodegeneration and Neuroinflammation. *Acta Neuropathol. Commun.* **2020**, *8*, 189. [CrossRef]
137. Yang, Y.; Li, T.; Li, Z.; Liu, N.; Yan, Y.; Liu, B. Role of Mitophagy in Cardiovascular Disease. *Aging Dis.* **2020**, *11*, 419. [CrossRef] [PubMed]
138. Millichap, L.E.; Damiani, E.; Tiano, L.; Hargreaves, I.P. Targetable Pathways for Alleviating Mitochondrial Dysfunction in Neurodegeneration of Metabolic and Non-Metabolic Diseases. *Int. J. Mol. Sci.* **2021**, *22*, 11444. [CrossRef] [PubMed]
139. Dehay, B.; Martinez-Vicente, M.; Caldwell, G.A.; Caldwell, K.A.; Yue, Z.; Cookson, M.R.; Klein, C.; Vila, M.; Bezard, E. Lysosomal Impairment in Parkinson's Disease. *Mov. Disord.* **2013**, *28*, 725–732. [CrossRef] [PubMed]
140. Shamoto-Nagai, M.; Maruyama, W.; Hashizume, Y.; Yoshida, M.; Osawa, T.; Riederer, P.; Naoi, M. In Parkinsonian Substantia Nigra, α-Synuclein Is Modified by Acrolein, a Lipid-Peroxidation Product, and Accumulates in the Dopamine Neurons with Inhibition of Proteasome Activity. *J. Neural Transm.* **2007**, *114*, 1559–1567. [CrossRef]
141. Girotti, A.W. Lipid Hydroperoxide Generation, Turnover, and Effector Action in Biological Systems. *J. Lipid Res.* **1998**, *39*, 1529–1542. [CrossRef]
142. Keane, P.C.; Kurzawa, M.; Blain, P.G.; Morris, C.M. Mitochondrial Dysfunction in Parkinson's Disease. *Park. Dis.* **2011**, *2011*, 1–18. [CrossRef]
143. Chen, X.J.; Butow, R.A. The Organization and Inheritance of the Mitochondrial Genome. *Nat. Rev. Genet.* **2005**, *6*, 815–825. [CrossRef]
144. Ide, T.; Tsutsui, H.; Hayashidani, S.; Kang, D.; Suematsu, N.; Nakamura, K.; Utsumi, H.; Hamasaki, N.; Takeshita, A. Mitochondrial DNA Damage and Dysfunction Associated With Oxidative Stress in Failing Hearts After Myocardial Infarction. *Circ. Res.* **2001**, *88*, 529–535. [CrossRef]

145. Dabravolski, S.A.; Khotina, V.A.; Sukhorukov, V.N.; Kalmykov, V.A.; Mikhaleva, L.M.; Orekhov, A.N. The Role of Mitochondrial DNA Mutations in Cardiovascular Diseases. *Int. J. Mol. Sci.* **2022**, *23*, 952. [CrossRef]
146. Qi, R.; Sammler, E.; Gonzalez-Hunt, C.P.; Barraza, I.; Pena, N.; Rouanet, J.P.; Naaldijk, Y.; Goodson, S.; Fuzzati, M.; Blandini, F.; et al. A Blood-Based Marker of Mitochondrial DNA Damage in Parkinson's Disease. *Sci. Transl. Med.* **2023**, *15*, eabo1557. [CrossRef]
147. Buneeva, O.; Fedchenko, V.; Kopylov, A.; Medvedev, A. Mitochondrial Dysfunction in Parkinson's Disease: Focus on Mitochondrial DNA. *Biomedicines* **2020**, *8*, 591. [CrossRef] [PubMed]
148. DeBalsi, K.L.; Hoff, K.E.; Copeland, W.C. Role of the Mitochondrial DNA Replication Machinery in Mitochondrial DNA Mutagenesis, Aging and Age-Related Diseases. *Ageing Res. Rev.* **2017**, *33*, 89–104. [CrossRef] [PubMed]
149. Mandavilli, B.S.; Ali, S.F.; Van Houten, B. DNA Damage in Brain Mitochondria Caused by Aging and MPTP Treatment. *Brain Res.* **2000**, *885*, 45–52. [CrossRef] [PubMed]
150. Dodson, M.W.; Guo, M. Pink1, Parkin, DJ-1 and Mitochondrial Dysfunction in Parkinson's Disease. *Curr. Opin. Neurobiol.* **2007**, *17*, 331–337. [CrossRef]
151. Castelo Rueda, M.P.; Raftopoulou, A.; Gögele, M.; Borsche, M.; Emmert, D.; Fuchsberger, C.; Hantikainen, E.M.; Vukovic, V.; Klein, C.; Pramstaller, P.P.; et al. Frequency of Heterozygous Parkin (PRKN) Variants and Penetrance of Parkinson's Disease Risk Markers in the Population-Based CHRIS Cohort. *Front. Neurol.* **2021**, *12*, 706145. [CrossRef]
152. Vizziello, M.; Borellini, L.; Franco, G.; Ardolino, G. Disruption of Mitochondrial Homeostasis: The Role of PINK1 in Parkinson's Disease. *Cells* **2021**, *10*, 3022. [CrossRef]
153. Ge, P.; Dawson, V.L.; Dawson, T.M. PINK1 and Parkin Mitochondrial Quality Control: A Source of Regional Vulnerability in Parkinson's Disease. *Mol. Neurodegener.* **2020**, *15*, 20. [CrossRef]
154. Wu, Y.; Jiang, T.; Hua, J.; Xiong, Z.; Dai, K.; Chen, H.; Li, L.; Peng, J.; Peng, X.; Zheng, Z.; et al. PINK1/Parkin-Mediated Mitophagy in Cardiovascular Disease: From Pathogenesis to Novel Therapy. *Int. J. Cardiol.* **2022**, *361*, 61–69. [CrossRef]
155. Rüb, C.; Wilkening, A.; Voos, W. Mitochondrial Quality Control by the Pink1/Parkin System. *Cell Tissue Res.* **2017**, *367*, 111–123. [CrossRef]
156. Moisoi, N.; Fedele, V.; Edwards, J.; Martins, L.M. Loss of PINK1 Enhances Neurodegeneration in a Mouse Model of Parkinson's Disease Triggered by Mitochondrial Stress. *Neuropharmacology* **2014**, *77*, 350–357. [CrossRef]
157. Noda, S.; Sato, S.; Fukuda, T.; Tada, N.; Uchiyama, Y.; Tanaka, K.; Hattori, N. Loss of Parkin Contributes to Mitochondrial Turnover and Dopaminergic Neuronal Loss in Aged Mice. *Neurobiol. Dis.* **2020**, *136*, 104717. [CrossRef] [PubMed]
158. Kubli, D.A.; Zhang, X.; Lee, Y.; Hanna, R.A.; Quinsay, M.N.; Nguyen, C.K.; Jimenez, R.; Petrosyan, S.; Murphy, A.N.; Gustafsson, Å.B. Parkin Protein Deficiency Exacerbates Cardiac Injury and Reduces Survival Following Myocardial Infarction. *J. Biol. Chem.* **2013**, *288*, 915–926. [CrossRef]
159. Billia, F.; Hauck, L.; Konecny, F.; Rao, V.; Shen, J.; Mak, T.W. PTEN-Inducible Kinase 1 (PINK1)/Park6 Is Indispensable for Normal Heart Function. *Proc. Natl. Acad. Sci. USA* **2011**, *108*, 9572–9577. [CrossRef] [PubMed]
160. Batelli, S.; Invernizzi, R.W.; Negro, A.; Calcagno, E.; Rodilossi, S.; Forloni, G.; Albani, D. The Parkinson's Disease-Related Protein DJ-1 Protects Dopaminergic Neurons in Vivo and Cultured Cells from Alpha-Synuclein and 6-Hydroxydopamine Toxicity. *Neurodegener. Dis.* **2015**, *15*, 13–23. [CrossRef]
161. Kim, R.H.; Smith, P.D.; Aleyasin, H.; Hayley, S.; Mount, M.P.; Pownall, S.; Wakeham, A.; You-Ten, A.J.; Kalia, S.K.; Horne, P.; et al. Hypersensitivity of DJ-1-Deficient Mice to 1-Methyl-4-Phenyl-1,2,3,6-Tetrahydropyrindine (MPTP) and Oxidative Stress. *Proc. Natl. Acad. Sci. USA* **2005**, *102*, 5215–5220. [CrossRef] [PubMed]
162. Repici, M.; Giorgini, F. DJ-1 in Parkinson's Disease: Clinical Insights and Therapeutic Perspectives. *J. Clin. Med.* **2019**, *8*, 1377. [CrossRef] [PubMed]
163. Tsoporis, J.N.; Drosatos, I.-A.; Gupta, S.; Amatullah, H.; Izhar, S.; Dos Santos, C.C.; Salpeas, V.; Rigopoulos, A.G.; Toumpoulis, I.K.; Triantafyllis, A.S.; et al. Cytoprotective Mechanisms of DJ-1: Implications in Cardiac Pathophysiology. *Molecules* **2021**, *26*, 3795. [CrossRef]
164. Dongworth, R.K.; Mukherjee, U.A.; Hall, A.R.; Astin, R.; Ong, S.-B.; Yao, Z.; Dyson, A.; Szabadkai, G.; Davidson, S.M.; Yellon, D.M.; et al. DJ-1 Protects against Cell Death Following Acute Cardiac Ischemia–Reperfusion Injury. *Cell Death Dis.* **2014**, *5*, e1082. [CrossRef]
165. Gallinat, A.; Mendieta, G.; Vilahur, G.; Padró, T.; Badimon, L. DJ-1 Administration Exerts Cardioprotection in a Mouse Model of Acute Myocardial Infarction. *Front. Pharmacol.* **2022**, *13*, 1002755. [CrossRef]
166. Tilokani, L.; Nagashima, S.; Paupe, V.; Prudent, J. Mitochondrial Dynamics: Overview of Molecular Mechanisms. *Essays Biochem.* **2018**, *62*, 341–360. [CrossRef]
167. Poznyak, A.V.; Kirichenko, T.V.; Borisov, E.E.; Shakhpazyan, N.K.; Kartuesov, A.G.; Orekhov, A.N. Mitochondrial Implications in Cardiovascular Aging and Diseases: The Specific Role of Mitochondrial Dynamics and Shifts. *Int. J. Mol. Sci.* **2022**, *23*, 2951. [CrossRef] [PubMed]
168. Li, A.; Gao, M.; Jiang, W.; Qin, Y.; Gong, G. Mitochondrial Dynamics in Adult Cardiomyocytes and Heart Diseases. *Front. Cell Dev. Biol.* **2020**, *8*, 584800. [CrossRef] [PubMed]

169. Jin, J.; Wei, X.; Zhi, X.; Wang, X.; Meng, D. Drp1-Dependent Mitochondrial Fission in Cardiovascular Disease. *Acta Pharmacol. Sin.* **2021**, *42*, 655–664. [CrossRef]
170. Vásquez-Trincado, C.; García-Carvajal, I.; Pennanen, C.; Parra, V.; Hill, J.A.; Rothermel, B.A.; Lavandero, S. Mitochondrial Dynamics, Mitophagy and Cardiovascular Disease. *J. Physiol.* **2016**, *594*, 509–525. [CrossRef]
171. Tong, M.; Zablocki, D.; Sadoshima, J. The Role of Drp1 in Mitophagy and Cell Death in the Heart. *J. Mol. Cell. Cardiol.* **2020**, *142*, 138–145. [CrossRef] [PubMed]
172. Hu, Q.; Zhang, H.; Gutiérrez Cortés, N.; Wu, D.; Wang, P.; Zhang, J.; Mattison, J.A.; Smith, E.; Bettcher, L.F.; Wang, M.; et al. Increased Drp1 Acetylation by Lipid Overload Induces Cardiomyocyte Death and Heart Dysfunction. *Circ. Res.* **2020**, *126*, 456–470. [CrossRef]
173. Portz, P.; Lee, M.K. Changes in Drp1 Function and Mitochondrial Morphology Are Associated with the α-Synuclein Pathology in a Transgenic Mouse Model of Parkinson's Disease. *Cells* **2021**, *10*, 885. [CrossRef]
174. Berthet, A.; Margolis, E.B.; Zhang, J.; Hsieh, I.; Zhang, J.; Hnasko, T.S.; Ahmad, J.; Edwards, R.H.; Sesaki, H.; Huang, E.J.; et al. Loss of Mitochondrial Fission Depletes Axonal Mitochondria in Midbrain Dopamine Neurons. *J. Neurosci.* **2014**, *34*, 14304–14317. [CrossRef]
175. Gao, X.-Y.; Yang, T.; Gu, Y.; Sun, X.-H. Mitochondrial Dysfunction in Parkinson's Disease: From Mechanistic Insights to Therapy. *Front. Aging Neurosci.* **2022**, *14*, 885500. [CrossRef]
176. Bastian, P.; Dulski, J.; Roszmann, A.; Jacewicz, D.; Kuban-Jankowska, A.; Slawek, J.; Wozniak, M.; Gorska-Ponikowska, M. Regulation of Mitochondrial Dynamics in Parkinson's Disease—Is 2-Methoxyestradiol a Missing Piece? *Antioxidants* **2021**, *10*, 248. [CrossRef]
177. Forte, M.; Schirone, L.; Ameri, P.; Basso, C.; Catalucci, D.; Modica, J.; Chimenti, C.; Crotti, L.; Frati, G.; Rubattu, S.; et al. The Role of Mitochondrial Dynamics in Cardiovascular Diseases. *Br. J. Pharmacol.* **2021**, *178*, 2060–2076. [CrossRef] [PubMed]
178. Chen, L.; Gong, Q.; Stice, J.P.; Knowlton, A.A. Mitochondrial OPA1, Apoptosis, and Heart Failure. *Cardiovasc. Res.* **2009**, *84*, 91–99. [CrossRef]
179. Papanicolaou, K.N.; Khairallah, R.J.; Ngoh, G.A.; Chikando, A.; Luptak, I.; O'Shea, K.M.; Riley, D.D.; Lugus, J.J.; Colucci, W.S.; Lederer, W.J.; et al. Mitofusin-2 Maintains Mitochondrial Structure and Contributes to Stress-Induced Permeability Transition in Cardiac Myocytes. *Mol. Cell. Biol.* **2011**, *31*, 1309–1328. [CrossRef] [PubMed]
180. Knowlton, A.A.; Chen, L.; Malik, Z.A. Heart Failure and Mitochondrial Dysfunction: The Role of Mitochondrial Fission/Fusion Abnormalities and New Therapeutic Strategies. *J. Cardiovasc. Pharmacol.* **2014**, *63*, 196–206. [CrossRef]
181. Uchikado, Y.; Ikeda, Y.; Ohishi, M. Current Understanding of the Pivotal Role of Mitochondrial Dynamics in Cardiovascular Diseases and Senescence. *Front. Cardiovasc. Med.* **2022**, *9*, 905072. [CrossRef] [PubMed]
182. Iannielli, A.; Bido, S.; Folladori, L.; Segnali, A.; Cancellieri, C.; Maresca, A.; Massimino, L.; Rubio, A.; Morabito, G.; Caporali, L.; et al. Pharmacological Inhibition of Necroptosis Protects from Dopaminergic Neuronal Cell Death in Parkinson's Disease Models. *Cell Rep.* **2018**, *22*, 2066–2079. [CrossRef]
183. Chen, Y.; Dorn, G.W. PINK1-Phosphorylated Mitofusin 2 Is a Parkin Receptor for Culling Damaged Mitochondria. *Science* **2013**, *340*, 471–475. [CrossRef]
184. Valdinocci, D.; Simões, R.F.; Kovarova, J.; Cunha-Oliveira, T.; Neuzil, J.; Pountney, D.L. Intracellular and Intercellular Mitochondrial Dynamics in Parkinson's Disease. *Front. Neurosci.* **2019**, *13*, 930. [CrossRef]
185. Su, Z.; Li, C.; Wang, H.; Zheng, M.; Chen, Q. Inhibition of DRP1-Dependent Mitochondrial Fission by Mdivi-1 Alleviates Atherosclerosis through the Modulation of M1 Polarization. *J. Transl. Med.* **2023**, *21*, 427. [CrossRef]
186. He, T.; Lin, X.; Su, A.; Zhang, Y.; Xing, Z.; Mi, L.; Wei, T.; Li, Z.; Wu, W. Mitochondrial Dysfunction-Targeting Therapeutics of Natural Products in Parkinson's Disease. *Front. Pharmacol.* **2023**, *14*, 1117337. [CrossRef]
187. Koklesova, L.; Liskova, A.; Samec, M.; Zhai, K.; AL-Ishaq, R.K.; Bugos, O.; Šudomová, M.; Biringer, K.; Pec, M.; Adamkov, M.; et al. Protective Effects of Flavonoids Against Mitochondriopathies and Associated Pathologies: Focus on the Predictive Approach and Personalized Prevention. *Int. J. Mol. Sci.* **2021**, *22*, 8649. [CrossRef] [PubMed]
188. Qi, X.; Qvit, N.; Su, Y.-C.; Mochly-Rosen, D. Novel Drp1 Inhibitor Diminishes Aberrant Mitochondrial Fission and Neurotoxicity. *J. Cell Sci.* **2012**, *126*, 789–802. [CrossRef]
189. Filichia, E.; Hoffer, B.; Qi, X.; Luo, Y. Inhibition of Drp1 Mitochondrial Translocation Provides Neural Protection in Dopaminergic System in a Parkinson's Disease Model Induced by MPTP. *Sci. Rep.* **2016**, *6*, 32656. [CrossRef] [PubMed]
190. Popov, L. Mitochondrial Biogenesis: An Update. *J. Cell. Mol. Medi* **2020**, *24*, 4892–4899. [CrossRef]
191. Jornayvaz, F.R.; Shulman, G.I. Regulation of Mitochondrial Biogenesis. *Essays Biochem.* **2010**, *47*, 69–84. [CrossRef] [PubMed]
192. Chen, C.; Turnbull, D.M.; Reeve, A.K. Mitochondrial Dysfunction in Parkinson's Disease—Cause or Consequence? *Biology* **2019**, *8*, 38. [CrossRef]
193. Sandhir, R.; Singhal, N.; Garg, P. Increasing Resveratrol Bioavailability: A Therapeutic Challenge Focusing on the Mitochondria. In *Mitochondrial Dysfunction and Nanotherapeutics*; Elsevier: Amsterdam, The Netherlands, 2021; pp. 349–384, ISBN 978-0-323-85666-9.
194. Garnier, A.; Fortin, D.; Deloménie, C.; Momken, I.; Veksler, V.; Ventura-Clapier, R. Depressed Mitochondrial Transcription Factors and Oxidative Capacity in Rat Failing Cardiac and Skeletal Muscles. *J. Physiol.* **2003**, *551*, 491–501. [CrossRef]
195. Schilling, J.; Kelly, D.P. The PGC-1 Cascade as a Therapeutic Target for Heart Failure. *J. Mol. Cell. Cardiol.* **2011**, *51*, 578–583. [CrossRef]
196. Riehle, C.; Abel, E.D. PGC-1 Proteins and Heart Failure. *Trends Cardiovasc. Med.* **2012**, *22*, 98–105. [CrossRef]

197. Karamanlidis, G.; Bautista-Hernandez, V.; Fynn-Thompson, F.; Del Nido, P.; Tian, R. Impaired Mitochondrial Biogenesis Precedes Heart Failure in Right Ventricular Hypertrophy in Congenital Heart Disease. *Circ. Heart Fail.* **2011**, *4*, 707–713. [CrossRef]
198. Oka, S.; Sabry, A.D.; Cawley, K.M.; Warren, J.S. Multiple Levels of PGC-1α Dysregulation in Heart Failure. *Front. Cardiovasc. Med.* **2020**, *7*, 2. [CrossRef]
199. Zheng, B.; Liao, Z.; Locascio, J.J.; Lesniak, K.A.; Roderick, S.S.; Watt, M.L.; Eklund, A.C.; Zhang-James, Y.; Kim, P.D.; Hauser, M.A.; et al. *PGC-1 α*, A Potential Therapeutic Target for Early Intervention in Parkinson's Disease. *Sci. Transl. Med.* **2010**, *2*, 52ra73. [CrossRef] [PubMed]
200. Lagouge, M.; Argmann, C.; Gerhart-Hines, Z.; Meziane, H.; Lerin, C.; Daussin, F.; Messadeq, N.; Milne, J.; Lambert, P.; Elliott, P.; et al. Resveratrol Improves Mitochondrial Function and Protects against Metabolic Disease by Activating SIRT1 and PGC-1α. *Cell* **2006**, *127*, 1109–1122. [CrossRef] [PubMed]
201. Li, X.; Feng, Y.; Wang, X.-X.; Truong, D.; Wu, Y.-C. The Critical Role of SIRT1 in Parkinson's Disease: Mechanism and Therapeutic Considerations. *Aging Dis.* **2020**, *11*, 1608. [CrossRef] [PubMed]
202. Li, P.; Song, X.; Zhang, D.; Guo, N.; Wu, C.; Chen, K.; Liu, Y.; Yuan, L.; Chen, X.; Huang, X. Resveratrol Improves Left Ventricular Remodeling in Chronic Kidney Disease via Sirt1-mediated Regulation of FoxO1 Activity and MnSOD Expression. *BioFactors* **2020**, *46*, 168–179. [CrossRef]
203. Dyck, G.; Raj, P.; Zieroth, S.; Dyck, J.; Ezekowitz, J. The Effects of Resveratrol in Patients with Cardiovascular Disease and Heart Failure: A Narrative Review. *Int. J. Mol. Sci.* **2019**, *20*, 904. [CrossRef]
204. Peng, K.; Tao, Y.; Zhang, J.; Wang, J.; Ye, F.; Dan, G.; Zhao, Y.; Cai, Y.; Zhao, J.; Wu, Q.; et al. Resveratrol Regulates Mitochondrial Biogenesis and Fission/Fusion to Attenuate Rotenone-Induced Neurotoxicity. *Oxidative Med. Cell. Longev.* **2016**, *2016*, 1–12. [CrossRef] [PubMed]
205. Su, C.-F.; Jiang, L.; Zhang, X.-W.; Iyaswamy, A.; Li, M. Resveratrol in Rodent Models of Parkinson's Disease: A Systematic Review of Experimental Studies. *Front. Pharmacol.* **2021**, *12*, 644219. [CrossRef]
206. Donniacuo, M.; Urbanek, K.; Nebbioso, A.; Sodano, L.; Gallo, L.; Altucci, L.; Rinaldi, B. Cardioprotective Effect of a Moderate and Prolonged Exercise Training Involves Sirtuin Pathway. *Life Sci.* **2019**, *222*, 140–147. [CrossRef]
207. Liu, Y.; Yan, T.; Chu, J.M.-T.; Chen, Y.; Dunnett, S.; Ho, Y.-S.; Wong, G.T.-C.; Chang, R.C.-C. The Beneficial Effects of Physical Exercise in the Brain and Related Pathophysiological Mechanisms in Neurodegenerative Diseases. *Lab. Investig.* **2019**, *99*, 943–957. [CrossRef]
208. Giorgi, C.; Marchi, S.; Pinton, P. The Machineries, Regulation and Cellular Functions of Mitochondrial Calcium. *Nat. Rev. Mol. Cell Biol.* **2018**, *19*, 713–730. [CrossRef]
209. Lai, L.; Qiu, H. The Physiological and Pathological Roles of Mitochondrial Calcium Uptake in Heart. *Int. J. Mol. Sci.* **2020**, *21*, 7689. [CrossRef]
210. Popoiu, T.-A.; Maack, C.; Bertero, E. Mitochondrial Calcium Signaling and Redox Homeostasis in Cardiac Health and Disease. *Front. Mol. Med.* **2023**, *3*, 1235188. [CrossRef] [PubMed]
211. Santulli, G.; Xie, W.; Reiken, S.R.; Marks, A.R. Mitochondrial Calcium Overload Is a Key Determinant in Heart Failure. *Proc. Natl. Acad. Sci. USA* **2015**, *112*, 11389–11394. [CrossRef] [PubMed]
212. Luongo, T.S.; Lambert, J.P.; Yuan, A.; Zhang, X.; Gross, P.; Song, J.; Shanmughapriya, S.; Gao, E.; Jain, M.; Houser, S.R.; et al. The Mitochondrial Calcium Uniporter Matches Energetic Supply with Cardiac Workload during Stress and Modulates Permeability Transition. *Cell Rep.* **2015**, *12*, 23–34. [CrossRef]
213. Petersen, C.E.; Sun, J.; Silva, K.; Kosmach, A.; Balaban, R.S.; Murphy, E. Increased Mitochondrial Free Ca2+ during Ischemia Is Suppressed, but Not Eliminated by, Germline Deletion of the Mitochondrial Ca2+ Uniporter. *Cell Rep.* **2023**, *42*, 112735. [CrossRef] [PubMed]
214. Wood-Kaczmar, A.; Deas, E.; Wood, N.W.; Abramov, A.Y. The Role of the Mitochondrial NCX in the Mechanism of Neurodegeneration in Parkinson's Disease. In *Sodium Calcium Exchange: A Growing Spectrum of Pathophysiological Implications*; Annunziato, L., Ed.; Advances in Experimental Medicine and Biology; Springer US: Boston, MA, USA, 2013; Volume 961, pp. 241–249, ISBN 978-1-4614-4755-9.
215. Scorziello, A.; Borzacchiello, D.; Sisalli, M.J.; Di Martino, R.; Morelli, M.; Feliciello, A. Mitochondrial Homeostasis and Signaling in Parkinson's Disease. *Front. Aging Neurosci.* **2020**, *12*, 100. [CrossRef]
216. Gandhi, S.; Wood-Kaczmar, A.; Yao, Z.; Plun-Favreau, H.; Deas, E.; Klupsch, K.; Downward, J.; Latchman, D.S.; Tabrizi, S.J.; Wood, N.W.; et al. PINK1-Associated Parkinson's Disease Is Caused by Neuronal Vulnerability to Calcium-Induced Cell Death. *Mol. Cell* **2009**, *33*, 627–638. [CrossRef]
217. Kostic, M.; Ludtmann, M.H.R.; Bading, H.; Hershfinkel, M.; Steer, E.; Chu, C.T.; Abramov, A.Y.; Sekler, I. PKA Phosphorylation of NCLX Reverses Mitochondrial Calcium Overload and Depolarization, Promoting Survival of PINK1-Deficient Dopaminergic Neurons. *Cell Rep.* **2015**, *13*, 376–386. [CrossRef]
218. Matuz-Mares, D.; González-Andrade, M.; Araiza-Villanueva, M.G.; Vilchis-Landeros, M.M.; Vázquez-Meza, H. Mitochondrial Calcium: Effects of Its Imbalance in Disease. *Antioxidants* **2022**, *11*, 801. [CrossRef]
219. McWilliams, T.G.; Prescott, A.R.; Allen, G.F.G.; Tamjar, J.; Munson, M.J.; Thomson, C.; Muqit, M.M.K.; Ganley, I.G. *Mito* -QC Illuminates Mitophagy and Mitochondrial Architecture in Vivo. *J. Cell Biol.* **2016**, *214*, 333–345. [CrossRef]
220. Ma, K.; Chen, G.; Li, W.; Kepp, O.; Zhu, Y.; Chen, Q. Mitophagy, Mitochondrial Homeostasis, and Cell Fate. *Front. Cell Dev. Biol.* **2020**, *8*, 467. [CrossRef] [PubMed]

221. Thomas, R.L.; Gustafsson, A.B. Mitochondrial Autophagy--an Essential Quality Control Mechanism for Myocardial Homeostasis. *Circ. J.* **2013**, *77*, 2449–2454. [CrossRef] [PubMed]
222. Shefa, U.; Jeong, N.; Song, I.; Chung, H.-J.; Kim, D.; Jung, J.; Huh, Y. Mitophagy Links Oxidative Stress Conditions and Neurodegenerative Diseases. *Neural Regen. Res.* **2019**, *14*, 749. [CrossRef]
223. Doblado, L.; Lueck, C.; Rey, C.; Samhan-Arias, A.K.; Prieto, I.; Stacchiotti, A.; Monsalve, M. Mitophagy in Human Diseases. *Int. J. Mol. Sci.* **2021**, *22*, 3903. [CrossRef] [PubMed]
224. Luo, H.; Zhang, R.; Krigman, J.; McAdams, A.; Ozgen, S.; Sun, N. A Healthy Heart and a Healthy Brain: Looking at Mitophagy. *Front. Cell Dev. Biol.* **2020**, *8*, 294. [CrossRef]
225. Bravo-San Pedro, J.M.; Kroemer, G.; Galluzzi, L. Autophagy and Mitophagy in Cardiovascular Disease. *Circ. Res.* **2017**, *120*, 1812–1824. [CrossRef]
226. Agarwal, S.; Muqit, M.M.K. PTEN-Induced Kinase 1 (PINK1) and Parkin: Unlocking a Mitochondrial Quality Control Pathway Linked to Parkinson's Disease. *Curr. Opin. Neurobiol.* **2022**, *72*, 111–119. [CrossRef]
227. Clark, E.H.; Vázquez De La Torre, A.; Hoshikawa, T.; Briston, T. Targeting Mitophagy in Parkinson's Disease. *J. Biol. Chem.* **2021**, *296*, 100209. [CrossRef]
228. Xiao, B.; Kuruvilla, J.; Tan, E.-K. Mitophagy and Reactive Oxygen Species Interplay in Parkinson's Disease. *npj Park. Dis.* **2022**, *8*, 135. [CrossRef]
229. Mizuno, Y.; Hattori, N.; Mori, H.; Suzuki, T.; Tanaka, K. Parkin and Parkinson s Disease. *Curr. Opin. Neurol.* **2001**, *14*, 477–482. [CrossRef] [PubMed]
230. Zhu, F.; Fan, M.; Xu, Z.; Cai, Y.; Chen, Y.; Yu, S.; Zeng, L. Neuroprotective effect of rapamycin against Parkinson's disease in mice. *Zhejiang Da Xue Xue Bao Yi Xue Ban.* **2018**, *47*, 465–472. [CrossRef] [PubMed]
231. Gao, G.; Chen, W.; Yan, M.; Liu, J.; Luo, H.; Wang, C.; Yang, P. Rapamycin Regulates the Balance between Cardiomyocyte Apoptosis and Autophagy in Chronic Heart Failure by Inhibiting mTOR Signaling. *Int. J. Mol. Med.* **2020**, *45*, 195–209. [CrossRef] [PubMed]
232. Seabright, A.P.; Fine, N.H.F.; Barlow, J.P.; Lord, S.O.; Musa, I.; Gray, A.; Bryant, J.A.; Banzhaf, M.; Lavery, G.G.; Hardie, D.G.; et al. AMPK Activation Induces Mitophagy and Promotes Mitochondrial Fission While Activating TBK1 in a PINK1-Parkin Independent Manner. *FASEB J.* **2020**, *34*, 6284–6301. [CrossRef]
233. Tian, Y.; Song, W.; Li, D.; Cai, L.; Zhao, Y. Resveratrol as A Natural Regulator Of Autophagy For Prevention And Treatment Of Cancer. *OncoTargets Ther.* **2019**, *12*, 8601–8609. [CrossRef]
234. De Santi, M.; Baldelli, G.; Diotallevi, A.; Galluzzi, L.; Schiavano, G.F.; Brandi, G. Metformin Prevents Cell Tumorigenesis through Autophagy-Related Cell Death. *Sci. Rep.* **2019**, *9*, 66. [CrossRef]
235. Herman, R.; Kravos, N.A.; Jensterle, M.; Janež, A.; Dolžan, V. Metformin and Insulin Resistance: A Review of the Underlying Mechanisms behind Changes in GLUT4-Mediated Glucose Transport. *Int. J. Mol. Sci.* **2022**, *23*, 1264. [CrossRef]
236. Alrouji, M.; Al-kuraishy, H.M.; Al-Gareeb, A.I.; Ashour, N.A.; Jabir, M.S.; Negm, W.A.; Batiha, G.E.-S. Metformin Role in Parkinson's Disease: A Double-Sword Effect. *Mol. Cell Biochem.* **2023**, *479*, 975–991. [CrossRef] [PubMed]
237. Li, J.Z.; Li, Y.R. Cardiovascular Protection by Metformin: Latest Advances in Basic and Clinical Research. *Cardiology* **2023**, *148*, 374–384. [CrossRef]
238. Jang, S.; Kang, H.T.; Hwang, E.S. Nicotinamide-Induced Mitophagy. *J. Biol. Chem.* **2012**, *287*, 19304–19314. [CrossRef]
239. Chen, A.; Kristiansen, C.K.; Hong, Y.; Kianian, A.; Fang, E.F.; Sullivan, G.J.; Wang, J.; Li, X.; Bindoff, L.A.; Liang, K.X. Nicotinamide Riboside and Metformin Ameliorate Mitophagy Defect in Induced Pluripotent Stem Cell-Derived Astrocytes With POLG Mutations. *Front. Cell Dev. Biol.* **2021**, *9*, 737304. [CrossRef] [PubMed]
240. Mischley, L.K.; Shankland, E.; Liu, S.Z.; Bhayana, S.; Fox, D.J.; Marcinek, D.J. ATP and NAD+ Deficiency in Parkinson's Disease. *Nutrients* **2023**, *15*, 943. [CrossRef] [PubMed]
241. Lei, L.; Zhang, X.; Lin, J.; Liang, Q.; Sohouli, M.H.; Izze da Silva Magalhães, E.; Fatahi, S.; Yang, L.; Xu, W.; Wang, X.; et al. Effects of NAD + Precursors on Blood Pressure, C-reactive Protein Concentration and Carotid Intima-media Thickness: A Meta-analysis of Randomized Controlled Trials. *Eur. J. Clin. Investig.* **2023**, *53*, e14078. [CrossRef]
242. Zhang, R.; Shen, Y.; Zhou, L.; Sangwung, P.; Fujioka, H.; Zhang, L.; Liao, X. Short-Term Administration of Nicotinamide Mononucleotide Preserves Cardiac Mitochondrial Homeostasis and Prevents Heart Failure. *J. Mol. Cell. Cardiol.* **2017**, *112*, 64–73. [CrossRef] [PubMed]
243. Metodiewa, D.; Kośka, C. Reactive Oxygen Species and Reactive Nitrogen Species: Relevance to Cyto(Neuro)Toxic Events and Neurologic Disorders. An Overview. *Neurotox. Res.* **1999**, *1*, 197–233. [CrossRef]
244. Guo, C.; Sun, L.; Chen, X.; Zhang, D. Oxidative Stress, Mitochondrial Damage and Neurodegenerative Diseases. *Neural Regen. Res.* **2013**, *8*, 2003–2014. [CrossRef]
245. Lambert, A.J.; Brand, M.D. Reactive Oxygen Species Production by Mitochondria. In *Mitochondrial DNA*; Stuart, J.A., Ed.; Methods in Molecular Biology; Humana Press: Totowa, NJ, USA, 2009; Volume 554, pp. 165–181, ISBN 978-1-934115-60-2.
246. Kirkinezos, I.G.; Bacman, S.R.; Hernandez, D.; Oca-Cossio, J.; Arias, L.J.; Perez-Pinzon, M.A.; Bradley, W.G.; Moraes, C.T. Cytochrome *c* Association with the Inner Mitochondrial Membrane Is Impaired in the CNS of G93A-SOD1 Mice. *J. Neurosci.* **2005**, *25*, 164–172. [CrossRef]
247. Chichuk, T.V.; Strashkevich, I.A.; Klebanov, G.I. Free radical mechanisms of low-intensive laser radiation. *Vestn. Ross. Akad. Med. Nauk.* **1999**, *2*, 27–32.

248. Samuni, A.M.; Lipman, A.; Barenholz, Y. Damage to Liposomal Lipids: Protection by Antioxidants and Cholesterol-Mediated Dehydration. *Chem. Phys. Lipids* **2000**, *105*, 121–134. [CrossRef]
249. Lang, J.K.; Vigo-Pelfrey, C. Quality Control of Liposomal Lipids with Special Emphasis on Peroxidation of Phospholipids and Cholesterol. *Chem. Phys. Lipids* **1993**, *64*, 19–29. [CrossRef]
250. Smeyne, M.; Smeyne, R.J. Glutathione Metabolism and Parkinson's Disease. *Free Radic. Biol. Med.* **2013**, *62*, 13–25. [CrossRef] [PubMed]
251. Wang, Y.-T.; Lin, H.-C.; Zhao, W.-Z.; Huang, H.-J.; Lo, Y.-L.; Wang, H.-T.; Lin, A.M.-Y. Acrolein Acts as a Neurotoxin in the Nigrostriatal Dopaminergic System of Rat: Involvement of α-Synuclein Aggregation and Programmed Cell Death. *Sci. Rep.* **2017**, *7*, 45741. [CrossRef] [PubMed]
252. Schaur, R.; Siems, W.; Bresgen, N.; Eckl, P. 4-Hydroxy-Nonenal—A Bioactive Lipid Peroxidation Product. *Biomolecules* **2015**, *5*, 2247–2337. [CrossRef]
253. Guéraud, F.; Atalay, M.; Bresgen, N.; Cipak, A.; Eckl, P.M.; Huc, L.; Jouanin, I.; Siems, W.; Uchida, K. Chemistry and Biochemistry of Lipid Peroxidation Products. *Free Radic. Res.* **2010**, *44*, 1098–1124. [CrossRef]
254. Pizzimenti, S.; Ciamporcero, E.; Daga, M.; Pettazzoni, P.; Arcaro, A.; Cetrangolo, G.; Minelli, R.; Dianzani, C.; Lepore, A.; Gentile, F.; et al. Interaction of Aldehydes Derived from Lipid Peroxidation and Membrane Proteins. *Front. Physiol.* **2013**, *4*, 242. [CrossRef]
255. Visanji, N.P.; Brooks, P.L.; Hazrati, L.-N.; Lang, A.E. The Prion Hypothesis in Parkinson's Disease: Braak to the Future. *Acta Neuropathol. Commun.* **2013**, *1*, 2. [CrossRef] [PubMed]
256. Gianazza, E.; Brioschi, M.; Fernandez, A.M.; Banfi, C. Lipoxidation in Cardiovascular Diseases. *Redox Biol.* **2019**, *23*, 101119. [CrossRef]
257. Paradies, G.; Petrosillo, G.; Paradies, V.; Ruggiero, F.M. Oxidative Stress, Mitochondrial Bioenergetics, and Cardiolipin in Aging. *Free Radic. Biol. Med.* **2010**, *48*, 1286–1295. [CrossRef] [PubMed]
258. Boveris, A.; Chance, B. The Mitochondrial Generation of Hydrogen Peroxide. General Properties and Effect of Hyperbaric Oxygen. *Biochem. J.* **1973**, *134*, 707–716. [CrossRef]
259. Conklin, D.J.; Guo, Y.; Jagatheesan, G.; Kilfoil, P.J.; Haberzettl, P.; Hill, B.G.; Baba, S.P.; Guo, L.; Wetzelberger, K.; Obal, D.; et al. Genetic Deficiency of Glutathione *S* -Transferase P Increases Myocardial Sensitivity to Ischemia–Reperfusion Injury. *Circ. Res.* **2015**, *117*, 437–449. [CrossRef]
260. Feroe, A.G.; Attanasio, R.; Scinicariello, F. Acrolein Metabolites, Diabetes and Insulin Resistance. *Environ. Res.* **2016**, *148*, 1–6. [CrossRef] [PubMed]
261. Pytel, E.; Jackowska, P.; Chwatko, G.; Olszewska-Banaszczyk, M.; Koter-Michalak, M.; Kubalczyk, P.; Broncel, M. Intensive Statin Therapy, Used Alone or in Combination with Ezetimibe, Improves Homocysteine Level and Lipid Peroxidation to a Similar Degree in Patients with Coronary Artery Diseases. *Pharmacol. Rep.* **2016**, *68*, 344–348. [CrossRef] [PubMed]
262. Kolamunne, R.T.; Dias, I.H.; Vernallis, A.B.; Grant, M.M.; Griffiths, H.R. Nrf2 Activation Supports Cell Survival during Hypoxia and Hypoxia/Reoxygenation in Cardiomyoblasts; the Roles of Reactive Oxygen and Nitrogen Species. *Redox Biol.* **2013**, *1*, 418–426. [CrossRef] [PubMed]
263. Gorelick, P.B.; Scuteri, A.; Black, S.E.; Decarli, C.; Greenberg, S.M.; Iadecola, C.; Launer, L.J.; Laurent, S.; Lopez, O.L.; Nyenhuis, D.; et al. Vascular Contributions to Cognitive Impairment and Dementia: A Statement for Healthcare Professionals from the American Heart Association/American Stroke Association. *Stroke* **2011**, *42*, 2672–2713. [CrossRef] [PubMed]
264. Brain, J.; Tully, P.J.; Turnbull, D.; Tang, E.; Greene, L.; Beach, S.; Siervo, M.; Stephan, B.C.M. Risk Factors for Dementia in the Context of Cardiovascular Disease: A Protocol of an Overview of Reviews. *PLoS ONE* **2022**, *17*, e0271611. [CrossRef]
265. De La Torre, J.C. Cardiovascular Risk Factors Promote Brain Hypoperfusion Leading to Cognitive Decline and Dementia. *Cardiovasc. Psychiatry Neurol.* **2012**, *2012*, 1–15. [CrossRef]
266. Moore, E.E.; Jefferson, A.L. Impact of Cardiovascular Hemodynamics on Cognitive Aging. *Arterioscler. Thromb. Vasc. Biol.* **2021**, *41*, 1255–1264. [CrossRef]
267. Goh, F.Q.; Kong, W.K.F.; Wong, R.C.C.; Chong, Y.F.; Chew, N.W.S.; Yeo, T.-C.; Sharma, V.K.; Poh, K.K.; Sia, C.-H. Cognitive Impairment in Heart Failure—A Review. *Biology* **2022**, *11*, 179. [CrossRef]
268. Sundbøll, J.; Horváth-Puhó, E.; Adelborg, K.; Schmidt, M.; Pedersen, L.; Bøtker, H.E.; Henderson, V.W.; Toft Sørensen, H. Higher Risk of Vascular Dementia in Myocardial Infarction Survivors. *Circulation* **2018**, *137*, 567–577. [CrossRef]
269. Sundbøll, J.; Szépligeti, S.K.; Szentkúti, P.; Adelborg, K.; Horváth-Puhó, E.; Pedersen, L.; Henderson, V.W.; Sørensen, H.T. Risk of Parkinson Disease and Secondary Parkinsonism in Myocardial Infarction Survivors. *J. Am. Heart Assoc.* **2022**, *11*, e022768. [CrossRef]
270. Siddall, H.K.; Yellon, D.M.; Ong, S.-B.; Mukherjee, U.A.; Burke, N.; Hall, A.R.; Angelova, P.R.; Ludtmann, M.H.R.; Deas, E.; Davidson, S.M.; et al. Loss of PINK1 Increases the Heart's Vulnerability to Ischemia-Reperfusion Injury. *PLoS ONE* **2013**, *8*, e62400. [CrossRef]
271. Carricarte Naranjo, C.; Marras, C.; Visanji, N.P.; Cornforth, D.J.; Sanchez-Rodriguez, L.; Schüle, B.; Goldman, S.M.; Estévez, M.; Stein, P.K.; Lang, A.E.; et al. Increased Markers of Cardiac Vagal Activity in Leucine-Rich Repeat Kinase 2-Associated Parkinson's Disease. *Clin. Auton. Res.* **2019**, *29*, 603–614. [CrossRef] [PubMed]
272. Navarro-Otano, J.; Gelpi, E.; Mestres, C.A.; Quintana, E.; Rauek, S.; Ribalta, T.; Santiago, V.; Tolosa, E. Alpha-Synuclein Aggregates in Epicardial Fat Tissue in Living Subjects without Parkinsonism. *Park. Relat. Disord.* **2013**, *19*, 27–31. [CrossRef] [PubMed]

273. Ma, L.-Y.; Liu, G.-L.; Wang, D.-X.; Zhang, M.-M.; Kou, W.-Y.; Feng, T. Alpha-Synuclein in Peripheral Tissues in Parkinson's Disease. *ACS Chem. Neurosci.* **2019**, *10*, 812–823. [CrossRef]
274. Wakabayashi, K.; Takahashi, H. Neuropathology of Autonomic Nervous System in Parkinson's Disease. *Eur. Neurol.* **1997**, *38*, 2–7. [CrossRef]

International Journal of
Molecular Sciences

MDPI

Review

Mitochondrial One-Carbon Metabolism and Alzheimer's Disease

Yizhou Yu * and L. Miguel Martins *

MRC Toxicology Unit, University of Cambridge, Gleeson Building, Tennis Court Road, Cambridge CB2 1QR, UK
* Correspondence: yzy21@cam.ac.uk (Y.Y.); lm795@cam.ac.uk (L.M.M.)

Abstract: Mitochondrial one-carbon metabolism provides carbon units to several pathways, including nucleic acid synthesis, mitochondrial metabolism, amino acid metabolism, and methylation reactions. Late-onset Alzheimer's disease is the most common age-related neurodegenerative disease, characterised by impaired energy metabolism, and is potentially linked to mitochondrial bioenergetics. Here, we discuss the intersection between the molecular pathways linked to both mitochondrial one-carbon metabolism and Alzheimer's disease. We propose that enhancing one-carbon metabolism could promote the metabolic processes that help brain cells cope with Alzheimer's disease-related injuries. We also highlight potential therapeutic avenues to leverage one-carbon metabolism to delay Alzheimer's disease pathology.

Keywords: Alzheimer's disease; mitochondria; one-carbon metabolism; folate

1. Introduction

Mitochondria are more than cellular powerhouses. Mitochondria act in their host cell as information-processing systems (reviewed in [1]). Mitochondria compartmentalise several biochemical pathways, including the oxidative phosphorylation (OXPHOS) system and a branch of folate-dependent one-carbon (1C) metabolism [2]. One-carbon metabolism is a process found in both prokaryotes [3] and eukaryotes [4]. In eukaryotes, 1C metabolism plays a fundamental role in metabolic pathways including nucleotide synthesis, DNA and protein methylation, and mitochondrial metabolism, which are linked to Alzheimer's disease (AD) risk.

The cause of AD remains debated. The familial forms of AD are mostly linked to the extracellular accumulation of amyloid-β peptides and the hyperphosphorylation of tau [4,5]. In contrast, late-onset AD can be more multifactorial [6,7], with a complex genetic architecture [8] that interacts with environmental factors [9]. Patients with AD exhibit increased DNA damage [10], mitochondrial dysfunction [11,12], dysregulated amino acid metabolism [13,14], and decreased DNA methylation levels [15]. Age is one of the greatest risk factors for AD. With age, several metabolic alterations are associated with an increase in AD severity [16]. Given the importance of 1C metabolism in healthy ageing, several studies have shown that increasing the expression of genes and the bioavailability of metabolites involved in 1C metabolism could lengthen health span and delay AD pathologies [17–21] and provide a basis for personalised medicine. In this review, we discuss the genetic, proteomic, and metabolic alterations in AD and the extent to which they are linked to mitochondrial 1C metabolism, with a particular focus on therapeutic opportunities for upregulating and enhancing 1C metabolism to prevent or delay AD pathology (Figure 1a). We focus on the mitochondrial component of 1C metabolism, given the availability of other reviews with a broader scope [2,22,23]. Our working hypothesis is that multiple hallmarks of AD, including Aβ accumulation, hyperphosphorylation of tau, and genetic risk factors, converge on mitochondrial dysfunction [24–27]. The upregulation of mitochondrial 1C metabolism could help neurons cope with these injuries and delay AD-related pathologies (Figure 1b).

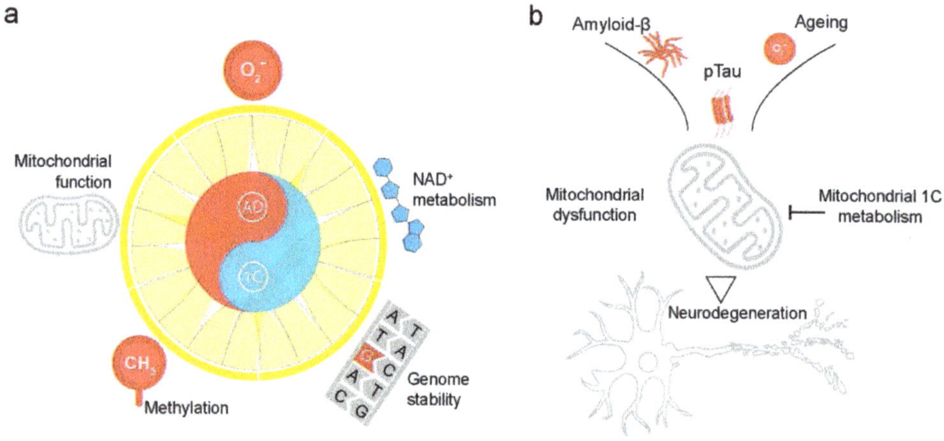

Figure 1. Links between mitochondrial 1C metabolism and AD. (**a**) An illustration of the 5 general cellular processes linked to both Alzheimer's disease (AD) (in red) and 1C metabolism (in blue), which are the main topics of this review (in grey): redox metabolism, NAD^+ metabolism, mitochondrial function, genome stability, and the methylation of DNA and proteins have been shown to be dysregulated in AD. (**b**) Working hypothesis on the potential of upregulating mitochondrial 1C metabolism to delay neurodegeneration in AD. AD-related pathologies such as the accumulation of toxic amyloid-β, hyperphosphorylated tau (pTau, and age-related accumulation of oxidative damage can lead to mitochondrial dysfunction and neurodegeneration. Upregulating mitochondrial 1C metabolism has the potential to alleviate AD-related damage and aid cells in coping with neurotoxic damage.

2. Folate 1C Metabolism: From Synthesis to Consumption

Folate is an essential metabolite in mitochondrial 1C metabolism and the generation of 1C donors. Folates are a group of molecules that share a common structure of three chemically distinct moieties: a pteridine ring, a para-aminobenzoic acid (PABA) linker, and one or more glutamates (Figure 2).

Folate, often referred to as vitamin B9, cannot be synthesised de novo in mammals, but it can be absorbed in the intestines from gut microbes or from ingested supplements or food as part of a normal diet [28,29]. In plants, folate synthesis is also compartmentalised: pterin and PABA precursors are made in the cytosol and plastids, respectively, and the assembly of folate from these precursors occurs in the mitochondria [30]. The term folate stems from the Latin word for leaf, folium, since folates are abundant in plant leaves [31]. Although substantial efforts have been made to increase folate production in plants [32], how much folate becomes bioavailable after the consumption of these plants remains uncertain. For instance, Mitchell and coworkers first purified folate in 1941. They noted that folate is present in animal tissues, green leaves, and mushrooms but not in processed foods [31], which suggests that folates can be lost in the processing of foods. Accordingly, folates are susceptible to UV photodegradation [33], light exposure [34], oxidation [35] and an acidic environment [35]. The folate synthesised by gut bacteria might thus constitute an important source.

Pioneering work from the Goldman group showed that cellular folate is imported by folate transporters in the plasma membrane [36] (Figure 3). Cells in the small intestine transport folate in the blood via the proton-coupled folate transporter (PCFT), coupled to the cotransport of proton ions [37]. Folate receptor α transports folate across the mammalian blood–brain barrier and choroid plexus into the brain and cerebrospinal fluids [38–41]. Autoantibodies against this receptor can block its function and have been shown to occur in psychiatric conditions [42–44].

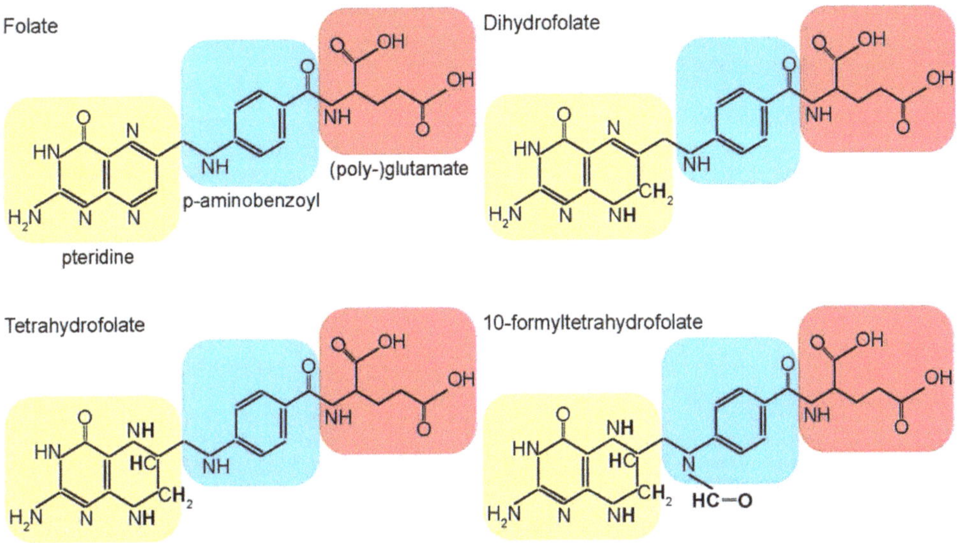

Figure 2. Structures of folate molecules. Folate molecules are composed of three distinct chemical components. At the core is a pterin heterocyclic ring (2-amino-4-hydroxy-pteridine, yellow), which is connected via a methylene bridge to a p-aminobenzoyl group (blue). This group is further linked through an amide bond to either a single glutamic acid molecule or a chain of glutamate residues (red). Folate molecules can carry one-carbon units in various oxidation states, which may be attached to the N_5 nitrogen atom of the pterin ring (see dihydrofolate and tetrahydrofolate for example) or the N_{10} nitrogen atom of the p-aminobenzoyl group (see 10-formyltetrahydrofolate for example). Different forms of folate molecules are shown, and the additional atoms compared to folate are in bold.

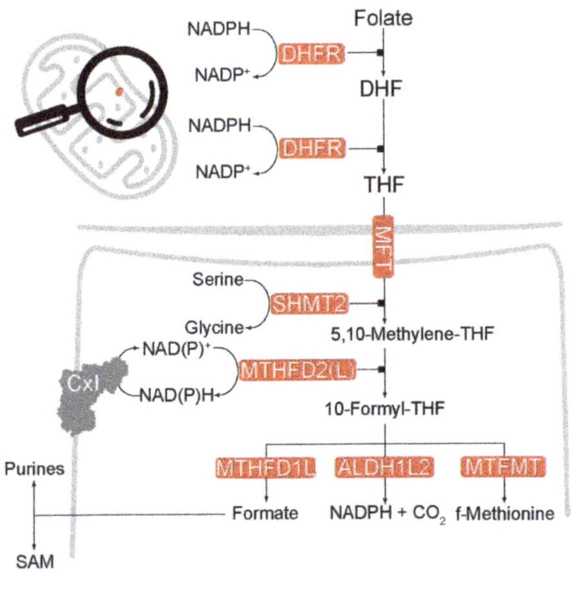

Figure 3. Pathway of mitochondrial 1C metabolism.

Reduced folate carrier (RFC), which is found in most cell types, mediates the transport of folate into the cell [45–47]. In the cytoplasm, dihydrofolate reductase (DHFR) metabolises folate to tetrahydrofolate (THF) while oxidising two molecules of nicotinamide adenine dinucleotide phosphate (NADPH) to $NADP^+$ [48] in a two-step process. THF participates in multiple metabolic processes such as the methylation of DNA and proteins. THF can also be imported into the mitochondria via mitochondrial folate transporters (MFTs) [49].

In mitochondria, serine hydroxymethyltransferase (SHMT2) catalyses the hydrolysis of THF to 5,10-methenyl-THF [50–52] (Figure 3). Subsequently, the NAD-dependent methylenetetrahydrofolate dehydrogenase-methenyltetrahydrofolate cyclohydrolase (Nmdmc), a bifunctional enzyme also known as mitochondrial methylenetetrahydrofolate dehydrogenase (MTHFD2/L), catalyses the formation of 10-formyl-THF from 5,10-methylene-THF by reducing either $NADP^+$ or NAD^+ to NADPH or NADH [53]. 10-Formyl-THF can have different fates. Mitochondrial 10-formyltetrahydrofolate dehydrogenase (ALDH1L2) can catalyse the oxidation of 10-formyl-THF to carbon dioxide (CO_2) while reducing $NADP^+$ to NADPH [54–56]. Mutations in ALDH1L2 are associated with neurological abnormalities [57] and an increase in reactive oxygen species [56]. Conversely, another methylenetetrahydrofolate dehydrogenase (MTHFD1L) directs the metabolites of mitochondrial 1C metabolism into the methyl and nucleotide biogenesis pathways by converting 10-formyl-THF to formate [58], which is transported into the cytosol to produce purines and methylate S-adenosylmethionine (SAM). The cytosolic component of 1C metabolism can potentially compensate for potential defects in the mitochondrial 1C pathway [59], suggesting some metabolic robustness.

Therefore, the folate-dependent 1C pathway fuels the synthesis of purines, contributes to the reduction of important redox co-factors $NAD(P)^+$ to NAD(P)H, and enables the synthesis of the main methylation factor, SAM. Due to the importance of folate 1C metabolism for cellular health, multiple countries, including the United States, have implemented regulations to supplement cereal grains used for wheat flour with folic acid as a strategy to increase the plasma folate levels in the human population [60].

Cells metabolise folate to generate 1C units and fuel 1C metabolism in the mitochondria. During mitochondrial 1C metabolism, dihydrofolate reductase (DHFR) reduces folate to dihydrofolate (DHF) and tetrahydrofolate (THF) while oxidising two molecules of NADPH to NADP+. Mitochondrial folate transporters (MTFs) import THF into mitochondria. Serine hydroxymethyltransferase (SHMT2), which is part of the mitochondrial glycine biosynthetic pathway, reduces THF to 5,10-methylene-THF, which is oxidised by methylenetetrahydrofolate reductase 2 (MTHFD2 or MTHFD2L) to 10-formyl-THF in a two-step process. 10-formyl-THF is used in different metabolic reactions, including the production of formates through methylenetetrahydrofolate dehydrogenase 1L (MTHFD1L), NADPH and CO_2 through aldehyde dehydrogenase 1, L2 (ALDH1L2), and the production of methionine through mitochondrial methionyl-tRNA formyltransferase (MTFMT). One-carbon metabolism-related proteins are distributed in the nuclear, mitochondrial, and cytoplasmic compartments [61]. Only the mitochondrial compartment of the 1C metabolism is shown in Figure 3.

3. Fuelling the Cellular Nucleotide Pool and Promoting Mitochondrial Biogenesis by Enhancing Mitochondrial 1C Metabolism

One-carbon metabolism plays a crucial role in replenishing pools of nucleotides (both purines and pyrimidines) to maintain substrate bioavailability for DNA repair. Specifically, 10-formyl-THF can be metabolised to inosine monophosphate (IMP) for de novo purine (adenosine and guanosine) synthesis.

Deficiencies in 1C metabolism can cause embryonic lethality or birth defects [62,63]. For example, impairment of 1C metabolism, such as through the suppression of SHMT1, causes neural tube closure defects through impaired nucleotide synthesis [64]. The replenishment of the nucleotide pool through deoxyuridine supplementation can prevent these defects [62], highlighting the role of 1C in nucleotide synthesis.

Various cellular processes in neurons, including nuclear DNA repair and the replication of mitochondrial DNA (mtDNA), rely on the availability of nucleotides [65]. Single-nucleus sequencing results from human post mortem brains showed that neurons accumulate approximately 20 genomic single-nucleotide variations per year, and neurons from patients with AD have significantly more DNA variations than those from age-matched controls [10]. During DNA repair, damaged nucleotides are removed and replaced by new nucleotides to restore the DNA sequence [66]. Oxidative damage to DNA creates oxidised DNA bases, of which deoxyguanosine oxidation to 7,8-dihydro-8-oxoguanosine (8-oxoG) is a major mutagenic event [67]. The DNA damage pattern in human neurons suggests that misrepaired damage to the deoxyguanosine nucleotide could be the cause of AD-related DNA mutations [10]. It is thus conceivable that an imbalanced nucleotide pool, such as a decreased availability of guanosine, could exacerbate the accumulation of somatic mutations in nuclear DNA through age and in AD (Figure 4). To test this hypothesis, it would be important to test the relative quantities of free nucleotides in patients with AD compared to controls, possibly using liquid chromatography-mass spectrometry (LC-MS). If there is indeed an imbalance in nucleotides, future research can investigate whether increasing nucleotide synthesis by upregulating 1C metabolism or taking deoxyguanosine as a supplement could delay AD pathology and decrease somatic mutations.

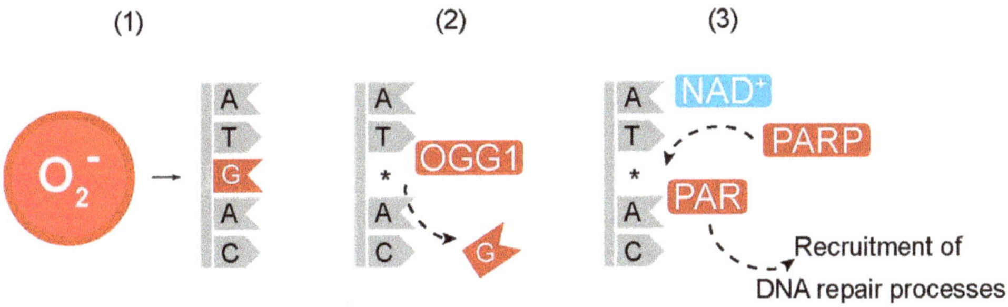

Figure 4. Links between mitochondrial 1C metabolism and DNA repair. Cellular stress can be caused by the accumulation of reactive oxygen species (ROS). High levels of ROS can damage DNA by converting deoxyguanosine to 8-oxo-2′-deoxyguanosine (8-oxo-dG) (1). 8-Oxoguanine glycosylase recognises and excises 8-oxo-dG, creating an apurinic site (AP site, indicated by an asterisk (2). The site where the nucleotide is lost is marked by an asterisk. Subsequently, poly(ADP-ribose) polymerases (PARPs) recognise the single-strand breaks produced from these excision processes (3). These enzymes catalyse the synthesis of poly(ADP-ribose) from NAD^+ using ATP at the site of DNA damage. Poly(ADP-ribose) polymers (PARs) subsequently act to recruit downstream DNA repair proteins.

An analysis of the intracellular pools of deoxyguanosine triphosphate indicated that this metabolite is concentrated in the mitochondrial matrix [68–71]. Deoxyguanosine kinase (DGUOK) is a mitochondrial enzyme that catalyses the first step of the phosphorylation of deoxyguanosine to its monophosphorylated form (dGMP). This first step in the phosphorylation of deoxyribonucleosides (dNs), such as deoxyguanosine, is the rate-limiting step in the salvage pathway of nucleotide synthesis [72]. Neurons are postmitotic cells that rely on the salvage biosynthetic pathway for nucleotide generation [73]. Mutations that impair DGUOK function cause mtDNA depletion syndrome [74], and a folate-mediated increase in nucleotide bioavailability through the de novo biosynthetic pathway leads to an increase in the mtDNA copy number [75]. Improving the mitochondrial function in models of AD by upregulating 1C metabolism might result in neuroprotection. Most cancer cells require an abundant nucleotide pool to sustain their high proliferation rate [76,77]. It is conceivable that in nonreplicating or postmitotic cells like neurons, the nucleotide pool could play a similar role in the replication of mtDNA and therefore sustain mitochondrial biogenesis. Mitochondria contain a streamlined genome in their circular mtDNA that encodes 13 proteins for energy production [78]. The replication of mtDNA is crucial for mitochondrial biogenesis [79], and an imbalance in the pool of nucleotides is linked to mtDNA depletion [80,81]. Additionally, a decrease in the number of mtDNA copies was observed in some patients with AD [82–84]. This observation supports Wallace's hypothesis, which suggests that mtDNA quantity and quality are measures of biological ageing and degenerative diseases [85]. Patients with mutations in DGUOK show a severe depletion of their nucleotide pools and a decrease in the enzymatic activities of mitochondrial-encoded respiratory complexes, leading to death before one year of age [80]. It is likely that the severe disease observed in these patients results from the depletion of their pools of nucleotides [80,81]. There are some results suggesting that post mortem brain samples from patients with AD also have altered levels of genes involved in nucleotide metabolism [86]. Ensuring an efficient flux of deoxyribonucleotides by enhancing mitochondrial 1C metabolism could thus ensure the presence of sufficient quantities of nucleotides to fuel mtDNA replication, promote mitochondrial biogenesis, and protect against AD pathology (Figure 4). This possibility is supported by the findings of a study showing that enhancing 1C metabolism via folate supplementation increased nucleotide bioavailability in vivo, increased mitochondrial biogenesis, and decreased neurodegeneration in Parkinson's disease models [75]. Future research is needed to systematically investigate the genes linked to nucleotide bioavailability and 1C metabolism.

mtDNA quantity and quality seem to vary across brain regions [82,87], among tissue types [88], and possibly among patients with AD. It is possible that, due to the multifaceted nature and high interindividual variability of AD pathology, only a subset of people could have insufficient mtDNA, while others have normal levels. Different cell types might have variable levels of mtDNA quality and quantity. We can also leverage advances in single-cell technologies to investigate mtDNA quantity and quality at the cellular level in the AD brain [88,89]. Taken together, future research could investigate the links among the levels of deoxynucleotides, DNA integrity, and mitochondrial biogenesis in individuals with AD and during ageing.

4. Role of 1C Metabolism in the Biosynthesis of Nucleotide-Containing Cofactors

In addition to acting as a direct substrate for DNA repair or synthesis, nucleotides or nucleotide derivatives can also act as cofactors for enzymatic reactions. Deoxyguanosine triphosphate (dGTP), for instance, binds to mitochondrial complex I [68,90] and could contribute to protein stability [91]. Mitochondrial complex I oxidises the reduced form of nicotinamide adenine dinucleotide (NADH) to NAD^+ while reducing ubiquinone to ubiquinol to transport protons across the mitochondrial inner membrane [92]. Patients with AD have lower mitochondrial complex I activity [11]; therefore, sufficient dGTP levels could improve the function of mitochondrial complex I by improving its stability in these patients.

The defects in complex I function [11,26] and lower NAD^+ levels in patients with AD indicate that the reduced activity of this respiratory complex could result in a decrease in NAD^+ levels. Ageing [93], neurodegenerative diseases such as AD [12,94], and epigenetic dysregulation [95,96] are all linked to decreased NAD^+ levels. NAD^+ and its phosphorylated form, $NADP^+$, are important cofactors in electron transfer and redox reactions. Increasing the NAD^+ levels in cells with defects in their mitochondrial electron transport chain rescues proliferative defects [97]. The introduction of an NADH dehydrogenase to increase the NAD^+/NADH ratio transgenically increases the lifespan of flies [98]. NAD^+ levels are also decreased in animal models of AD [12,99,100]. The restoration of NAD^+ levels has shown promising effects in animal models of neurodegeneration [12,99,101–103], and these approaches are currently being tested in clinical trials [104]. Taken together, this significant body of evidence indicates that increasing NAD^+ metabolism could be a viable strategy for delaying AD onset or mitigating AD symptoms by improving mitochondrial function.

Feeding fly models of Parkinson's disease associated with a loss of mitochondrial function with folic acid showed increased NAD^+ levels, resulting in neuroprotection [75], which highlights the importance of 1C metabolism as a source of NAD^+. Given the role of 1C metabolism in purine metabolism, boosting the mitochondrial 1C pathway may increase the pools of adenine used to make NAD^+. In cellular and animal models, nicotinamide mononucleotide adenylyltransferase transfers the adenosine moiety of ATP to nicotinamide mononucleotide to form NAD^+ [105,106]. NAD^+ can also be synthesised from adenosine monophosphate [107,108]. It is thus conceivable that enhancing 1C pathway activity could replenish the NAD^+ pool in AD. Several enzymes of the mitochondrial 1C pathway play a role in NAD^+ homeostasis. The oxidation of formyl-THF to CO_2 and THF by the ALDH1L2 enzyme leads to the production of mitochondrial NADPH (Figure 3). NADPH can directly support the antioxidant defence system, as glutathione reductase utilises NADPH to recycle oxidised glutathione back to its reduced form. Increasing NADPH also led to a decrease in oxidative stress and an increase in health span in mice [109]. Upon mitochondrial complex I deficiency, serine catabolism through 1C metabolism can fuel the generation of NADH [50]. The generation of NADH is mediated by mitochondrial MTHFD2 (L), which acts upstream of ALDH1L2 [50]. As the upregulation of the fly orthologue of MTHFD2(L) was shown to improve mitochondrial function and rescue neurodegeneration in fly models of Parkinson's disease [110], it would be important to test whether its action in the upregulation of ALDH1L2 and MTHFD2(L) in fly models of AD would also result in neuroprotection. Taken together, we propose that increasing 1C metabolism could protect against AD pathologies by increasing NAD^+ levels and boosting mitochondrial function, in the context of ageing and AD, which are both linked to a decrease in mitochondrial health [111].

Increasing NAD^+ levels through the 1C pathway could also act to promote DNA repair. The levels of the DNA repair proteins poly(ADP-ribose) polymerases (PARPs) are increased in patients with AD [12,103,112]. PARPs catalyses the formation of ADP-ribose polymers from NAD^+ to protein acceptors, and higher PARP activity has been described as important for maintaining genome stability across the life span in several model organisms [113]. Patients with AD have been shown to have increased DNA damage [114], which can activate PARPs [115,116] to maintain genome integrity. However, increased PARP activity could be detrimental to cellular function either by excessively lowering the bioavailability of NAD^+ for other enzymes, such as sirtuins, or by lowering ATP levels and depleting cellular energy stores. An abundant pool of NAD^+ might also be important for the ability of PARPs to protect cells from DNA damage [117]. Accordingly, a decrease in NAD^+ levels may impair PARP function and compromise the accurate storage of cellular information stored in their DNA. The associations among NAD^+ levels, PARP activity, genome integrity, and DNA repair processes in AD remain to be investigated.

5. Role of 1C Metabolism in Epigenetic and Post-Translational Modifications of Proteins

In addition to preserving the fidelity of the genome by supplying cofactors for DNA repair enzymes, 1C metabolism also provides methyl groups for the methylation of nuclear DNA and mtDNA. Methylation, as an epigenetic modification, can regulate gene expression and maintain cellular identity. One-carbon metabolism provides the methyl groups necessary for DNA methylation reactions through the synthesis of SAM, a major donor of methyl groups. The levels of SAM are decreased in the brains of patients with AD [118]. SAM is generated from methionine, an amino acid obtained from dietary sources, and ATP through the mitochondrial 1C pathway [119]. Methionine adenosyltransferase, an enzyme involved in 1C metabolism, catalyses the conversion of methionine to SAM, facilitating the transfer of methyl groups to DNA and other substrates. Changes in DNA methylation are linked to lifespan and ageing [120,121]. The importance of preserving accurate DNA methylation patterns is important in the contexts of AD [122,123] and ageing, as defects in this process can contribute to disease onset and age-related functional decline.

Reprogramming somatic cells into pluripotent stem cells by expressing Yamanaka factors also requires 1C metabolism to maintain efficiency [124,125]. It is therefore conceivable that increasing methyl donor or genetic variations in 1C genes could be linked to DNA methylation. Clinical studies showed that genetic mutations that impair the function of MTHFR, a gene involved in 1C metabolism, are linked to lower levels of DNA methylation [126]. Dietary supplementation with folic acid is linked to higher levels of DNA methylation [126,127]. Ageing [120,128] and AD [123,129,130] are linked to lower levels of DNA methylation globally. Dietary supplementation with SAM in mouse models of AD rescued AD pathologies [131,132], indicating a causal link between SAM levels and AD pathology. The observation that feeding SAM orally in a mouse model of AD increased methylation in the brain suggests that SAM can cross the blood–brain barrier [131] and thus be used as a dietary supplement for patients with AD. However, detailed pharmacokinetic measurements of SAM in animal models and patients with AD would be required to determine whether the dietary intake of SAM could increase the levels of bioactive SAM in the brain.

mtDNA has low or no methylation [133]. However, some studies have reported that mtDNA can be methylated by DNA methyltransferases (DNMTs) [134–136]. The levels of mtDNA methylation are altered in both animal models of AD [137] and some patients with AD [15,122,138–140]. The D-loop region of the mitochondrial genome regulates the replication of mtDNA and its transcription [141–144] and is methylated in both model animals and humans [145,146]. Both the hypo- and hypermethylation of the D loop have been observed in AD [138,140,147]. This variation in the degree of methylation might be explained by variations in disease stage or the brain area used for the analysis. DNMT3a activity can alter the mtDNA 5-methylcytosine levels [148], both of which are changed in AD [149]. The levels of 5-hydroxymethylcytosine in the mtDNA were decreased in aged animals compared to their younger counterparts, in line with changes in the mRNA levels of the enzymes involved in this methylation [150]. The functional consequences linked to the methylation of mtDNA patterns, including D-loop methylation, on mitochondrial dynamics remain underinvestigated. The overexpression of the DNA methyltransferase 1 variant with a mitochondrially targeted sequence (mtDNMT1) led to the specific upregulation of ND1 mRNA levels [136]. ND1, a subunit of mitochondrial complex I, is essential for initiating complex I assembly [151]. It is possible that altering mtDNA methylation through mtDNMT1 could regulate mitochondrial gene expression and rescue mitochondrial dysfunction in AD.

In addition to the methylation of mtDNA, the methylation status of the NADH dehydrogenase 5 RNA transcript is elevated in cells treated with Aβ and patients with AD. This increased methylation leads to translational repression and mitochondrial dysfunction in AD [152]. A global investigation of N6-methyladenosine levels in a mouse model of AD showed that RNA methylation is elevated in the mouse model [153]. Consistently, enzymes involved in RNA methylation are also differentially expressed in AD [154,155]. Interestingly, mechanistic target of rapamycin complex 1 (mTORC1), which has been linked to AD risk and longevity, is also a key regulator of RNA modification through the addition of N6-methyladenosine [156–159]. mTORC1 introduces an N6-methyladenosine modification to MXD2, which results in its degradation [160,161]. MXD2 is a negative regulator of cMYC, and its degradation causes an increase in cMYC activity and a global upregulation of translation [160,161]. Endoplasmic reticulum stress, which is associated with translational shutdown, is prevalent in individuals with AD [162]. Increasing mTORC1-dependent translational upregulation could thus be a potential avenue to reverse translational stress in AD.

Protein methylation is a type of post-translational modification that can play an important role in regulating protein function. The bioavailability of the 1C donor SAM is critical to mitochondrial function as it enables mitochondrial complex I assembly and iron-sulphur cluster biosynthesis [163]. Arginine methyltransferase NDUFAF7 methylates arginine 85 of NDUFS2, a complex I subunit that facilitates the assembly of complex I [164,165] in a

SAM-dependent manner [163]. Impairment of complex I activity can lead to ROS production and neurodegeneration, and patients with AD have impaired complex I activity in the brain [11,26]. Facilitating complex I assembly through 1C metabolism could potentially alleviate AD progression. More widely, the methylation of other proteins involved in AD could also be linked to neuronal function. For instance, the microtubule-associated protein tau can undergo extensive post-translational modifications. Tau phosphorylation increases its propensity to aggregate [166]. On the other hand, methylation of tau has been detected in the brains of patients with AD [167], and biochemical analyses have indicated that increased methylation decreases the propensity of tau to aggregate and protects against its neurotoxic effects [168]. Future work could leverage advances in mass spectrometry to unbiasedly examine the difference in the protein methylome between patients with AD and controls [169].

6. Therapeutic Opportunities and Novel Methods of Enhancing Mitochondrial 1C Metabolism

Based on previous observations that increasing mitochondrial 1C metabolism could delay AD phenotypes at multiple omic levels, research on the effect of supplementation with the precursor metabolite folate on AD pathology has shown encouraging results. Here, we discuss various results and limitations on the potential of using folate as a therapy for AD, focusing on clinical data.

The reference range for the concentration of folate in plasma or serum in humans typically spans from 13.5 to 45.3 nM [170,171]. Despite several countries adopting regulations on folic acid fortification [172], patients with AD have lower folate levels in their plasma than controls [18]. Dietary supplementation with more than 400 μg of folate per day in patients with AD slowed their cognitive decline [173–175]. There are, however, numerous results that show a lack of association between folate supplementation and the suppression of AD pathology [176–178], suggesting some potentially heterogeneous effects of folate supplementation.

Understanding these discrepancies is key for evaluating the therapeutic potential of increasing mitochondrial 1C metabolism to delay AD pathology. A potential issue with studies investigating the link between folate intake and subsequent AD risk using epidemiological methods [176,177] would be reverse causation: it is possible that individuals with increased frailty or AD risk could be self-medicating by taking folic acid supplements. Randomised clinical trials to test the efficacy of dietary supplementation with folates compared to a placebo would address this shortcoming. However, in a clinical trial of the effect of folic acid supplementation on individuals with mild cognitive impairments, it was reported that the effect of folate supplementation on improving cognition was not statistically significant [179]. Another putative explanation for the lack of efficacy of folate dietary intake might result from individual differences in the capacity to absorb and metabolise folate. Several proteins, including folate receptors, reduce folate carriers and proton-coupled folate transporters [180–183] and regulate the transport of folate in different tissues, including the blood–brain barrier and the intestine. Differences in the expression levels of these folate transporters might exist in patients with AD, which could alter the efficiency of folate transport across the blood–brain barrier in individual patients. For instance, the vitamin D receptor regulates the expression of folate transporters, and treating mice with the active form of vitamin D increased the transport of folate in the brain [184]. Previous research showed that patients with AD have lower vitamin D levels than healthy controls [185], which could result in the lower expression of folate transporters. Characterising the expression of folate transporters in patients with AD could inform whether taking folate orally would be sufficient to increase mitochondrial 1C metabolism in the brain. Since vitamin D might play a role in the transport of folate, it would be informative to reanalyse the epidemiological data on folate intake, while accounting for serum vitamin D concentrations. The hypothesis would thus be that folate and vitamin D combined supplementation could have an increased beneficial effect on preserving cognitive health in patients with AD compared to the effects of folate supplementation alone.

Folate is metabolised intracellularly into more biologically active molecules such as THF or SAM through mitochondrial 1C metabolism. The transcripts encoding for the components of 1C metabolism such as *DHFR* are altered post mortem [186]. Additionally, post mortem AD brains have increased signs of an unfolded protein response [187], suggesting a decreased level of translation [188]. It is thus possible that in some patients with AD, defects in 1C metabolic pathways prevent the efficient metabolism of folate. Enhancing mitochondrial 1C metabolism directly with the supplementation of the 1C donor THF or other forms of folates could be a viable strategy to bypass such defects.

Another potential approach to increase folate delivery in patients with AD is the use of gut bacteria that produce a range of different folate products including the more metabolically ready DHF and THF [29,189]. Pioneering studies on the identification and function of folates have mostly relied on bacterial sources. Folate derived from yeast was used to treat tropical macrocytic anaemia in humans [190,191]. Folate was also first detected in *Streptococcus lactis* [31]. These observations suggest that microbes containing the metabolic pathways involved in folate synthesis can excrete forms of folate that are more metabolically active to be absorbed by the gut. An important question remains as to whether the microbes that contain genes for de novo folate synthesis still produce folate in the human gut. The caecum and colon of rats fed human milk containing Bifidobacterium, a folate producer, were engrafted with this bacterial strain. This resulted in increased plasma folate levels in these animals [192]. In humans, the supplementation with Bifidobacterium (*Bifidobacterium adolescentis* DSM 18350, *Bifidobacterium adolescentis* DSM 18352, and *Bifidobacterium pseudocatenulatum* DSM 18353) was linked to increases in folate levels and faecal Bifidobacterium count. We suggest that manipulating the gut microbiome and feeding animal models with bacteria that produce different forms of folates could be a viable alternative to dietary folate intake to enhance mitochondrial 1C metabolism in the host.

Taken together, upregulating mitochondrial 1C metabolism through pharmacological and probiotic methods could be beneficial for patients with AD. We envisage that patients could adopt these treatments in addition to existing AD treatments such as cholinesterase inhibitors (reviewed in [193]) and antibody-based therapies [194].

7. Conclusions and Outlook

Here, we focused on the potential mechanistic links between mitochondrial 1C metabolism and AD. We propose that upregulating 1C metabolism is a potential therapeutic approach for countering the neurodegeneration in AD by improving mitochondrial health. Mitochondrial 1C plays vital roles in cellular and organismal functions. These roles range from maintaining mitochondrial function to ensuring normal foetal development in vertebrates. We reason that leveraging the increasing amount of multimodal data, such as genomic, transcriptomic, methylomic, proteomic, and metabolomic data, from different human tissues, to explore novel approaches to increase 1C metabolism could result in new approaches to promote healthy ageing. These insights could also elucidate the interindividual differences in mitochondrial 1C metabolism, which could inform the design of personalised treatments for neurodegenerative diseases such as AD.

8. Perspectives

1. Mitochondrial 1C metabolism plays a central role in various biochemical processes, including mitochondrial function, nucleotide synthesis, amino acid metabolism, and epigenetic regulation. These processes are intertwined with the mechanisms of ageing and the onset of AD.
2. Mitochondrial 1C reactions produce 1C units while synthesising coenzymes such as NADPH. Mitochondrial 1C metabolism differs in cell-type and disease-specific

contexts. Defects in this metabolic pathway lead to multiple repercussions, such as imbalances in crucial metabolites, oxidative stress, and defects in DNA repair.

3. Further research on the causal effects of genes and metabolites in the 1C pathway could elucidate healthy ageing trajectories and the mechanisms of AD.

Author Contributions: Conceptualisation, Y.Y. and L.M.M.; original draft preparation, Y.Y.; review and editing, Y.Y. and L.M.M.; project administration, L.M.M.; funding acquisition, L.M.M. All authors have read and agreed to the published version of the manuscript.

Funding: This research was funded by the UK Medical Research Council, intramural project MC_UU_00025/3 (RG94521).

Conflicts of Interest: Y.Y. is an inventor on a filed patent that is related to enhancing folate one-carbon metabolism to protect against Alzheimer's disease. Y.Y. is a co-founder and holds equity in Healthspan Biotics. L.M.M. declares no conflict of interests.

References

1. Picard, M.; Shirihai, O.S. Mitochondrial Signal Transduction. *Cell Metab.* **2022**, *34*, 1620–1653. [CrossRef] [PubMed]
2. Ducker, G.S.; Rabinowitz, J.D. One-Carbon Metabolism in Health and Disease. *Cell Metab.* **2017**, *25*, 27–42. [CrossRef] [PubMed]
3. Kleerebezemab, M.; Hols, P.; Hugenholtz, J. Lactic Acid Bacteria as a Cell Factory: Rerouting of Carbon Metabolism in Lactococcus Lactis by Metabolic Engineering. *Enzym. Microb. Technol.* **2000**, *26*, 840–848. [CrossRef] [PubMed]
4. Tibbetts, A.S.; Appling, D.R. Compartmentalization of Mammalian Folate-Mediated One-Carbon Metabolism. *Annu. Rev. Nutr.* **2010**, *30*, 57–81. [CrossRef] [PubMed]
5. Trojanowski, J.Q. Tauists, Baptists, Syners, Apostates, and New Data. *Ann. Neurol.* **2002**, *52*, 263–265. [CrossRef] [PubMed]
6. Storandt, M.; Head, D.; Fagan, A.M.; Holtzman, D.M.; Morris, J.C. Toward a Multifactorial Model of Alzheimer Disease. *Neurobiol. Aging* **2012**, *33*, 2262–2271. [CrossRef] [PubMed]
7. Knopman, D.S.; Amieva, H.; Petersen, R.C.; Chételat, G.; Holtzman, D.M.; Hyman, B.T.; Nixon, R.A.; Jones, D.T. Alzheimer Disease. *Nat. Rev. Dis. Primer* **2021**, *7*, 33. [CrossRef]
8. Bellenguez, C.; Küçükali, F.; Jansen, I.E.; Kleineidam, L.; Moreno-Grau, S.; Amin, N.; Naj, A.C.; Campos-Martin, R.; Grenier-Boley, B.; Andrade, V.; et al. New Insights into the Genetic Etiology of Alzheimer's Disease and Related Dementias. *Nat. Genet.* **2022**, *54*, 412–436. [CrossRef]
9. Livingston, G.; Huntley, J.; Sommerlad, A.; Ames, D.; Ballard, C.; Banerjee, S.; Brayne, C.; Burns, A.; Cohen-Mansfield, J.; Cooper, C.; et al. Dementia Prevention, Intervention, and Care: 2020 Report of the Lancet Commission. *Lancet* **2020**, *396*, 413–446. [CrossRef]
10. Miller, M.B.; Huang, A.Y.; Kim, J.; Zhou, Z.; Kirkham, S.L.; Maury, E.A.; Ziegenfuss, J.S.; Reed, H.C.; Neil, J.E.; Rento, L.; et al. Somatic Genomic Changes in Single Alzheimer's Disease Neurons. *Nature* **2022**, *604*, 714–722. [CrossRef]
11. Venkataraman, A.V.; Mansur, A.; Rizzo, G.; Bishop, C.; Lewis, Y.; Kocagoncu, E.; Lingford-Hughes, A.; Huiban, M.; Passchier, J.; Rowe, J.B.; et al. Widespread Cell Stress and Mitochondrial Dysfunction Occur in Patients with Early Alzheimer's Disease. *Sci. Transl. Med.* **2022**, *14*, eabk1051. [CrossRef] [PubMed]
12. Yu, Y.; Fedele, G.; Celardo, I.; Loh, S.H.Y.; Martins, L.M. Parp Mutations Protect from Mitochondrial Toxicity in Alzheimer's Disease. *Cell Death Dis.* **2021**, *12*, 651. [CrossRef]
13. Fekkes, D.; van der Cammen, T.J.M.; van Loon, C.P.M.; Verschoor, C.; van Harskamp, F.; de Koning, I.; Schudel, W.J.; Pepplinkhuizen, L. Abnormal Amino Acid Metabolism in Patients with Early Stage Alzheimer Dementia. *J. Neural Transm.* **1998**, *105*, 287–294. [CrossRef] [PubMed]
14. Trushina, E.; Dutta, T.; Persson, X.-M.T.; Mielke, M.M.; Petersen, R.C. Identification of Altered Metabolic Pathways in Plasma and CSF in Mild Cognitive Impairment and Alzheimer's Disease Using Metabolomics. *PLoS ONE* **2013**, *8*, e63644. [CrossRef]
15. De Jager, P.L.; Srivastava, G.; Lunnon, K.; Burgess, J.; Schalkwyk, L.C.; Yu, L.; Eaton, M.L.; Keenan, B.T.; Ernst, J.; McCabe, C.; et al. Alzheimer's Disease: Early Alterations in Brain DNA Methylation at ANK1, BIN1, RHBDF2 and Other Loci. *Nat. Neurosci.* **2014**, *17*, 1156–1163. [CrossRef] [PubMed]
16. López-Otín, C.; Blasco, M.A.; Partridge, L.; Serrano, M.; Kroemer, G. Hallmarks of Aging: An Expanding Universe. *Cell* **2023**, *186*, 243–278. [CrossRef] [PubMed]
17. Coppedè, F.; Grossi, E.; Buscema, M.; Migliore, L. Application of Artificial Neural Networks to Investigate One-Carbon Metabolism in Alzheimer's Disease and Healthy Matched Individuals. *PLoS ONE* **2013**, *8*, e74012. [CrossRef] [PubMed]
18. Zhang, X.; Bao, G.; Liu, D.; Yang, Y.; Li, X.; Cai, G.; Liu, Y.; Wu, Y. The Association Between Folate and Alzheimer's Disease: A Systematic Review and Meta-Analysis. *Front. Neurosci.* **2021**, *15*, 661198. [CrossRef] [PubMed]
19. Naj, A.C.; Beecham, G.W.; Martin, E.R.; Gallins, P.J.; Powell, E.H.; Konidari, I.; Whitehead, P.L.; Cai, G.; Haroutunian, V.; Scott, W.K.; et al. Dementia Revealed: Novel Chromosome 6 Locus for Late-Onset Alzheimer Disease Provides Genetic Evidence for Folate-Pathway Abnormalities. *PLoS Genet.* **2010**, *6*, e1001130. [CrossRef]

20. Yu, S.; Jang, Y.; Paik, D.; Lee, E.; Park, J.-J. Nmdmc Overexpression Extends Drosophila Lifespan and Reduces Levels of Mitochondrial Reactive Oxygen Species. *Biochem. Biophys. Res. Commun.* **2015**, *465*, 845–850. [CrossRef]
21. Dayon, L.; Guiraud, S.P.; Corthésy, J.; Da Silva, L.; Migliavacca, E.; Tautvydaitė, D.; Oikonomidi, A.; Moullet, B.; Henry, H.; Métairon, S.; et al. One-Carbon Metabolism, Cognitive Impairment and CSF Measures of Alzheimer Pathology: Homocysteine and Beyond. *Alzheimers Res. Ther.* **2017**, *9*, 43. [CrossRef] [PubMed]
22. Lionaki, E.; Ploumi, C.; Tavernarakis, N. One-Carbon Metabolism: Pulling the Strings behind Aging and Neurodegeneration. *Cells* **2022**, *11*, 214. [CrossRef] [PubMed]
23. Coppedè, F. One-Carbon Epigenetics and Redox Biology of Neurodegeneration. *Free Radic. Biol. Med.* **2021**, *170*, 19–33. [CrossRef] [PubMed]
24. Reddy, P.H.; Beal, M.F. Amyloid Beta, Mitochondrial Dysfunction and Synaptic Damage: Implications for Cognitive Decline in Aging and Alzheimer's Disease. *Trends Mol. Med.* **2008**, *14*, 45–53. [CrossRef] [PubMed]
25. Simonovitch, S.; Schmukler, E.; Masliah, E.; Pinkas-Kramarski, R.; Michaelson, D.M. The Effects of APOE4 on Mitochondrial Dynamics and Proteins in Vivo. *J. Alzheimers Dis. JAD* **2019**, *70*, 861–875. [CrossRef] [PubMed]
26. Terada, T.; Therriault, J.; Kang, M.S.P.; Savard, M.; Pascoal, T.A.; Lussier, F.; Tissot, C.; Wang, Y.-T.; Benedet, A.; Matsudaira, T.; et al. Mitochondrial Complex I Abnormalities Is Associated with Tau and Clinical Symptoms in Mild Alzheimer's Disease. *Mol. Neurodegener.* **2021**, *16*, 28. [CrossRef] [PubMed]
27. Cheng, Y.; Bai, F. The Association of Tau With Mitochondrial Dysfunction in Alzheimer's Disease. *Front. Neurosci.* **2018**, *12*, 163. [CrossRef] [PubMed]
28. Mulligan, J.E.; Greene, G.W.; Caldwell, M. Sources of Folate and Serum Folate Levels in Older Adults. *J. Am. Diet. Assoc.* **2007**, *107*, 495–499. [CrossRef] [PubMed]
29. Rossi, M.; Amaretti, A.; Raimondi, S. Folate Production by Probiotic Bacteria. *Nutrients* **2011**, *3*, 118–134. [CrossRef]
30. Hanson, A.D.; Gregory, J.F. Folate Biosynthesis, Turnover, and Transport in Plants. *Annu. Rev. Plant Biol.* **2011**, *62*, 105–125. [CrossRef]
31. Mitchell, H.K.; Snell, E.E.; Williams, R.J. Journal of the American Chemical Society, Vol. 63, 1941: The concentration of "folic acid" by Herschel K. Mitchell, Esmond E. Snell, and Roger J. Williams. *Nutr. Rev.* **1988**, *46*, 324–325. [CrossRef]
32. Hossain, T.; Rosenberg, I.; Selhub, J.; Kishore, G.; Beachy, R.; Schubert, K. Enhancement of Folates in Plants through Metabolic Engineering. *Proc. Natl. Acad. Sci. USA* **2004**, *101*, 5158–5163. [CrossRef] [PubMed]
33. Off, M.K.; Steindal, A.E.; Porojnicu, A.C.; Juzeniene, A.; Vorobey, A.; Johnsson, A.; Moan, J. Ultraviolet Photodegradation of Folic Acid. *J. Photochem. Photobiol. B* **2005**, *80*, 47–55. [CrossRef] [PubMed]
34. Stokstad, E.L.R.; Fordham, D.; de Grunigen, A. The Inactivation of Pteroylglutamic Acid (Liver Lactobacillus Casei Factor) by Light. *J. Biol. Chem.* **1947**, *167*, 877–878. [CrossRef] [PubMed]
35. Liang, X.S.; Zhao, F.Q.; Hao, L.X. Research on Stability of Synthetic Folic Acid. *Adv. Mater. Res.* **2013**, *781–784*, 1215–1218. [CrossRef]
36. Zhao, R.; Diop-Bove, N.; Visentin, M.; Goldman, I.D. Mechanisms of Membrane Transport of Folates into Cells and Across Epithelia. *Annu. Rev. Nutr.* **2011**, *31*, 177–201. [CrossRef] [PubMed]
37. Qiu, A.; Jansen, M.; Sakaris, A.; Min, S.H.; Chattopadhyay, S.; Tsai, E.; Sandoval, C.; Zhao, R.; Akabas, M.H.; Goldman, I.D. Identification of an Intestinal Folate Transporter and the Molecular Basis for Hereditary Folate Malabsorption. *Cell* **2006**, *127*, 917–928. [CrossRef]
38. Spector, R.; Johanson, C.E. REVIEW: Vitamin Transport and Homeostasis in Mammalian Brain: Focus on Vitamins B and E. *J. Neurochem.* **2007**, *103*, 425–438. [CrossRef] [PubMed]
39. Suh, J.R.; Herbig, A.K.; Stover, P.J. New Perspectives on Folate Catabolism. *Annu. Rev. Nutr.* **2001**, *21*, 255–282. [CrossRef]
40. Spector, R.; Lorenzo, A.V. Folate Transport by the Choroid Plexus in Vitro. *Science* **1975**, *187*, 540–542. [CrossRef]
41. Spector, R.; Lorenzo, A.V. Folate Transport in the Central Nervous System. *Am. J. Physiol.* **1975**, *229*, 777–782. [CrossRef] [PubMed]
42. Ramaekers, V.T.; Thöny, B.; Sequeira, J.M.; Ansseau, M.; Philippe, P.; Boemer, F.; Bours, V.; Quadros, E.V. Folinic Acid Treatment for Schizophrenia Associated with Folate Receptor Autoantibodies. *Mol. Genet. Metab.* **2014**, *113*, 307–314. [CrossRef]
43. Frye, R.E.; Sequeira, J.M.; Quadros, E.V.; James, S.J.; Rossignol, D.A. Cerebral Folate Receptor Autoantibodies in Autism Spectrum Disorder. *Mol. Psychiatry* **2013**, *18*, 369–381. [CrossRef] [PubMed]
44. Sadighi, Z.; Butler, I.J.; Koenig, M.K. Adult-Onset Cerebral Folate Deficiency. *Arch. Neurol.* **2012**, *69*, 778–779. [CrossRef] [PubMed]
45. Whetstine, J.R.; Flatley, R.M.; Matherly, L.H. The Human Reduced Folate Carrier Gene Is Ubiquitously and Differentially Expressed in Normal Human Tissues: Identification of Seven Non-Coding Exons and Characterization of a Novel Promoter. *Biochem. J.* **2002**, *367*, 629–640. [CrossRef]
46. Matherly, L.H. Molecular and Cellular Biology of the Human Reduced Folate Carrier. *Prog. Nucleic Acid Res. Mol. Biol.* **2001**, *67*, 131–162. [CrossRef] [PubMed]
47. Witt, T.L.; Stapels, S.E.; Matherly, L.H. Restoration of Transport Activity by Co-Expression of Human Reduced Folate Carrier Half-Molecules in Transport-Impaired K562 Cells: Localization of a Substrate Binding Domain to Transmembrane Domains 7-12. *J. Biol. Chem.* **2004**, *279*, 46755–46763. [CrossRef] [PubMed]
48. Chen, M.J.; Shimada, T.; Moulton, A.D.; Cline, A.; Humphries, R.K.; Maizel, J.; Nienhuis, A.W. The Functional Human Dihydrofolate Reductase Gene. *J. Biol. Chem.* **1984**, *259*, 3933–3943. [CrossRef] [PubMed]

49. Cybulski, R.L.; Fisher, R.R. Uptake of Oxidized Folates by Rat Liver Mitochondria. *Biochim. Biophys. Acta BBA Biomembr.* **1981**, *646*, 329–333. [CrossRef]
50. Yang, L.; Garcia Canaveras, J.C.; Chen, Z.; Wang, L.; Liang, L.; Jang, C.; Mayr, J.A.; Zhang, Z.; Ghergurovich, J.M.; Zhan, L.; et al. Serine Catabolism Feeds NADH When Respiration Is Impaired. *Cell Metab.* **2020**, *31*, 809–821.e6. [CrossRef]
51. Stover, P.; Schirch, V. Serine Hydroxymethyltransferase Catalyzes the Hydrolysis of 5,10-Methenyltetrahydrofolate to 5-Formyltetrahydrofolate. *J. Biol. Chem.* **1990**, *265*, 14227–14233. [CrossRef] [PubMed]
52. Minton, D.R.; Nam, M.; McLaughlin, D.J.; Shin, J.; Bayraktar, E.C.; Alvarez, S.W.; Sviderskiy, V.O.; Papagiannakopoulos, T.; Sabatini, D.M.; Birsoy, K.; et al. Serine Catabolism by SHMT2 Is Required for Proper Mitochondrial Translation Initiation and Maintenance of Formylmethionyl tRNAs. *Mol. Cell* **2018**, *69*, 610–621.e5. [CrossRef] [PubMed]
53. Shin, M.; Momb, J.; Appling, D.R. Human Mitochondrial MTHFD2 Is a Dual Redox Cofactor-Specific Methylenetetrahydrofolate Dehydrogenase/Methenyltetrahydrofolate Cyclohydrolase. *Cancer Metab.* **2017**, *5*, 11. [CrossRef] [PubMed]
54. Strickland, K.C.; Krupenko, N.I.; Dubard, M.E.; Hu, C.J.; Tsybovsky, Y.; Krupenko, S.A. Enzymatic Properties of ALDH1L2, a Mitochondrial 10-Formyltetrahydrofolate Dehydrogenase. *Chem. Biol. Interact.* **2011**, *191*, 129–136. [CrossRef] [PubMed]
55. Krupenko, N.I.; Dubard, M.E.; Strickland, K.C.; Moxley, K.M.; Oleinik, N.V.; Krupenko, S.A. ALDH1L2 Is the Mitochondrial Homolog of 10-Formyltetrahydrofolate Dehydrogenase. *J. Biol. Chem.* **2010**, *285*, 23056–23063. [CrossRef] [PubMed]
56. Hennequart, M.; Pilley, S.E.; Labuschagne, C.F.; Coomes, J.; Mervant, L.; Driscoll, P.C.; Legrave, N.M.; Lee, Y.; Kreuzaler, P.; Macintyre, B.; et al. ALDH1L2 Regulation of Formate, Formyl-Methionine, and ROS Controls Cancer Cell Migration and Metastasis. *Cell Rep.* **2023**, *42*, 112562. [CrossRef] [PubMed]
57. Sarret, C.; Ashkavand, Z.; Paules, E.; Dorboz, I.; Pediaditakis, P.; Sumner, S.; Eymard-Pierre, E.; Francannet, C.; Krupenko, N.I.; Boespflug-Tanguy, O.; et al. Deleterious Mutations in ALDH1L2 Suggest a Novel Cause for Neuro-Ichthyotic Syndrome. *Npj Genom. Med.* **2019**, *4*, 17. [CrossRef] [PubMed]
58. Pike, S.T.; Rajendra, R.; Artzt, K.; Appling, D.R. Mitochondrial C1-Tetrahydrofolate Synthase (MTHFD1L) Supports the Flow of Mitochondrial One-Carbon Units into the Methyl Cycle in Embryos. *J. Biol. Chem.* **2010**, *285*, 4612–4620. [CrossRef] [PubMed]
59. Ducker, G.S.; Chen, L.; Morscher, R.J.; Ghergurovich, J.M.; Esposito, M.; Teng, X.; Kang, Y.; Rabinowitz, J.D. Reversal of Cytosolic One-Carbon Flux Compensates for Loss of the Mitochondrial Folate Pathway. *Cell Metab.* **2016**, *23*, 1140–1153. [CrossRef] [PubMed]
60. Jacques, P.F.; Selhub, J.; Bostom, A.G.; Wilson, P.W.F.; Rosenberg, I.H. The Effect of Folic Acid Fortification on Plasma Folate and Total Homocysteine Concentrations. *N. Engl. J. Med.* **1999**, *340*, 1449–1454. [CrossRef]
61. Fox, J.T.; Stover, P.J. Chapter 1 Folate-Mediated One-Carbon Metabolism. In *Vitamins & Hormones*; Folic Acid and Folates; Academic Press: Cambridge, MA, USA, 2008; Volume 79, pp. 1–44.
62. Martiniova, L.; Field, M.S.; Finkelstein, J.L.; Perry, C.A.; Stover, P.J. Maternal Dietary Uridine Causes, and Deoxyuridine Prevents, Neural Tube Closure Defects in a Mouse Model of Folate-Responsive Neural Tube Defects. *Am. J. Clin. Nutr.* **2015**, *101*, 860–869. [CrossRef] [PubMed]
63. Blom, H.J.; Shaw, G.M.; den Heijer, M.; Finnell, R.H. Neural Tube Defects and Folate: Case Far from Closed. *Nat. Rev. Neurosci.* **2006**, *7*, 724–731. [CrossRef] [PubMed]
64. Beaudin, A.E.; Abarinov, E.V.; Noden, D.M.; Perry, C.A.; Chu, S.; Stabler, S.P.; Allen, R.H.; Stover, P.J. Shmt1 and de Novo Thymidylate Biosynthesis Underlie Folate-Responsive Neural Tube Defects in Mice1234. *Am. J. Clin. Nutr.* **2011**, *93*, 789–798. [CrossRef] [PubMed]
65. Reichard, P. Interactions Between Deoxyribonucleotide and Dna Synthesis. *Annu. Rev. Biochem.* **1988**, *57*, 349–374. [CrossRef] [PubMed]
66. Lindahl, T. Instability and Decay of the Primary Structure of DNA. *Nature* **1993**, *362*, 709–715. [CrossRef] [PubMed]
67. Shibutani, S.; Takeshita, M.; Grollman, A.P. Insertion of Specific Bases during DNA Synthesis Past the Oxidation-Damaged Base 8-oxodG. *Nature* **1991**, *349*, 431–434. [CrossRef] [PubMed]
68. Molina-Granada, D.; González-Vioque, E.; Dibley, M.G.; Cabrera-Pérez, R.; Vallbona-Garcia, A.; Torres-Torronteras, J.; Sazanov, L.A.; Ryan, M.T.; Cámara, Y.; Martí, R. Most Mitochondrial dGTP Is Tightly Bound to Respiratory Complex I through the NDUFA10 Subunit. *Commun. Biol.* **2022**, *5*, 620. [CrossRef] [PubMed]
69. Song, S.; Pursell, Z.F.; Copeland, W.C.; Longley, M.J.; Kunkel, T.A.; Mathews, C.K. DNA Precursor Asymmetries in Mammalian Tissue Mitochondria and Possible Contribution to Mutagenesis through Reduced Replication Fidelity. *Proc. Natl. Acad. Sci. USA* **2005**, *102*, 4990–4995. [CrossRef]
70. Ferraro, P.; Franzolin, E.; Pontarin, G.; Reichard, P.; Bianchi, V. Quantitation of Cellular Deoxynucleoside Triphosphates. *Nucleic Acids Res.* **2010**, *38*, e85. [CrossRef]
71. Wheeler, L.J.; Mathews, C.K. Nucleoside Triphosphate Pool Asymmetry in Mammalian Mitochondria. *J. Biol. Chem.* **2011**, *286*, 16992–16996. [CrossRef]
72. Johansson, M.; Karlsson, A. Cloning and Expression of Human Deoxyguanosine Kinase cDNA. *Proc. Natl. Acad. Sci. USA* **1996**, *93*, 7258–7262. [CrossRef] [PubMed]
73. Arnér, E.S.; Eriksson, S. Mammalian Deoxyribonucleoside Kinases. *Pharmacol. Ther.* **1995**, *67*, 155–186. [CrossRef] [PubMed]
74. Freisinger, P.; Fütterer, N.; Lankes, E.; Gempel, K.; Berger, T.M.; Spalinger, J.; Hoerbe, A.; Schwantes, C.; Lindner, M.; Santer, R.; et al. Hepatocerebral Mitochondrial DNA Depletion Syndrome Caused by Deoxyguanosine Kinase (DGUOK) Mutations. *Arch. Neurol.* **2006**, *63*, 1129–1134. [CrossRef] [PubMed]

75. Tufi, R.; Gandhi, S.; de Castro, I.P.; Lehmann, S.; Angelova, P.R.; Dinsdale, D.; Deas, E.; Plun-Favreau, H.; Nicotera, P.; Abramov, A.Y.; et al. Enhancing Nucleotide Metabolism Protects against Mitochondrial Dysfunction and Neurodegeneration in a PINK1 Model of Parkinson's Disease. *Nat. Cell Biol.* **2014**, *16*, 157–166. [CrossRef]
76. Zhang, W.C.; Shyh-Chang, N.; Yang, H.; Rai, A.; Umashankar, S.; Ma, S.; Soh, B.S.; Sun, L.L.; Tai, B.C.; Nga, M.E.; et al. Glycine Decarboxylase Activity Drives Non-Small Cell Lung Cancer Tumor-Initiating Cells and Tumorigenesis. *Cell* **2012**, *148*, 259–272. [CrossRef]
77. Kunz, B.A.; Kohalmi, S.E. Modulation of Mutagenesis by Deoxyribonucleotide Levels. *Annu. Rev. Genet.* **1991**, *25*, 339–359. [CrossRef] [PubMed]
78. Chen, X.J.; Butow, R.A. The Organization and Inheritance of the Mitochondrial Genome. *Nat. Rev. Genet.* **2005**, *6*, 815–825. [CrossRef] [PubMed]
79. Jornayvaz, F.R.; Shulman, G.I. Regulation of Mitochondrial Biogenesis. *Essays Biochem.* **2010**, *47*, 69–84. [CrossRef] [PubMed]
80. Mandel, H.; Szargel, R.; Labay, V.; Elpeleg, O.; Saada, A.; Shalata, A.; Anbinder, Y.; Berkowitz, D.; Hartman, C.; Barak, M.; et al. The Deoxyguanosine Kinase Gene Is Mutated in Individuals with Depleted Hepatocerebral Mitochondrial DNA. *Nat. Genet.* **2001**, *29*, 337–341. [CrossRef]
81. Nishino, I.; Spinazzola, A.; Hirano, M. Thymidine Phosphorylase Gene Mutations in MNGIE, a Human Mitochondrial Disorder. *Science* **1999**, *283*, 689–692. [CrossRef]
82. Rodríguez-Santiago, B.; Casademont, J.; Nunes, V. Is Mitochondrial DNA Depletion Involved in Alzheimer's Disease? *Eur. J. Hum. Genet.* **2001**, *9*, 279–285. [CrossRef] [PubMed]
83. Klein, H.-U.; Trumpff, C.; Yang, H.-S.; Lee, A.J.; Picard, M.; Bennett, D.A.; De Jager, P.L. Characterization of Mitochondrial DNA Quantity and Quality in the Human Aged and Alzheimer's Disease Brain. *Mol. Neurodegener.* **2021**, *16*, 75. [CrossRef] [PubMed]
84. Andrews, S.J.; Goate, A.M. Mitochondrial DNA Copy Number Is Associated with Cognitive Impairment. *Alzheimers Dement.* **2020**, *16*, e047543. [CrossRef]
85. Wallace, D.C. Mitochondrial Genetics: A Paradigm for Aging and Degenerative Diseases? *Science* **1992**, *256*, 628–632. [CrossRef] [PubMed]
86. Pesini, A.; Iglesias, E.; Bayona-Bafaluy, M.P.; Garrido-Pérez, N.; Meade, P.; Gaudó, P.; Jiménez-Salvador, I.; Andrés-Benito, P.; Montoya, J.; Ferrer, I.; et al. Brain Pyrimidine Nucleotide Synthesis and Alzheimer Disease. *Aging* **2019**, *11*, 8433–8462. [CrossRef] [PubMed]
87. Thubron, E.B.; Rosa, H.S.; Hodges, A.; Sivaprasad, S.; Francis, P.T.; Pienaar, I.S.; Malik, A.N. Regional Mitochondrial DNA and Cell-Type Changes in Post-Mortem Brains of Non-Diabetic Alzheimer's Disease Are Not Present in Diabetic Alzheimer's Disease. *Sci. Rep.* **2019**, *9*, 11386. [CrossRef] [PubMed]
88. Ludwig, L.S.; Lareau, C.A.; Ulirsch, J.C.; Christian, E.; Muus, C.; Li, L.H.; Pelka, K.; Ge, W.; Oren, Y.; Brack, A.; et al. Lineage Tracing In Humans Enabled By Mitochondrial Mutations And Single Cell Genomics. *Cell* **2019**, *176*, 1325–1339.e22. [CrossRef] [PubMed]
89. Lareau, C.A.; Ludwig, L.S.; Muus, C.; Gohil, S.H.; Zhao, T.; Chiang, Z.; Pelka, K.; Verboon, J.M.; Luo, W.; Christian, E.; et al. Massively Parallel Single-Cell Mitochondrial DNA Genotyping and Chromatin Profiling. *Nat. Biotechnol.* **2021**, *39*, 451–461. [CrossRef] [PubMed]
90. Grba, D.N.; Chung, I.; Bridges, H.R.; Agip, A.-N.A.; Hirst, J. Investigation of Hydrated Channels and Proton Pathways in a High-Resolution Cryo-EM Structure of Mammalian Complex I. *Sci. Adv.* **2023**, *9*, eadi1359. [CrossRef]
91. Agip, A.-N.A.; Blaza, J.N.; Bridges, H.R.; Viscomi, C.; Rawson, S.; Muench, S.P.; Hirst, J. CryoEM Structures of Complex I from Mouse Heart Mitochondria in Two Biochemically-Defined States. *Nat. Struct. Mol. Biol.* **2018**, *25*, 548–556. [CrossRef]
92. Hirst, J. Mitochondrial Complex I. *Annu. Rev. Biochem.* **2013**, *82*, 551–575. [CrossRef]
93. Covarrubias, A.J.; Perrone, R.; Grozio, A.; Verdin, E. NAD+ Metabolism and Its Roles in Cellular Processes during Ageing. *Nat. Rev. Mol. Cell Biol.* **2021**, *22*, 119–141. [CrossRef] [PubMed]
94. Lehmann, S.; Loh, S.H.Y.; Martins, L.M. Enhancing NAD+ Salvage Metabolism Is Neuroprotective in a PINK1 Model of Parkinson's Disease. *Biol. Open* **2017**, *6*, 141–147. [CrossRef]
95. Imai, S.; Guarente, L. It Takes Two to Tango: NAD^+ and Sirtuins in Aging/Longevity Control. *Npj Aging Mech. Dis.* **2016**, *2*, 16017. [CrossRef]
96. Imai, S.; Armstrong, C.M.; Kaeberlein, M.; Guarente, L. Transcriptional Silencing and Longevity Protein Sir2 Is an NAD-Dependent Histone Deacetylase. *Nature* **2000**, *403*, 795–800. [CrossRef] [PubMed]
97. Titov, D.V.; Cracan, V.; Goodman, R.P.; Peng, J.; Grabarek, Z.; Mootha, V.K. Complementation of Mitochondrial Electron Transport Chain by Manipulation of the NAD+/NADH Ratio. *Science* **2016**, *352*, 231–235. [CrossRef]
98. Sanz, A.; Soikkeli, M.; Portero-Otín, M.; Wilson, A.; Kemppainen, E.; McIlroy, G.; Ellilä, S.; Kemppainen, K.K.; Tuomela, T.; Lakanmaa, M.; et al. Expression of the Yeast NADH Dehydrogenase Ndi1 in Drosophila Confers Increased Lifespan Independently of Dietary Restriction. *Proc. Natl. Acad. Sci. USA* **2010**, *107*, 9105–9110. [CrossRef] [PubMed]
99. Hou, Y.; Lautrup, S.; Cordonnier, S.; Wang, Y.; Croteau, D.L.; Zavala, E.; Zhang, Y.; Moritoh, K.; O'Connell, J.F.; Baptiste, B.A.; et al. NAD+ Supplementation Normalizes Key Alzheimer's Features and DNA Damage Responses in a New AD Mouse Model with Introduced DNA Repair Deficiency. *Proc. Natl. Acad. Sci. USA* **2018**, *115*, E1876–E1885. [CrossRef]
100. Katsyuba, E.; Romani, M.; Hofer, D.; Auwerx, J. NAD + Homeostasis in Health and Disease. *Nat. Metab.* **2020**, *2*, 9–31. [CrossRef]

101. Araki, T.; Sasaki, Y.; Milbrandt, J. Increased Nuclear NAD Biosynthesis and SIRT1 Activation Prevent Axonal Degeneration. *Science* **2004**, *305*, 1010–1013. [CrossRef]
102. Gong, B.; Pan, Y.; Vempati, P.; Zhao, W.; Knable, L.; Ho, L.; Wang, J.; Sastre, M.; Ono, K.; Sauve, A.A.; et al. Nicotinamide Riboside Restores Cognition through an Upregulation of Proliferator-Activated Receptor-γ Coactivator 1α Regulated β-Secretase 1 Degradation and Mitochondrial Gene Expression in Alzheimer's Mouse Models. *Neurobiol. Aging* **2013**, *34*, 1581–1588. [CrossRef] [PubMed]
103. Turunc Bayrakdar, E.; Uyanikgil, Y.; Kanit, L.; Koylu, E.; Yalcin, A. Nicotinamide Treatment Reduces the Levels of Oxidative Stress, Apoptosis, and PARP-1 Activity in Aβ(1-42)-Induced Rat Model of Alzheimer's Disease. *Free Radic. Res.* **2014**, *48*, 146–158. [CrossRef] [PubMed]
104. Orr, M.E.; Kotkowski, E.; Bair-Kelps, D.; Romo, T.; Espinoza, S.; Musi, N.; Powers, B.; San Antonio Claude D. Pepper Center. Results from a Pilot Study: The Effects of Nicotinamide Riboside on Mild Cognitive Impairment. *Alzheimers Dement.* **2020**, *16*, e044746. [CrossRef]
105. Emanuelli, M.; Carnevali, F.; Lorenzi, M.; Raffaelli, N.; Amici, A.; Ruggieri, S.; Magni, G. Identification and Characterization of YLR328W, the Saccharomyces Cerevisiae Structural Gene Encoding NMN Adenylyltransferase. Expression and Characterization of the Recombinant Enzyme. *FEBS Lett.* **1999**, *455*, 13–17. [CrossRef] [PubMed]
106. Raffaelli, N.; Sorci, L.; Amici, A.; Emanuelli, M.; Mazzola, F.; Magni, G. Identification of a Novel Human Nicotinamide Mononucleotide Adenylyltransferase. *Biochem. Biophys. Res. Commun.* **2002**, *297*, 835–840. [CrossRef]
107. Lee, J.; Churchil, H.; Choi, W.-B.; Lynch, J.E.; Roberts, F.E.; Volante, R.P.; Reider, P.J. A Chemical Synthesis of Nicotinamide Adenine Dinucleotide (NAD^+). *Chem. Commun.* **1999**, 729–730. [CrossRef]
108. Walt, D.R.; Rios-Mercadillo, V.M.; Auge, J.; Whitesides, G.M. Synthesis of Nicotinamide Adenine Dinucleotide (NAD) from Adenosine Monophosphate (AMP). *J. Am. Chem. Soc.* **1980**, *102*, 7805–7806. [CrossRef]
109. Nóbrega-Pereira, S.; Fernandez-Marcos, P.J.; Brioche, T.; Gomez-Cabrera, M.C.; Salvador-Pascual, A.; Flores, J.M.; Viña, J.; Serrano, M. G6PD Protects from Oxidative Damage and Improves Healthspan in Mice. *Nat. Commun.* **2016**, *7*, 10894. [CrossRef] [PubMed]
110. Celardo, I.; Lehmann, S.; Costa, A.C.; Loh, S.H.; Miguel Martins, L. dATF4 Regulation of Mitochondrial Folate-Mediated One-Carbon Metabolism Is Neuroprotective. *Cell Death Differ.* **2017**, *24*, 638–648. [CrossRef]
111. Verdin, E. NAD+ in Aging, Metabolism, and Neurodegeneration. *Science* **2015**, *350*, 1208–1213. [CrossRef]
112. Abeti, R.; Duchen, M.R. Activation of PARP by Oxidative Stress Induced by β-Amyloid: Implications for Alzheimer's Disease. *Neurochem. Res.* **2012**, *37*, 2589–2596. [CrossRef] [PubMed]
113. Grube, K.; Bürkle, A. Poly(ADP-Ribose) Polymerase Activity in Mononuclear Leukocytes of 13 Mammalian Species Correlates with Species-Specific Life Span. *Proc. Natl. Acad. Sci. USA* **1992**, *89*, 11759–11763. [CrossRef] [PubMed]
114. Miller, M.B.; Reed, H.C.; Walsh, C.A. Brain Somatic Mutation in Aging and Alzheimer's Disease. *Annu. Rev. Genom. Hum. Genet.* **2021**, *22*, 239–256. [CrossRef] [PubMed]
115. Langelier, M.-F.; Planck, J.L.; Roy, S.; Pascal, J.M. Structural Basis for DNA Damage–Dependent Poly(ADP-Ribosyl)Ation by Human PARP-1. *Science* **2012**, *336*, 728–732. [CrossRef] [PubMed]
116. Zandarashvili, L.; Langelier, M.-F.; Velagapudi, U.K.; Hancock, M.A.; Steffen, J.D.; Billur, R.; Hannan, Z.M.; Wicks, A.J.; Krastev, D.B.; Pettitt, S.J.; et al. Structural Basis for Allosteric PARP-1 Retention on DNA Breaks. *Science* **2020**, *368*, eaax6367. [CrossRef] [PubMed]
117. Wilk, A.; Hayat, F.; Cunningham, R.; Li, J.; Garavaglia, S.; Zamani, L.; Ferraris, D.M.; Sykora, P.; Andrews, J.; Clark, J.; et al. Extracellular NAD+ Enhances PARP-Dependent DNA Repair Capacity Independently of CD73 Activity. *Sci. Rep.* **2020**, *10*, 651. [CrossRef] [PubMed]
118. Morrison, L.D.; Smith, D.D.; Kish, S.J. Brain S-Adenosylmethionine Levels Are Severely Decreased in Alzheimer's Disease. *J. Neurochem.* **1996**, *67*, 1328–1331. [CrossRef] [PubMed]
119. Newman, A.C.; Maddocks, O.D.K. Serine and Functional Metabolites in Cancer. *Trends Cell Biol.* **2017**, *27*, 645–657. [CrossRef] [PubMed]
120. Lu, A.T.; Fei, Z.; Haghani, A.; Robeck, T.R.; Zoller, J.A.; Li, C.Z.; Lowe, R.; Yan, Q.; Zhang, J.; Vu, H.; et al. Universal DNA Methylation Age across Mammalian Tissues. *Nat. Aging* **2023**, *3*, 1144–1166. [CrossRef]
121. Horvath, S. DNA Methylation Age of Human Tissues and Cell Types. *Genome Biol.* **2013**, *14*, 3156. [CrossRef]
122. Silva, T.C.; Young, J.I.; Zhang, L.; Gomez, L.; Schmidt, M.A.; Varma, A.; Chen, X.S.; Martin, E.R.; Wang, L. Cross-Tissue Analysis of Blood and Brain Epigenome-Wide Association Studies in Alzheimer's Disease. *Nat. Commun.* **2022**, *13*, 4852. [CrossRef] [PubMed]
123. Chouliaras, L.; Mastroeni, D.; Delvaux, E.; Grover, A.; Kenis, G.; Hof, P.R.; Steinbusch, H.W.M.; Coleman, P.D.; Rutten, B.P.F.; van den Hove, D.L.A. Consistent Decrease in Global DNA Methylation and Hydroxymethylation in the Hippocampus of Alzheimer's Disease Patients. *Neurobiol. Aging* **2013**, *34*, 2091–2099. [CrossRef] [PubMed]
124. Kovatcheva, M.; Melendez, E.; Chondronasiou, D.; Pietrocola, F.; Bernad, R.; Caballe, A.; Junza, A.; Capellades, J.; Holguín-Horcajo, A.; Prats, N.; et al. Vitamin B12 Is a Limiting Factor for Induced Cellular Plasticity and Tissue Repair. *Nat. Metab.* **2023**, *5*, 1911–1930. [CrossRef] [PubMed]
125. Hernandez-Benitez, R.; Wang, C.; Shi, L.; Ouchi, Y.; Zhong, C.; Hishida, T.; Liao, H.-K.; Magill, E.A.; Memczak, S.; Soligalla, R.D.; et al. Intervention with Metabolites Emulating Endogenous Cell Transitions Accelerates Muscle Regeneration in Young and Aged Mice. *Cell Rep. Med.* **2024**, *5*, 101449. [CrossRef]

126. Shelnutt, K.P.; Kauwell, G.P.A.; Gregory, J.F.; Maneval, D.R.; Quinlivan, E.P.; Theriaque, D.W.; Henderson, G.N.; Bailey, L.B. Methylenetetrahydrofolate Reductase 677C→T Polymorphism Affects DNA Methylation in Response to Controlled Folate Intake in Young Women. *J. Nutr. Biochem.* **2004**, *15*, 554–560. [CrossRef] [PubMed]
127. Kim, Y.-I.; Baik, H.W.; Fawaz, K.; Knox, T.; Lee, Y.M.; Norton, R.; Libby, E.; Mason, J.B. Effects of Folate Supplementation on Two Provisional Molecular Markers of Colon Cancer: A Prospective, Randomized trial11The Content of This Publication Does Not Necessarily Reflect the Views or Policies of the US Department of Agriculture, nor Does Mention of Trade Names, Commercial Products, or Organizations Imply Endorsement by the US Government. *Am. J. Gastroenterol.* **2001**, *96*, 184–195. [CrossRef]
128. Wilson, V.L.; Smith, R.A.; Ma, S.; Cutler, R.G. Genomic 5-Methyldeoxycytidine Decreases with Age. *J. Biol. Chem.* **1987**, *262*, 9948–9951. [CrossRef] [PubMed]
129. Bakulski, K.M.; Dolinoy, D.C.; Sartor, M.A.; Paulson, H.L.; Konen, J.R.; Lieberman, A.P.; Albin, R.L.; Hu, H.; Rozek, L.S. Genome-Wide DNA Methylation Differences between Late-Onset Alzheimer's Disease and Cognitively Normal Controls in Human Frontal Cortex. *J. Alzheimers Dis. JAD* **2012**, *29*, 571–588. [CrossRef] [PubMed]
130. Mastroeni, D.; Grover, A.; Delvaux, E.; Whiteside, C.; Coleman, P.D.; Rogers, J. Epigenetic Changes in Alzheimer's Disease: Decrements in DNA Methylation. *Neurobiol. Aging* **2010**, *31*, 2025–2037. [CrossRef]
131. Do Carmo, S.; Hanzel, C.E.; Jacobs, M.L.; Machnes, Z.; Iulita, M.F.; Yang, J.; Yu, L.; Ducatenzeiler, A.; Danik, M.; Breuillaud, L.S.; et al. Rescue of Early Bace-1 and Global DNA Demethylation by S-Adenosylmethionine Reduces Amyloid Pathology and Improves Cognition in an Alzheimer's Model. *Sci. Rep.* **2016**, *6*, 34051. [CrossRef]
132. Fuso, A.; Nicolia, V.; Cavallaro, R.A.; Scarpa, S. DNA Methylase and Demethylase Activities Are Modulated by One-Carbon Metabolism in Alzheimer's Disease Models. *J. Nutr. Biochem.* **2011**, *22*, 242–251. [CrossRef]
133. Guitton, R.; Nido, G.S.; Tzoulis, C. No Evidence of Extensive Non-CpG Methylation in mtDNA. *Nucleic Acids Res.* **2022**, *50*, 9190–9194. [CrossRef]
134. Devall, M.; Smith, R.G.; Jeffries, A.; Hannon, E.; Davies, M.N.; Schalkwyk, L.; Mill, J.; Weedon, M.; Lunnon, K. Regional Differences in Mitochondrial DNA Methylation in Human Post-Mortem Brain Tissue. *Clin. Epigenetics* **2017**, *9*, 47. [CrossRef] [PubMed]
135. Huang, C.-H.; Chang, M.-C.; Lai, Y.-C.; Lin, C.-Y.; Hsu, C.-H.; Tseng, B.-Y.; Hsiao, C.K.; Lu, T.-P.; Yu, S.-L.; Hsieh, S.-T.; et al. Mitochondrial DNA Methylation Profiling of the Human Prefrontal Cortex and Nucleus Accumbens: Correlations with Aging and Drug Use. *Clin. Epigenetics* **2022**, *14*, 79. [CrossRef] [PubMed]
136. Shock, L.S.; Thakkar, P.V.; Peterson, E.J.; Moran, R.G.; Taylor, S.M. DNA Methyltransferase 1, Cytosine Methylation, and Cytosine Hydroxymethylation in Mammalian Mitochondria. *Proc. Natl. Acad. Sci. USA* **2011**, *108*, 3630–3635. [CrossRef]
137. Xu, Y.; Xu, L.; Han, M.; Liu, X.; Li, F.; Zhou, X.; Wang, Y.; Bi, J. Altered Mitochondrial DNA Methylation and Mitochondrial DNA Copy Number in an APP/PS1 Transgenic Mouse Model of Alzheimer Disease. *Biochem. Biophys. Res. Commun.* **2019**, *520*, 41–46. [CrossRef] [PubMed]
138. Stoccoro, A.; Siciliano, G.; Migliore, L.; Coppedè, F. Decreased Methylation of the Mitochondrial D-Loop Region in Late-Onset Alzheimer's Disease. *J. Alzheimers Dis.* **2017**, *59*, 559–564. [CrossRef]
139. Ding, B.; Zhang, X.; Wan, Z.; Tian, F.; Ling, J.; Tan, J.; Peng, X. Characterization of Mitochondrial DNA Methylation of Alzheimer's Disease in Plasma Cell-Free DNA. *Diagnostics* **2023**, *13*, 2351. [CrossRef]
140. Blanch, M.; Mosquera, J.L.; Ansoleaga, B.; Ferrer, I.; Barrachina, M. Altered Mitochondrial DNA Methylation Pattern in Alzheimer Disease–Related Pathology and in Parkinson Disease. *Am. J. Pathol.* **2016**, *186*, 385–397. [CrossRef]
141. Kasamatsu, H.; Robberson, D.L.; Vinograd, J. A Novel Closed-Circular Mitochondrial DNA with Properties of a Replicating Intermediate. *Proc. Natl. Acad. Sci. USA* **1971**, *68*, 2252–2257. [CrossRef]
142. Doda, J.N.; Wright, C.T.; Clayton, D.A. Elongation of Displacement-Loop Strands in Human and Mouse Mitochondrial DNA Is Arrested near Specific Template Sequences. *Proc. Natl. Acad. Sci. USA* **1981**, *78*, 6116–6120. [CrossRef]
143. Fish, J.; Raule, N.; Attardi, G. Discovery of a Major D-Loop Replication Origin Reveals Two Modes of Human mtDNA Synthesis. *Science* **2004**, *306*, 2098–2101. [CrossRef]
144. Holt, I.J.; Lorimer, H.E.; Jacobs, H.T. Coupled Leading- and Lagging-Strand Synthesis of Mammalian Mitochondrial DNA. *Cell* **2000**, *100*, 515–524. [CrossRef]
145. Stoccoro, A.; Coppedè, F. Mitochondrial DNA Methylation and Human Diseases. *Int. J. Mol. Sci.* **2021**, *22*, 4594. [CrossRef]
146. Coppedè, F. Mitochondrial DNA Methylation and Mitochondria-Related Epigenetics in Neurodegeneration. *Neural Regen. Res.* **2023**, *19*, 405–406. [CrossRef]
147. Stoccoro, A.; Baldacci, F.; Ceravolo, R.; Giampietri, L.; Tognoni, G.; Siciliano, G.; Migliore, L.; Coppedè, F. Increase in Mitochondrial D-Loop Region Methylation Levels in Mild Cognitive Impairment Individuals. *Int. J. Mol. Sci.* **2022**, *23*, 5393. [CrossRef]
148. Chestnut, B.A.; Chang, Q.; Price, A.; Lesuisse, C.; Wong, M.; Martin, L.J. Epigenetic Regulation of Motor Neuron Cell Death through DNA Methylation. *J. Neurosci.* **2011**, *31*, 16619–16636. [CrossRef]
149. Wong, M.; Gertz, B.; Chestnut, B.A.; Martin, L.J. Mitochondrial DNMT3A and DNA Methylation in Skeletal Muscle and CNS of Transgenic Mouse Models of ALS. *Front. Cell. Neurosci.* **2013**, *7*, 279. [CrossRef]
150. Dzitoyeva, S.; Chen, H.; Manev, H. Effect of Aging on 5-Hydroxymethylcytosine in Brain Mitochondria. *Neurobiol. Aging* **2012**, *33*, 2881–2891. [CrossRef]
151. Sánchez-Caballero, L.; Guerrero-Castillo, S.; Nijtmans, L. Unraveling the Complexity of Mitochondrial Complex I Assembly: A Dynamic Process. *Biochim. Biophys. Acta BBA Bioenerg.* **2016**, *1857*, 980–990. [CrossRef]

152. Jörg, M.; Plehn, J.E.; Kristen, M.; Lander, M.; Walz, L.; Lietz, C.; Wijns, J.; Pichot, F.; Rojas-Charry, L.; Wirtz Martin, K.M.; et al. N1-Methylation of Adenosine (m1A) in ND5 mRNA Leads to Complex I Dysfunction in Alzheimer's Disease. *Mol. Psychiatry* 2024, *ahead of print*. [CrossRef]
153. Han, M.; Liu, Z.; Xu, Y.; Liu, X.; Wang, D.; Li, F.; Wang, Y.; Bi, J. Abnormality of m6A mRNA Methylation Is Involved in Alzheimer's Disease. *Front. Neurosci.* **2020**, *14*, 98. [CrossRef]
154. Hui, Y.; Ma, Q.; Zhou, X.-R.; Wang, H.; Dong, J.-H.; Gao, L.-N.; Zhang, T.; Li, Y.-Y.; Gong, T. Immunological Characterization and Diagnostic Models of RNA N6-Methyladenosine Regulators in Alzheimer's Disease. *Sci. Rep.* **2023**, *13*, 14588. [CrossRef]
155. Shafik, A.M.; Zhang, F.; Guo, Z.; Dai, Q.; Pajdzik, K.; Li, Y.; Kang, Y.; Yao, B.; Wu, H.; He, C.; et al. N6-Methyladenosine Dynamics in Neurodevelopment and Aging, and Its Potential Role in Alzheimer's Disease. *Genome Biol.* **2021**, *22*, 17. [CrossRef]
156. Mannick, J.B.; Lamming, D.W. Targeting the Biology of Aging with mTOR Inhibitors. *Nat. Aging* **2023**, *3*, 642–660. [CrossRef]
157. Perluigi, M.; Di Domenico, F.; Barone, E.; Butterfield, D.A. mTOR in Alzheimer Disease and Its Earlier Stages: Links to Oxidative Damage in the Progression of This Dementing Disorder. *Free Radic. Biol. Med.* **2021**, *169*, 382–396. [CrossRef]
158. Talboom, J.S.; Velazquez, R.; Oddo, S. The Mammalian Target of Rapamycin at the Crossroad between Cognitive Aging and Alzheimer's Disease. *Npj Aging Mech. Dis.* **2015**, *1*, 15008. [CrossRef]
159. Tang, H.-W.; Weng, J.-H.; Lee, W.X.; Hu, Y.; Gu, L.; Cho, S.; Lee, G.; Binari, R.; Li, C.; Cheng, M.E.; et al. mTORC1-Chaperonin CCT Signaling Regulates m6A RNA Methylation to Suppress Autophagy. *Proc. Natl. Acad. Sci. USA* **2021**, *118*, e2021945118. [CrossRef]
160. Cho, S.; Lee, G.; Pickering, B.F.; Jang, C.; Park, J.H.; He, L.; Mathur, L.; Kim, S.-S.; Jung, S.; Tang, H.-W.; et al. mTORC1 Promotes Cell Growth via m6A-Dependent mRNA Degradation. *Mol. Cell* **2021**, *81*, 2064–2075.e8. [CrossRef]
161. Villa, E.; Sahu, U.; O'Hara, B.P.; Ali, E.S.; Helmin, K.A.; Asara, J.M.; Gao, P.; Singer, B.D.; Ben-Sahra, I. mTORC1 Stimulates Cell Growth through SAM Synthesis and m6A mRNA-Dependent Control of Protein Synthesis. *Mol. Cell* **2021**, *81*, 2076–2093.e9. [CrossRef]
162. Ajoolabady, A.; Lindholm, D.; Ren, J.; Pratico, D. ER Stress and UPR in Alzheimer's Disease: Mechanisms, Pathogenesis, Treatments. *Cell Death Dis.* **2022**, *13*, 706. [CrossRef] [PubMed]
163. Schober, F.A.; Moore, D.; Atanassov, I.; Moedas, M.F.; Clemente, P.; Végvári, Á.; Fissi, N.E.; Filograna, R.; Bucher, A.-L.; Hinze, Y.; et al. The One-Carbon Pool Controls Mitochondrial Energy Metabolism via Complex I and Iron-Sulfur Clusters. *Sci. Adv.* **2021**, *7*, eabf0717. [CrossRef] [PubMed]
164. Zurita Rendón, O.; Silva Neiva, L.; Sasarman, F.; Shoubridge, E.A. The Arginine Methyltransferase NDUFAF7 Is Essential for Complex I Assembly and Early Vertebrate Embryogenesis. *Hum. Mol. Genet.* **2014**, *23*, 5159–5170. [CrossRef] [PubMed]
165. Rhein, V.F.; Carroll, J.; Ding, S.; Fearnley, I.M.; Walker, J.E. NDUFAF7 Methylates Arginine 85 in the NDUFS2 Subunit of Human Complex I. *J. Biol. Chem.* **2013**, *288*, 33016–33026. [CrossRef] [PubMed]
166. Shi, Y.; Zhang, W.; Yang, Y.; Murzin, A.G.; Falcon, B.; Kotecha, A.; van Beers, M.; Tarutani, A.; Kametani, F.; Garringer, H.J.; et al. Structure-Based Classification of Tauopathies. *Nature* **2021**, *598*, 359–363. [CrossRef] [PubMed]
167. Thomas, S.N.; Funk, K.E.; Wan, Y.; Liao, Z.; Davies, P.; Kuret, J.; Yang, A.J. Dual Modification of Alzheimer's Disease PHF-Tau Protein by Lysine Methylation and Ubiquitylation: A Mass Spectrometry Approach. *Acta Neuropathol.* **2012**, *123*, 105–117. [CrossRef] [PubMed]
168. Funk, K.E.; Thomas, S.N.; Schafer, K.N.; Cooper, G.L.; Liao, Z.; Clark, D.J.; Yang, A.J.; Kuret, J. Lysine Methylation Is an Endogenous Post-Translational Modification of Tau Protein in Human Brain and a Modulator of Aggregation Propensity. *Biochem. J.* **2014**, *462*, 77–88. [CrossRef] [PubMed]
169. Guo, A.; Gu, H.; Zhou, J.; Mulhern, D.; Wang, Y.; Lee, K.A.; Yang, V.; Aguiar, M.; Kornhauser, J.; Jia, X.; et al. Immunoaffinity Enrichment and Mass Spectrometry Analysis of Protein Methylation. *Mol. Cell. Proteom.* **2014**, *13*, 372–387. [CrossRef] [PubMed]
170. Galukande, M.; Jombwe, J.; Fualal, J.; Baingana, R.; Gakwaya, A. Reference Values for Serum Levels of Folic Acid and Vitamin B12 in a Young Adult Ugandan Population. *Afr. Health Sci.* **2011**, *11*, 240–243.
171. Bailey, L.B. Folate Status Assessment. *J. Nutr.* **1990**, *120*, 1508–1511. [CrossRef]
172. Lawrence, M.A.; Chai, W.; Kara, R.; Rosenberg, I.H.; Scott, J.; Tedstone, A. Examination of Selected National Policies towards Mandatory Folic Acid Fortification. *Nutr. Rev.* **2009**, *67*, S73–S78. [CrossRef] [PubMed]
173. Corrada, M.M.; Kawas, C.H.; Hallfrisch, J.; Muller, D.; Brookmeyer, R. Reduced Risk of Alzheimer's Disease with High Folate Intake: The Baltimore Longitudinal Study of Aging. *Alzheimers Dement. J. Alzheimers Assoc.* **2005**, *1*, 11–18. [CrossRef] [PubMed]
174. Luchsinger, J.A.; Tang, M.-X.; Miller, J.; Green, R.; Mayeux, R. Relation of Higher Folate Intake to Lower Risk of Alzheimer Disease in the Elderly. *Arch. Neurol.* **2007**, *64*, 86–92. [CrossRef] [PubMed]
175. Chen, H.; Liu, S.; Ji, L.; Wu, T.; Ji, Y.; Zhou, Y.; Zheng, M.; Zhang, M.; Xu, W.; Huang, G. Folic Acid Supplementation Mitigates Alzheimer's Disease by Reducing Inflammation: A Randomized Controlled Trial. *Mediat. Inflamm.* **2016**, *2016*, 5912146. [CrossRef] [PubMed]
176. Morris, M.C.; Evans, D.A.; Schneider, J.A.; Tangney, C.C.; Bienia, J.L.; Aggarwal, N.T. Dietary Folate and Vitamins B-12 and B-6 Not Associated with Incident Alzheimer's Disease. *J. Alzheimers Dis. JAD* **2006**, *9*, 435–443. [CrossRef] [PubMed]
177. Nelson, C.; Wengreen, H.J.; MUNGER, R.G.; CORCORAN, C.D. Dietary Folate, Vitamin B-12, Vitamin B-6 and Incident Alzheimer's Disease: The Cache County Memory, Health, and Aging Study. *J. Nutr. Health Aging* **2009**, *13*, 899–905. [CrossRef] [PubMed]

178. Clarke, R.; Bennett, D.; Parish, S.; Lewington, S.; Skeaff, M.; Eussen, S.J.P.M.; Lewerin, C.; Stott, D.J.; Armitage, J.; Hankey, G.J.; et al. Effects of Homocysteine Lowering with B Vitamins on Cognitive Aging: Meta-Analysis of 11 Trials with Cognitive Data on 22,000 Individuals. *Am. J. Clin. Nutr.* **2014**, *100*, 657–666. [CrossRef] [PubMed]
179. Kwok, T.; Wu, Y.; Lee, J.; Lee, R.; Yung, C.Y.; Choi, G.; Lee, V.; Harrison, J.; Lam, L.; Mok, V. A Randomized Placebo-Controlled Trial of Using B Vitamins to Prevent Cognitive Decline in Older Mild Cognitive Impairment Patients. *Clin. Nutr.* **2020**, *39*, 2399–2405. [CrossRef] [PubMed]
180. Alam, C.; Kondo, M.; O'Connor, D.L.; Bendayan, R. Clinical Implications of Folate Transport in the Central Nervous System. *Trends Pharmacol. Sci.* **2020**, *41*, 349–361. [CrossRef]
181. Grapp, M.; Wrede, A.; Schweizer, M.; Hüwel, S.; Galla, H.-J.; Snaidero, N.; Simons, M.; Bückers, J.; Low, P.S.; Urlaub, H.; et al. Choroid Plexus Transcytosis and Exosome Shuttling Deliver Folate into Brain Parenchyma. *Nat. Commun.* **2013**, *4*, 2123. [CrossRef]
182. Zhao, R.; Aluri, S.; Goldman, I.D. The Proton-Coupled Folate Transporter (PCFT-SLC46A1) and the Syndrome of Systemic and Cerebral Folate Deficiency of Infancy: Hereditary Folate Malabsorption. *Mol. Asp. Med.* **2017**, *53*, 57–72. [CrossRef]
183. Sangha, V.; Hoque, M.T.; Henderson, J.T.; Bendayan, R. Novel Localization of Folate Transport Systems in the Murine Central Nervous System. *Fluids Barriers CNS* **2022**, *19*, 92. [CrossRef]
184. Alam, C.; Aufreiter, S.; Georgiou, C.J.; Hoque, M.T.; Finnell, R.H.; O'Connor, D.L.; Goldman, I.D.; Bendayan, R. Upregulation of Reduced Folate Carrier by Vitamin D Enhances Brain Folate Uptake in Mice Lacking Folate Receptor Alpha. *Proc. Natl. Acad. Sci. USA* **2019**, *116*, 17531–17540. [CrossRef]
185. Littlejohns, T.J.; Henley, W.E.; Lang, I.A.; Annweiler, C.; Beauchet, O.; Chaves, P.H.M.; Fried, L.; Kestenbaum, B.R.; Kuller, L.H.; Langa, K.M.; et al. Vitamin D and the Risk of Dementia and Alzheimer Disease. *Neurology* **2014**, *83*, 920–928. [CrossRef]
186. Mathys, H.; Davila-Velderrain, J.; Peng, Z.; Gao, F.; Mohammadi, S.; Young, J.Z.; Menon, M.; He, L.; Abdurrob, F.; Jiang, X.; et al. Single-Cell Transcriptomic Analysis of Alzheimer's Disease. *Nature* **2019**, *570*, 332–337. [CrossRef]
187. Hoozemans, J.J.M.; Veerhuis, R.; Van Haastert, E.S.; Rozemuller, J.M.; Baas, F.; Eikelenboom, P.; Scheper, W. The Unfolded Protein Response Is Activated in Alzheimer's Disease. *Acta Neuropathol.* **2005**, *110*, 165–172. [CrossRef]
188. Popovic, R.; Celardo, I.; Yu, Y.; Costa, A.C.; Loh, S.H.Y.; Martins, L.M. Combined Transcriptomic and Proteomic Analysis of Perk Toxicity Pathways. *Int. J. Mol. Sci.* **2021**, *22*, 4598. [CrossRef]
189. Bermingham, A.; Derrick, J.P. The Folic Acid Biosynthesis Pathway in Bacteria: Evaluation of Potential for Antibacterial Drug Discovery. *BioEssays* **2002**, *24*, 637–648. [CrossRef]
190. Rosenberg, I.H. A History of the Isolation and Identification of Folic Acid (Folate). *Ann. Nutr. Metab.* **2012**, *61*, 231–235. [CrossRef]
191. Wills, L. Treatment of "Pernicious Anaemia of Pregnancy" and "Tropical Anaemia". *Br. Med. J.* **1931**, *1*, 1059–1064. [CrossRef]
192. Krause, L.J.; Forsberg, C.W.; O'Connor, D.L. Feeding Human Milk to Rats Increases Bifidobacterium in the Cecum and Colon Which Correlates with Enhanced Folate Status. *J. Nutr.* **1996**, *126*, 1505–1511. [CrossRef] [PubMed]
193. Stanciu, G.D.; Luca, A.; Rusu, R.N.; Bild, V.; Beschea Chiriac, S.I.; Solcan, C.; Bild, W.; Ababei, D.C. Alzheimer's Disease Pharmacotherapy in Relation to Cholinergic System Involvement. *Biomolecules* **2019**, *10*, 40. [CrossRef] [PubMed]
194. van Dyck, C.H.; Swanson, C.J.; Aisen, P.; Bateman, R.J.; Chen, C.; Gee, M.; Kanekiyo, M.; Li, D.; Reyderman, L.; Cohen, S.; et al. Lecanemab in Early Alzheimer's Disease. *N. Engl. J. Med.* **2023**, *388*, 9–21. [CrossRef] [PubMed]

International Journal of
Molecular Sciences

MDPI

Review

Exploring the Role of Surface and Mitochondrial ATP-Sensitive Potassium Channels in Cancer: From Cellular Functions to Therapeutic Potentials

Dong-Oh Moon

Department of Biology Education, Daegu University, 201, Daegudae-ro, Gyeongsan-si 38453, Gyeongsangbuk-do, Republic of Korea; domoon@daegu.ac.kr; Tel.: +82-53-850-6992

Abstract: ATP-sensitive potassium (KATP) channels are found in plasma membranes and mitochondria. These channels are a type of ion channel that is regulated by the intracellular concentration of adenosine triphosphate (ATP) and other nucleotides. In cell membranes, they play a crucial role in linking metabolic activity to electrical activity, especially in tissues like the heart and pancreas. In mitochondria, KATP channels are involved in protecting cells against ischemic damage and regulating mitochondrial function. This review delves into the role of KATP channels in cancer biology, underscoring their critical function. Notably responsive to changes in cellular metabolism, KATP channels link metabolic states to electrical activity, a feature that becomes particularly significant in cancer cells. These cells, characterized by uncontrolled growth, necessitate unique metabolic and signaling pathways, differing fundamentally from normal cells. Our review explores the intricate roles of KATP channels in influencing the metabolic and ionic balance within cancerous cells, detailing their structural and operational mechanisms. We highlight the channels' impact on cancer cell survival, proliferation, and the potential of KATP channels as therapeutic targets in oncology. This includes the challenges in targeting these channels due to their widespread presence in various tissues and the need for personalized treatment strategies. By integrating molecular biology, physiology, and pharmacology perspectives, the review aims to enhance the understanding of cancer as a complex metabolic disease and to open new research and treatment avenues by focusing on KATP channels. This comprehensive approach provides valuable insights into the potential of KATP channels in developing innovative cancer treatments.

Keywords: KATP channel; cancer; mitochondria; potassium

1. Introduction

KATP channels are crucial in controlling cell functions across various tissues such as the heart, pancreas, and brain. Their distinctive characteristic lies in their responsiveness to the cell's metabolic condition, particularly to alterations in ATP/ADP ratios, thereby linking cellular metabolism with electrical activities [1,2]. Recent research has increasingly highlighted the important role of KATP channels in the field of oncology.

Cancer cells are known for their rampant growth and proliferation, necessitating unique metabolic processes and signaling pathways, unlike normal cells. KATP channels' capacity to influence membrane potential and the pathways of intracellular signaling is vital in comprehending the physiology of cancer cells [3,4]. This review is focused on dissecting the complex roles of KATP channels within cancer cells, examining their impact on the distinct metabolic and ionic makeup of tumor environments.

Initially, we will investigate the fundamental architecture and operational mechanisms of KATP channels, emphasizing their regulatory functions. Subsequently, the focus will shift to their evolving significance in oncology, exploring how changes in their expression and functionality can affect cancer cell endurance, growth, and spread. The review will also discuss current studies on the potential of KATP channels as targets in cancer therapies, including the associated challenges and prospects.

Incorporating insights from molecular biology, physiology, and pharmacology, this thorough analysis aims to present an integrated perspective on the role of KATP channels in cancer. This contributes to the broader understanding of cancer as a multifaceted metabolic disorder. By elucidating the complex interactions between KATP channels and cancer cells, this review seeks to pave the way for new research and treatment approaches in combating cancer.

2. Biological Functions of Potassium

Potassium (K^+) is an essential electrolyte that maintains cell membrane potential, regulates fluid balance, supports nerve and muscle function, including heart rhythm, and contributes to overall electrolyte and acid–base balance in the body. This review emphasizes the diverse and vital roles of K^+ in cancer cell physiology, encompassing its impact on glycolysis, cell cycle progression, apoptosis, and metastasis.

K^+ is crucial for regulating glycolysis in cancer cells, with hexokinase I and II overexpression initiating glucose metabolism critical for cancer cell growth [5,6]. The activity of hexokinase II, influenced by intracellular K^+ levels affected by plasma membrane K^+ channels such as Kv1.3, modulates glycolytic activity [7]. Pyruvate, the end product of glycolysis, either enters the TCA cycle or converts to lactic acid based on oxygen availability [8]. Pyruvate kinase, particularly its PKM2 isoform, acts as a metabolic switch in cancer cells, promoting lactic acid production. K^+ and other monovalent cations' influence on PK, including PKM2, highlights K^+ channels' significant role in cancer metabolism.

K^+ plays a pivotal role in the regulation of the cell cycle, being a key intracellular ion essential for maintaining the electrochemical gradient across cell membranes. During the G1 phase of the cell cycle, membrane hyperpolarization occurs, a process significantly influenced by growth factors like IGF-1. These growth factors interact with receptor tyrosine kinases (RTKs), such as IGF-1R, triggering pathways like extracellular signal-regulated kinase1/2 (ERK) and Phosphoinositide 3-kinase (PI_3K). This activation leads to an increase in the expression and activity of various K^+ channels, including Kv channels and calcium (Ca^{2+})-activated K^+ channels. The resulting hyperpolarization of the membrane establishes an electrical gradient that promotes Ca^{2+} influx through channels such as Ca^{2+} release-activated Ca^{2+} (CRAC) channel1, CRAC3, transient receptor potential canonical 1 (TRPC1), and TRPV6. This influx of Ca^{2+} further regulates the activity and expression of Ca^{2+}-activated K^+ channels, sustaining the hyperpolarized state and enhancing Ca^{2+} entry. The elevation in intracellular Ca^{2+} levels activates Ca^{2+}-dependent signaling enzymes, impacting the expression and activity of transcription factors like FOS, JUN, NFAT, and C-MYC. This sequence of events triggers the expression of cyclins and CDKs while inhibiting CDK inhibitor proteins, including p27KIP1 and p21waf1/cip1 [9–11]. Additionally, K^+ is instrumental in controlling cell volume, which is crucial for cell cycle progression. For example, the Eag2 channels regulate the expression of cyclin B1 through the p38 MAP kinase pathway during the M phase of the cell cycle, demonstrating another dimension of K^+'s role in cell cycle regulation [12].

K^+ plays a crucial role in apoptosis by regulating enzymatic activities essential for cellular breakdown. High intracellular K^+ levels inhibit enzymes like nucleases, necessary for DNA degradation during apoptosis, with inhibition occurring at normal cellular K^+ concentrations (around 150 mM) [13]. K^+ also affects caspase activation, where physiological levels of K+ inhibit apoptotic enzyme cascades. Apoptotic cells exhibit a significant K^+ concentration reduction to about 35 mM, leading to enzyme activation involved in apoptosis [13]. This K^+ efflux is associated with cell shrinkage, a characteristic of apoptosis, facilitating the activation of apoptosis-inducing enzymes [14]. Experiments involving K^+ depletion and K^+ channel overexpression have confirmed apoptosis induction across various cell types.

In cancer cells, the modulation of K^+ channels present a potential therapeutic target. The involvement of these channels in apoptosis varies according to cancer type, channel type, and their regulation by factors influencing cell death or survival. Overall, K^+'s role in apoptosis, particularly through its effects on enzymatic activities and cell volume regulation, offers novel insight into the mechanisms of apoptosis regulation. This understanding has significant implications for developing therapeutic strategies targeting K^+ channels in cancer treatment.

In the context of cancer metastasis, the role of K^+ is critically linked to its influence on cell migration and invasion, which are key processes in the metastatic cascade. This aspect of cancer progression is not only crucial but often determines the lethality of the disease. Metastasis is responsible for over 90% of cancer-related deaths, with cell migration playing a central role in this process by enabling the spread of primary tumor cells to distant sites in the body [15]. The migration of cancer cells is characterized by dynamic changes in cell volume, which are crucial for the movement of cells. The leading edge of a migratory cell extends by increasing its volume, which is facilitated by the influx of ions and water. K^+ channels play a role in this process by helping to regulate the cell volume at both the leading and trailing edges of the cell. During cell migration, K^+ channels exhibit a polarized subcellular distribution. This distribution is essential for the localized hydrodynamic changes in the cell. At the cell's trailing edge, Ca^{2+} entry activates Ca^{2+}-activated K^+ channels, leading to K^+ efflux [16]. This efflux is part of the mechanism that reduces cell volume at the trailing edge, a critical step for cell motility. K^+ channels work in coordination with Cl- channels, Na^+ channels, and Na^+-K^+-Cl^- cotransporters to maintain ionic and water homeostasis during cell migration. This coordinated activity is crucial for the local changes in cell volume that drive the protrusion and retraction of the cell's leading and trailing edges, respectively. The precise function of certain K^+ channels, such as Kir4.2, situated at the leading edge of migrating cells [17], remains a subject of ongoing research. However, it is hypothesized that K^+ influx through Kir channels at the leading edge could occur due to a local reversal of the K^+ electrochemical gradient. The direction of K^+ flow through these channels, whether inward or outward, depends on the local electrochemical gradient and is crucial for understanding their precise role in cell migration and metastasis. The movement of cancer cells through tissues requires the degradation of extracellular matrix proteins. K^+ channels, by regulating the cell volume and maintaining the ionic balance, indirectly facilitate these processes, aiding in tumor cell invasion. Figure 1 depicts the physiological role of K^+ in various cellular processes.

The functions of K^+ as outlined above are mediated by a variety of K^+ channels. K^+ channels are primarily classified into four distinct groups based on their structural characteristics and functional roles: voltage-gated (Kv), calcium-activated (KCa), inwardly rectifying (Kir), and two-pore-domain (K2P) potassium channels. Within the inner mitochondrial membrane, several specialized types have been identified, including mitochondrial KATP channels, mitochondrial large-conductance calcium-activated potassium (mitoBKCa) channels, mitochondrial voltage-dependent potassium (mitoKv1.3) channels, and twin-pore TASK-3 potassium channels. The discovery of the mitochondrial KATP channel was first made in liver mitochondria, with subsequent findings in various tissues such as the heart, brain, kidney, skeletal muscle, human T lymphocytes, and even amoeba mitochondria. This article will focus on the significance of KATP channels within cancer cells, underscoring their distinct functionality among the diverse potassium channel types.

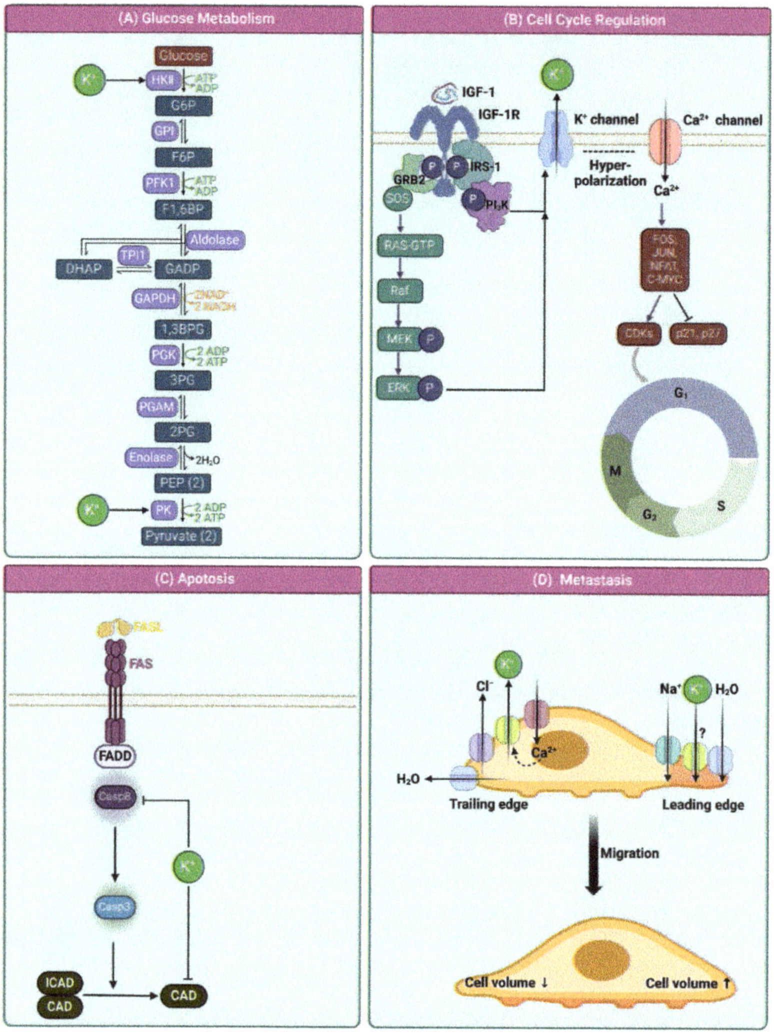

Figure 1. Schematic Representation of Potassium's (K^+) Role in Various Cellular Processes. (**A**) K^+ interaction with hexokinase II (HKII) initiates glycolysis by converting glucose to glucose-6-phosphate (G6P). This segment traces the glycolytic pathway, showing the influence of K^+ on key metabolic enzymes, including pyruvate kinase (PK), leading to pyruvate production and its metabolic outcomes in varying oxygen conditions. (**B**) The role of K^+ in cell cycle regulation is depicted, beginning with the engagement of insulin-like growth factor 1 (IGF-1) with its receptor IGF-1R. Activation of PI_3K/Akt and RAS/ERK pathways leads to K^+ channel-mediated membrane hyperpolarization, affecting Ca^{2+} uptake and activating transcription factors that govern cell cycle progression. (**C**) K^+ is depicted as an inhibitor of apoptosis, where elevated K^+ levels suppress the activation of caspase-8 (Casp8) and the CAD enzyme, highlighting its role in inhibiting the apoptotic process. (**D**) K^+'s control over cell volume changes during cancer cell migration is shown, with a focus on the polarized distribution of K^+ channels and other ion channels at the cellular edges. The coordination of these channels is critical for facilitating cell migration, a vital process in cancer metastasis. The question mark indicates that the exact potassium channel is not known. Cartoon in Figure 1 was created with BioRender.com.

3. Structure and Regulation of KATP Channels

Plasma membrane KATP channels play a pivotal role in various tissues, acting as key mediators between cellular metabolic activity and membrane excitability. These channels are formed as hetero-octameric complexes, composed of four inward rectifier K^+ channel subunits (Kir6.1 or Kir6.2, corresponding to genes KCNJ8 and KCNJ11, respectively) and four sulfonylurea receptor subunits (SUR1 or SUR2, associated with genes ABCC8 and ABCC9, respectively). The process of alternative splicing of ABCC9 gives rise to unique SUR2A and SUR2B subunits, which differ in their carboxyl terminal amino acid sequences. The spatial relationship of KCNJ8 with ABCC9 on chromosome 12 and of KCNJ11 with ABCC8 on chromosome 11 indicates a likely co-regulation and gene duplication phenomenon [18]. Each Kir6 unit encompasses two membrane-spanning domains surrounding a pore loop, crucial for K^+ selectivity. These units feature a significant cytoplasmic domain at the amino and carboxyl ends. The SUR subunits, part of the ATP-binding cassette superfamily, consist of 17 transmembrane domains along with two intracellular nucleotide-binding folds. These elements together establish two adenine nucleotide-binding sites, ABS1 and ABS2, at their interface [19,20].

The understanding of mitochondrial KATP channels has evolved over time, reflecting their complex nature and the ongoing research in this field. Initially, it was believed that these mitochondrial channels shared structural similarities with their plasma membrane counterparts, possibly being variants of the same family. Early studies suggested that subunits Kir6.1 or Kir6.2, which are characteristic of plasma membrane KATP channels, might also form the mitochondrial channels. However, this view has been challenged by more recent research. Subsequent investigations pointed towards the ROMK2 potassium channel, a variant of the renal outer medullary potassium channel, as a likely structural component of mitochondrial KATP channels [21,22]. This was a significant development, highlighting the distinct characteristics of mitochondrial channels. Furthermore, recent breakthroughs identified the CCDC51 gene as responsible for producing the pore-forming subunit of the mitochondrial KATP channel [23]. This finding was crucial in understanding the channel's structure and function. The channel's inhibition by glibenclamide, an antidiabetic drug, led to speculation about the involvement of the glibenclamide receptor (SUR) as a component of the channel. This hypothesis was confirmed by the discovery that CCDC51 interacts with mitochondrial SUR, encoded by the ABCB8 gene. This interaction forms a channel with the established pharmacological properties of mitochondrial KATP channels. Another intriguing aspect of mitochondrial KATP channels is the suggested involvement of ATP synthase subunits or respiratory chain components in their formation. This hypothesis gained support from observations that the channel is sensitive to specific modulators and inhibitors. It indicates that the F1FO segment of ATP synthase might facilitate potassium flux, functioning similarly for both potassium and hydrogen ions [24]. These findings underscore the possibility that mitochondrial ATP-sensitive potassium flux might be mediated by a variety of proteins, each contributing to the channel's multifaceted role in cellular physiology. The structures of plasma membrane KATP channels and mitochondrial KATP channels are shown in Figure 2.

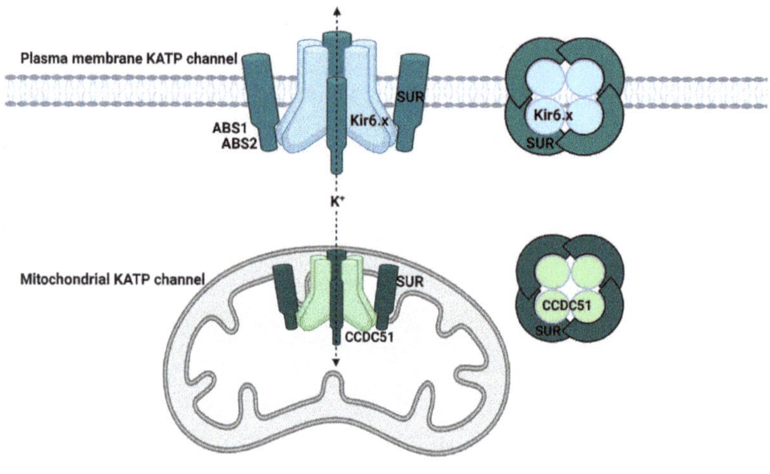

Figure 2. Structural Comparison of Plasma Membrane and Mitochondrial KATP Channels. The plasma membrane KATP channel is depicted as a hetero-octameric complex, with four inward rectifier K^+ channel subunits (Kir6.x) and four sulfonylurea receptor subunits (SUR), which together modulate cellular metabolism and membrane excitability. These channels are shown with two transmembrane domains and a central pore loop, flanked by significant cytoplasmic domains, essential for potassium ion selectivity. The SUR subunits exhibit 17 transmembrane domains and two nucleotide-binding folds, forming adenine nucleotide-binding sites (ABS1 and ABS2). In contrast, the mitochondrial KATP channel, formed by the interaction of CCDC51 with mitochondrial SUR (encoded by ABCB8), highlights a unique structure divergent from the plasma membrane counterpart. Cartoon in Figure 2 was created with BioRender.com.

4. Mechanisms of Opening and Closing of KATP Channels

The regulation of plasma membrane KATP channels' opening and closing is primarily governed by ATP and ADP levels but also influenced by various other physiological factors, including phosphatidylinositol 4,5-bisphosphate (PIP_2), long-chain acyl-CoA molecules, and intracellular pH levels. This review delves into these diverse regulatory elements and explores how they collectively modulate KATP channel activation, particularly in the context of cancer cell physiology.

Plasma membrane KATP channels are inhibited by intracellular ATP, with binding occurring on the Kir6 subunit [25,26]. The inhibition is not due to phosphorylation but direct binding to the channel, with ATP analogues also inhibiting channel activity. In the absence of Mg^{2+}, binding of ADP to SUR blocks KATP channel activity with lower affinity than ATP, highlighting the importance of electrostatic interactions with phosphate moieties of ATP [27,28]. Cancer cells undergo significant metabolic reprogramming, which includes a marked change in their ATP/ADP ratio. In normal cells, the adenine nucleotide translocator (ANT) facilitates the electrogenic exchange of ATP for ADP within mitochondria, a process closely linked to the mitochondrial membrane potential ($\Delta\Psi$). This exchange maintains a high cytosolic ATP/ADP ratio [29]. In contrast, cancer cells exhibit a significant decrease in this ratio owing to a switch to a different ATP/ADP exchange mechanism. Cancer cells predominantly utilize the ATP-Mg^{2+}/phosphate carrier (AMPC) for ATP/ADP exchange, as opposed to ANT used in normal cells. AMPC differs from ANT in its ability to facilitate the net uptake of adenine nucleotides, essential for mitochondrial biogenesis, and is notably upregulated in cancer cells [30,31]. The non-electrogenic nature of exchange via AMPC leads to substantially lower ATP/ADP ratios in the cytosol of cancer cells, contributing to the characteristic aerobic glycolysis and lactate production, a phenomenon known as the Warburg metabolic phenotype [32]. The decreased ATP/ADP ratio in cancer cells has several repercussions, one of which is the potential activation of KATP channels. These channels are sensitive to intracellular ATP and ADP levels and play a critical role in various cellular processes. In the context of cancer, the reduced ATP/ADP ratio could lead to the activation of KATP channels, affecting cellular functions such as ion transport, membrane potential regulation, and possibly influencing cellular proliferation and survival mechanisms. Furthermore, the lower ATP/ADP ratios in cancer cells result in diminished stimulation of mitochondrial oxidative phosphorylation, favoring glycolysis over oxidative phosphorylation for ATP production. This shift in energy metabolism, however, does not seem to impede the growth and proliferation of cancer cells. The energy requirements for vital cellular processes like protein and nucleic acid synthesis in eukaryotic cancer cells are akin to those in prokaryotes, where natural ATP/ADP ratios are relatively low [33,34]. The alteration in ATP/ADP ratios in cancer cells, stemming from a switch in ATP/ADP exchange mechanisms, not only underscores the metabolic flexibility of cancer cells but also highlights potential targets for therapeutic intervention, such as the KATP channels. Understanding how these channels are regulated in the context of cancer metabolism and how they contribute to cancer cell physiology could open new avenues for cancer treatment strategies.

PIP_2 is a crucial regulator of plasma membrane KATP channel activity, particularly influencing the Kir6.2 subunit. The binding of PIP_2 to Kir6.2 facilitates the opening of KATP channels, a mechanism that appears to be conserved in Kir6.1 channels, underscoring the fundamental role of phospholipid binding and channel gating processes [35,36]. In the context of cancer cell signaling, PIP_2 serves as a key substrate for generating second messengers, such as diacylglycerol (DAG) and inositol 1,4,5-trisphosphate (IP_3), through the activation of phospholipase C (PLC). The dysregulation of PLC, leading to altered PIP_2 metabolism, is a common feature in various oncogenic pathways [37]. This alteration in PIP_2 levels is also intricately linked to the PI_3K/AKT signaling pathway, often hyperactivated in cancers. The phosphorylation of phosphoinositides, including the conversion of PIP_2 to its phosphorylated form PIP_3, is modulated by oncogenic drivers like PI_3K and tumor suppressors such as PTEN. PTEN acts as a phosphatase that converts PIP_3 back to PIP_2, with its loss or mutation leading to elevated PIP_3 levels and subsequent aberrant activation of downstream signaling pathways that contribute to tumorigenesis [38]. Consequently, in cancer cells, where PIP_2 levels are frequently upregulated, KATP channels are more likely to be in an activated state, suggesting a potential link between altered PIP_2 metabolism and KATP channel activity in the cancerous milieu.

Long-chain acyl-coA (LC-CoA) molecules, which are intermediates in the β-oxidation of fatty acids, are known to activate plasma membrane KATP channels by interacting with the same residues on the Kir6.2 subunit as PIP_2 [39,40]. In cancer cells, there is often a significant reprogramming of lipid metabolism, characterized by an increase in fatty acid synthesis and uptake to support rapid cell proliferation. This metabolic shift results in an accumulation of fatty acid intermediates like acyl-CoA molecules. Carracedo et al. have illustrated the pivotal role of lipid metabolism in cancer, emphasizing the synthesis and degradation of fatty acids, which subsequently influence the levels of acyl-CoA [41]. Consequently, the elevated presence of LC-CoA molecules in cancer cells is likely to contribute to the activation of KATP channels.

The activity of plasma membrane KATP channels is also influenced by the intracellular pH levels [42,43]. At a molecular level, the sensitivity of KATP channels to ATP is modulated by changes in pH. Studies involving the Kir6.2 subunit of these channels have identified critical amino acids, specifically Thr71 and His175, that are believed to be key in the channel's pH sensitivity [44,45]. However, the precise mechanism by which these amino acids interact with protons and influence ATP-dependent channel gating remains an area of active research. Given the tendency of cancer cells to have a lower pH compared to normal cells, a consequence of their reliance on glycolysis for energy [46], there is a likelihood of increased KATP channel activity in these cells. The shift towards glycolysis in cancer cells, a process referred to as the Warburg effect, leads to increased production of lactic acid, thereby reducing the intracellular pH. This enhanced activity could play a role in the unique physiological behaviors observed in cancer cells, including their growth and survival mechanisms. Understanding this relationship between intracellular pH and KATP channel function could provide new insights into cancer cell biology and potential therapeutic targets.

Plasma membrane KATP channels are subject to regulation by phosphorylation. Specifically, Protein Kinase A (PKA) plays a key role in modulating the activity of these channels in smooth muscle and pancreatic tissues. The Kir6.2 subunit of the KATP channel contains two sites known to be targeted by PKA phosphorylation. When phosphorylated, these sites enhance the probability of the channel remaining open, altering its functional state [47,48]. Cancer cells often exhibit abnormal signaling via G protein-coupled receptors (GPCRs), leading to elevated cyclic AMP (cAMP) levels and consequent PKA activation. This aberration in GPCR signaling can stem from overexpression, mutations, or dysregulated control of these receptors, influencing adenylate cyclase (AC) activity and impacting downstream pathways [49].

In addition to PKA, Protein Kinase C (PKC) also regulates plasma membrane KATP channel activity. PKC achieves this through the phosphorylation of a conserved T180 residue on the Kir6.2 subunit [50,51]. In the context of cancer, PKC activation is often driven by increased diacylglycerol (DAG) and Ca^{2+} levels, common in dysregulated signal transduction pathways characteristic of malignancies. This increase in DAG may be a result of either heightened activity of phospholipase C (PLC) or changes in lipid metabolism typically observed in cancer cells [52]. The role of PKC in cancer is complex, with different isoforms playing either oncogenic or tumor-suppressive roles, depending on their expression and mutation status. Additionally, alterations in RTKs signaling, frequently observed in various cancers, can lead to PKC activation, thereby influencing cellular processes like proliferation, survival, and migration.

A notable distinction in the regulatory mechanisms of mitochondrial KATP channels, compared to their plasma membrane counterparts, is their activation in low-ATP conditions [23,53]. This is an adaptive response observed not only in cardiac tissues during ischemia but also in cancer cells, where a similar energy deficit can occur due to hypoxic conditions. The opening of mitochondrial KATP channels during energy scarcity helps to maintain cellular homeostasis. In the case of heart muscle cells, the onset of ischemia leads to a dip in ATP levels, which triggers the opening of these mitochondrial KATP channels. This event might be followed by a change in the mitochondrial membrane potential, which likely activates voltage-regulated potassium channels [54,55]. Furthermore, with ATP levels down, ion pumps may fail, causing an increase in cell calcium levels. The surge in calcium during ischemia and subsequent return of blood flow could overload the mitochondria with calcium, especially when oxygen is restored, potentially activating calcium-sensitive potassium channels [56]. This process is crucial as it facilitates the maintenance of ionic balance and cellular protection under stress. Unlike plasma membrane KATP channels, which are generally inhibited by a decrease in ATP, their mitochondrial equivalents are designed to respond to such energetic crises by opening, which underscores their role in cellular survival mechanisms. Moreover, the low-ATP condition induced by ischemia, a commonality shared with cancer cells experiencing hypoxia, underscores the universality of this protective response across different cell types. The metabolic stress in cancerous tissues can similarly activate mitochondrial KATP channels, suggesting a potential target for therapeutic intervention. Aside from ATP concentration, mitochondrial KATP channels are influenced by a host of other factors. These include the mitochondrial membrane potential, intracellular pH, and the presence of reactive oxygen species (ROS) [53,57]. Each of these factors can modulate the activity of mitochondrial KATP channels, contributing to their complex role in cell physiology. For instance, a change in the mitochondrial membrane potential could activate or deactivate these channels, while a more acidic intracellular pH, a result of anaerobic glycolysis and ATP hydrolysis, may modify their sensitivity. Additionally, an increase in ROS during reperfusion, when oxygen is reintroduced, has been noted to stimulate these channels, suggesting a multifaceted regulatory system that responds to a variety of cellular conditions. Figure 3 presents a model of the regulatory mechanisms governing the opening and closing of KATP channels.

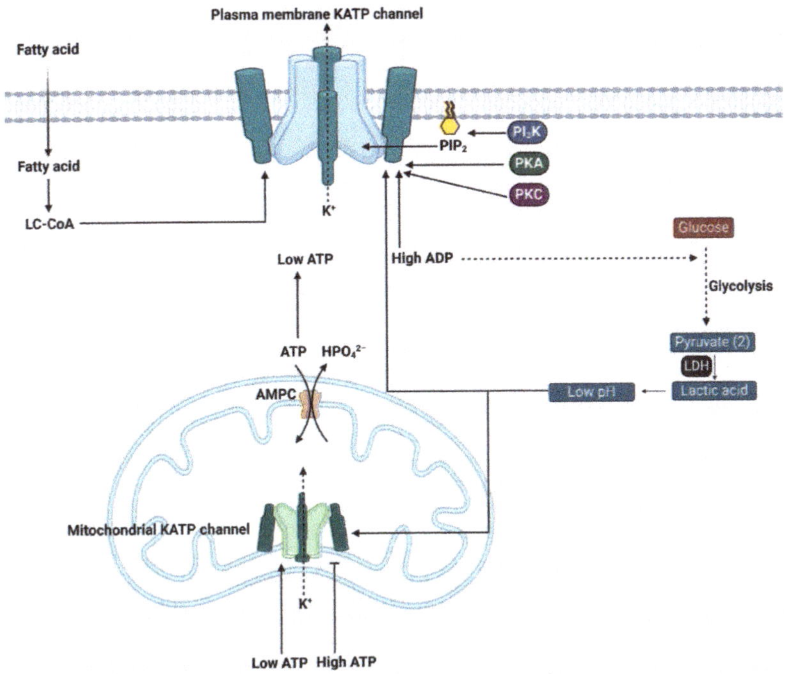

Figure 3. KATP Channel Regulation in Cell Metabolism. High concentration of ATP inhibits plasma membrane KATP channels at the Kir6 subunit, while ADP shows lower-affinity interaction at the SUR subunit, reflecting the distinctive ATP/ADP ratios in cells. PIP_2 binding to Kir6.2 activates KATP channels, with further modulation by PKA and PKC phosphorylation amid cancerous signaling irregularities. Long-chain acyl-CoA molecules, elevated due to cancer cell lipid metabolism, also trigger KATP channel activation. Additionally, KATP channel activity is influenced by intracellular pH through specific amino acid interactions on Kir6.2, relevant in the acidic environment of cells from lactate production. Mitochondrial KATP channels are modulated by intracellular ATP levels, where a decrease prompts opening, and by pH changes, with acidity influencing their activity. Cartoon in Figure 3 was created with BioRender.com.

5. Changes in Expression or Mutation of Genes Constituting KATP Channels in Cancer Cells

Understanding the expression and mutations of KATP channel genes in cancer cells is vital for assessing disease progression, developing targeted therapies, enabling personalized medicine, understanding drug resistance mechanisms, identifying diagnostic and prognostic biomarkers, and gaining insights into cancer metabolism.

Research has demonstrated varying expression patterns of the ABCC8 and ABCC9 genes, crucial in forming KATP channels, across different cancer types. Notably, ABCC8 gene expression exhibits both downregulation and upregulation in cancers such as pancreatic, breast, lung, and colorectal. This review will further explore the varied expression changes in ABCC8 and ABCC9 in a range of cancers, highlighting their potential impact on cancer behavior and treatment responses.

Mohelnikova-Duchonova and colleagues, in their study employing quantitative real-time PCR (qPCR) on tissue samples from 32 patients undergoing surgery for pancreatic adenocarcinoma (PDAC), observed downregulation in the expression of the ABCC8 gene [58]. Hlaváč et al. conducted transcript level analysis of 49 human ABC transporters and immunoblotting for protein expression on post-treatment tumor and non-neoplastic tissue samples from 68 breast carcinoma patients, along with an independent series of

100 pretreatment patients, revealing downregulation of ABCC8 in breast carcinoma [59]. Wang et al. analyzed the FPKM dataset from the TCGA-LUAD database, using 535 lung adenocarcinoma (LUAD) samples and 59 paracancerous samples, and found downregulation of ABCC8 in lung adenocarcinoma [60]. Hlavata et al. conducted quantitative real-time polymerase chain reaction (qRT-PCR) on tissue samples from colorectal carcinoma (CRC) patients, revealing downregulation of ABCC8 in colorectal carcinoma [61]. Conversely, Huang et al. utilized immunocytochemistry and Western blot techniques on human glioma cell lines (U87 and U251), glioma biopsies, and a mice tumor model and observed upregulation of ABCC8 in glioma, impacting cell proliferation and ERK activity [62]. Mao X. et al. analyzed the mRNA expression of ABCC family members in 882 gastric cancer (GC) patients and found upregulation of ABCC8 in gastric cancer [63]. Xiao et al. conducted gene expression analysis using databases on Pancreatic Endocrine Neoplasms (PanNETs) tissues and found upregulation in ABCC8 in PanNETs [64].

Research focusing on the modulation of ABCC8 expression in cancer cells is currently insufficient. Earlier studies have concentrated on understanding the regulatory mechanisms of ABCC8 expression, specifically in pancreatic β-cells within diabetic models [65,66]. Key transcription factors such as Sp1, FoxA2/HNF3β, Beta2/NeuroD, and STAT3 have been recognized as vital regulators of ABCC8 transcription in these cells [67,68]. In the realm of the central nervous system (CNS), studies have shown that hypoxia or ischemia instigates an increase in ABCC8 expression, a process closely related to SP1 activation by hypoxia-inducible factor 1α (Hif1α) [69]. Sp1 is known to initiate ABCC8 transcription across various species [66,69], and targeted inhibition or genetic downregulation of Hif has been found to mitigate brain ischemia/hypoxia by reducing SUR1 overexpression [70,71]. In cancer cells, hypoxia often occurs due to rapid tumor growth surpassing blood vessel development, leading to a reduction in oxygen supply. This decrease in oxygen is likely to stabilize Hif1α, which in turn is expected to activate SP1 and subsequently induce ABCC8 in response to the hypoxic state. Additionally, the activation of ABCC8 transcription in the CNS via the NF-κB pathway, triggered by TNFα, plays a significant role, with NF-κB binding sites present in the ABCC8 promoter regions of both rats and humans [72]. In brain endothelial cells, TNFα exposure, acting as an NF-κB stimulator, enhances ABCC8 mRNA and SUR1 protein levels [73]. Moreover, TLR4 pathway activation in microglia leads to an increase in ABCC8 mRNA and protein levels in the CNS [74,75]. Based on insights from studies in pancreatic beta cells and the CNS, it is hypothesized that ABCC8 expression in cancer cells may be significantly influenced by mechanisms involving hypoxia and inflammation, mediated by TNF-α and TLR signaling. Concurrently, cancer-related inflammation, often a result of interactions between tumor cells and the immune system, prompts the secretion of various factors that stimulate immune cells to produce TNF-α. This cytokine is speculated to activate the NF-κB pathway, playing a pivotal role in inflammatory responses and the regulation of ABCC8 expression in cancer cells. Furthermore, TLR signaling within cancer tissues, often initiated by the recognition of tumor-associated antigens or damage-associated molecular patterns (DAMPs) released from stressed or dying cancer cells, is expected to be an additional factor influencing ABCC8 expression. The mechanism that controls the expression of the ABCC8 gene in cancer cells is illustrated in Figure 4.

Next, this review will examine the findings from research on mutations in the ABCC8 gene. Xiao et al. undertook an extensive mutation analysis using databases focused on PanNETs tissues. This investigation led to the discovery of a notable mutation in the ABCC8 gene specific to PanNETs [64]. In a case study presented by Calton et al., genetic analysis of a child diagnosed with hepatoblastoma revealed a recessive mutation in the ABCC8 gene [76]. Additionally, this study identified UPD 11p15, a genetic abnormality, in both the pancreas and liver of the patient. Further advancing understanding, Soucek et al. [77]. conducted comprehensive exome sequencing in breast cancer patients. Their approach, which involved next-generation sequencing, specifically targeted the ABCC8 and ABCD2 genes. Remarkably, they uncovered 113 genetic mutations within these genes, including a range of frameshifts and missense alterations, shedding new light on the genetic landscape of breast cancer.

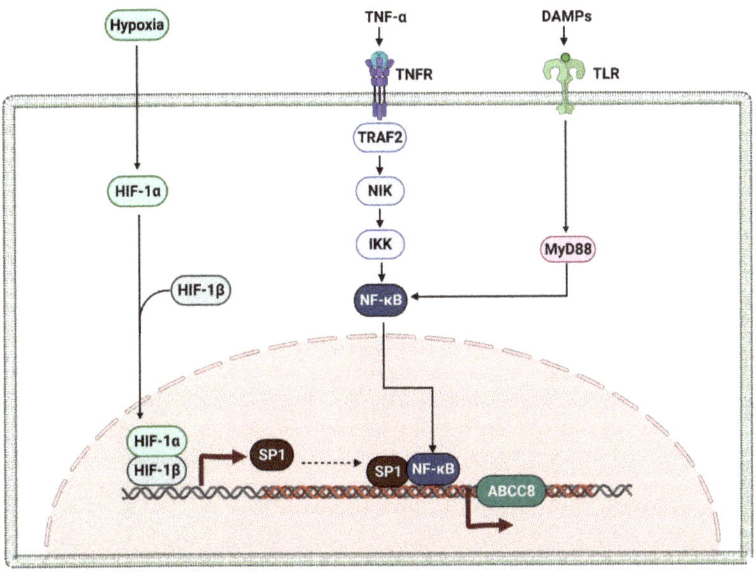

Figure 4. Regulation of ABCC8 Expression in Hypoxic and Inflammatory Conditions. Hypoxia-induced stabilization of HIF-1α interacts with HIF-1β, initiating ABCC8 transcription via SP1 activation. In parallel, TNF-α engagement with TNFR triggers the NF-κB signaling pathway, enhancing ABCC8 expression. Additionally, TLR4 activation by DAMPs, leading to MyD88 involvement, further influences ABCC8 transcription. These interconnected pathways underscore the complexity of ABCC8 regulation in the cancer microenvironment, driven by hypoxia and inflammation commonly associated with tumor progression. Cartoon in Figure 4 was created with BioRender.com.

Regarding investigations into the expression of the ABCC9 gene, Vázquez-Sánchez et al. conducted research on cervical cancer, analyzing both cell lines and human biopsy samples. Their methodology involved reverse transcription polymerase chain reaction and immunochemistry. The findings highlighted upregulation of ABCC9 in cervical cancer [4]. Mao et al. undertook an extensive study with 882 gastric cancer (GC) patients. Their focus was on the mRNA expression of the ABCC family, including ABCC9. The results indicated upregulation of ABCC9 in gastric cancer [63]. In another study by Mao et al., the emphasis was on epithelial ovarian cancer (EOC). They employed quantitative real-time PCR to analyze ABC and SLC transporter genes in EOC tissues, revealing upregulation of ABCC9 in epithelial ovarian cancer [78]. However, contrary to the above results indicating upregulation of ABCC9 expression in various cancers, there have also been reports of studies showing its downregulation. For instance, Zhang et al. reported downregulation of ABCC9 in triple-negative breast cancer based on differential expression and methylation analysis of the tissue [79]. Similarly, Demidenko et al. found downregulation of ABCC9 in prostate cancer, as determined through gene expression profiling and methylation analysis of prostate cancer tissue [80]. Additionally, mutations in ABCC9 have been documented in diverse cancers such as large granular lymphocyte leukemia, endometrial, and gastric cancers (Cheon et al. [81], Le Gallo et al. [82], Zhang et al. [83]), expanding our understanding of its genetic variability in oncogenesis.

In another notable study, Warnecke-Eberz et al. identified upregulation of the KCNJ8 gene in biopsies from patients with locally advanced esophageal squamous cell carcinoma (ESCC), employing genome microarray and TaqMan low-density array techniques for their analysis [84]. Furthermore, research conducted by Zhang et al. revealed upregulation of the KCNJ11 gene via NF-κB signaling in hepatocellular carcinoma (HCC), a finding observed across multiple

HCC cell lines, including Hep3B, MHCC-97H, MHCC-97L, Huh7, SUN-423, and HepG2. This study utilized data mining of the TCGA cohort to arrive at its conclusions [85].

In our final topic, we delve into the gene expression of CCDC51, a key component of mitochondrial KATP channels. The body of research specifically focusing on the CCDC51 gene is quite scarce. However, a significant piece of research employing analysis of both RNA and protein levels has provided insight into the CCDC51 gene, which encodes a subunit integral to the mitochondrial KATP channels. This study utilized existing datasets to ascertain that CCDC51 is actively transcribed and translated across a wide array of tissues in both humans and mice, indicating a fundamental role in cellular physiology [86,87]. Further detailed examination through immunofluorescence assays has shed light on the spatial expression pattern of the CCDC51 protein within cells. These assays revealed a precise localization, with the protein consistently present on the inner mitochondrial membrane [23,88]. This finding is notable as it underscores the specificity of CCDC51's role in mitochondrial function. Moreover, the same assays have verified that the outer mitochondrial membrane lacks CCDC51 protein presence, which suggests selective involvement in the inner mitochondrial mechanisms. This selective localization is particularly evident in HeLa cells, a line of human cervical cancer cells, thereby providing a window into the gene's functional dynamics in a cancerous context. The information discussed thus far is concisely summarized in Table 1 for ease of reference.

Table 1. Variations in Expression and Mutations of KATP Channel Genes (ABCC8, ABCC9, KCNJ8, and KCNJ11) Across Different Cancer Types.

Cancer Cell Type	Model	Research Method	Expression or Mutation	Ref.
Pancreatic Adenocarcinoma (PDAC)	Patient tissue samples (32 surgically treated PDAC patients)	Quantitative Real-Time PCR (qPCR)	Downregulation of ABCC8 in PDAC tumors	[58]
Breast Carcinoma	Post-treatment tumor and non-neoplastic tissue samples from 68 patients; independent series of 100 pretreatment patients	Transcript level analysis of 49 human ABC transporters; immunoblotting for protein expression	Downregulation of ABCC8 in Breast Carcinoma	[59]
Lung Adenocarcinoma (LUAD)	Patient samples (535 LUAD samples and 59 paracancerous samples from TCGA database)	Analysis using FPKM dataset from TCGA-LUAD	Downregulation of ABCC8 in LUAD cancer	[60]
Colorectal Carcinoma (CRC)	Tissue samples from CRC patients	Quantitative real-time polymerase chain reaction (qRTPCR)	Downregulation of ABCC8 in CRC	[61]
Glioma	Human glioma cell lines (U87 and U251), glioma biopsies, and a mice tumor model	Immunocytochemistry, Western blot	Upregulation of ABCC8 in Glioma	[62]
Gastric Cancer (GC)	882 GC patients	Analysis of mRNA expression of ABCC family members in GC patients	Upregulation of ABCC8 in GC	[63]
Pancreatic Endocrine Neoplasms (PanNETs)	PanNET tissues	Gene expression analysis and mutation identification using databases	Upregulation and Mutation in ABCC8 in PanNETs	[64]
Hepatoblastoma	Case study of a child with hepatoblastoma	Genetic testing for ABCC8 mutation and UPD 11p15	ABCC8 recessive mutation and UPD 11p15 in pancreas and liver	[76]

Table 1. *Cont.*

Cancer Cell Type	Model	Research Method	Expression or Mutation	Ref.
Breast Cancer	Exome sequencing in breast cancer patients	Next-generation sequencing of ABCC8 and ABCD2 genes	113 genetic mutation in ABCC8 and ABCD2, including frameshifts and missense alterations	[77]
Cervical Cancer	Cervical cancer cell lines and human biopsies	Reverse transcription polymerase chain reaction and immunochemistry	Upregulation of ABCC9 in Cervical Cancer	[4]
Gastric Cancer (GC)	882 GC patients	Analysis of mRNA expression of ABCC family members in GC patients	Upregulation of ABCC9 in GC	[63]
Epithelial Ovarian Cancer (EOC)	EOC tissue	Quantitative real-time PCR of ABC and SLC transporter genes in EOC	Upregulation of ABCC9 in EOC	[78]
Triple-negative Breast Cancer	Triple-negative Breast Cancer tissue	Differential expression and methylation analysis	Downregulation of ABCC9 in Breast Cancer	[79]
Prostate Cancer	Prostate Cancer tissue	Gene expression profiling and methylation analysis	Downregulation of ABCC9 in Prostate Cancer	[80]
Large Granular Lymphocyte (LGL) Leukemia	105 (LGL) Leukemia patients	Whole-exome and transcriptome sequencing	ABCC9 Mutation: Identified as a recurrently mutated putative driver	[81]
Endometrial Cancer	Frozen primary tumor tissues	Whole-exome sequencing	ABCC9 Mutation: 6% of serous tumors	[82]
Gastric Cancer (GC)	Genomic variant analysis with TCGA database	Prognosis model construction based on TCGA gastric cancer data	ABCC9 Mutation	[83]
Esophageal cancer	Patients with locally advanced squamous cell carcinoma of the esophagus (ESCC) biopsies	Genome microarray and TaqMan low-density array	Upregulation of KCNJ8	[84]
Hepatocellular carcinoma (HCC)	HCC cell lines Hep3B, MHCC-97H, MHCC-97L, Huh7, SUN-423, and HepG2	Data mining TCGA cohort	Upregulation of KCNJ11 via NF-κB signaling	[85]
Human cervical cancer	Cell lines HeLa	Immunofluorescence assay	Expression of CCDC51 on mitochondrial inner membrane	[23]

6. Cancer Cell Growth and KATP Channel

The regulation of membrane potential, essential for cell cycle progression, involves adaptations in membrane permeability. K^+ conductance is a key factor in setting the resting membrane potential across various cell types. Unlike the quick action potentials in neurons, cell cycle-related changes in potential are more gradual, a result of alterations in K^+ conductance [89,90]. In lymphocytes and Schwann cells, research indicates that blocking K^+ channels can lead to a halt in the cell cycle or reduce proliferation [91,92]. Studies on embryonic retinal cells have shown alterations in K^+ channel composition during the G1 phase [93]. Furthermore, in mouse oocytes, K^+ channel activity appears to be partly governed by the cytoplasmic cell-cycle clock, suggesting a role in cell division beyond nuclear controls [94]. This implies K^+ channels' involvement in cell-cycle checkpoint signaling and the integration of cellular clocks. K^+ channels also influence the entry of Ca^{2+} into cells, pivotal for cell proliferation and other key physiological processes [95,96]. The current understanding extends beyond K^+ currents alone as emerging evidence points to specific channels impacting cell proliferation through non-standard mechanisms like protein interactions and voltage-induced conformations.

This review focuses on the role of KATP channels in cell cycle progression and cancer cell proliferation. KATP channels, linking cellular metabolism to membrane excitability, are gaining attention for their involvement in tumor growth and cancer cell proliferation. However, this role is still being unraveled. For instance, Scarth et al. observed a crucial role for KATP channels in cervical carcinogenesis related to human papillomaviruses (HPVs), with a noted upregulation in the SUR1 component in HPV-positive cervical cancer cells, correlated with E7 oncoprotein activity. Blocking these channels significantly reduced cell proliferation, suggesting a new avenue for HPV-related cervical cancer treatment [97]. Ru et al. found that KATP channel blockers reduced proliferation and tumor growth in U87-MG human glioma cells, hinting at a Ca^{2+}-dependent mechanism [98]. Huang et al. also noted higher KATP channel expression in glioma tissues compared to normal ones. Their inhibition lessened glioma cell proliferation and tumor formation in animal models, indicating the potential of KATP channel blockers in glioma therapy [62]. Klimatcheva et al. identified a KATP channel in MCF-7 human breast cancer cells, essential for G1 phase progression, presenting new targets for breast cancer treatment [99]. Wondergem et al. discovered that the sulfonylurea receptor and KATP channels regulate cell growth in human bladder carcinoma (HTB-9) cells. Glibenclamide, a KATP channel blocker, effectively reduced cell proliferation, underscoring the role of the channel role in cancer cell growth mechanisms [100]. Wonderlin et al. reported that membrane potential changes in MCF-7 cells during the cell cycle, likely related to K^+ permeability, are linked to cell cycle progression in breast cancer cells [101]. These studies collectively emphasize the significant role of KATP channels in various cancers, particularly in cell cycle progression and proliferation. The specific mechanisms, including their impact on intracellular Ca^{2+} signaling and potential activation of the MAPK/ERK pathway, remain areas of active research. This growing body of evidence opens up new possibilities for cancer therapy targeting KATP channels. Further comprehensive research is needed to fully understand and exploit KATP channels as therapeutic targets in cancer.

Exploring the function of mitochondrial KATP channels, Angela Paggio's research offers crucial insights, particularly in cancer cell biology. Paggio's team employed Crispr/Cas9 to specifically target the CCDC51 gene in HeLa cells, which is vital for these channels. This gene deletion led to a disruption of ATP-dependent potassium movements within the mitochondria, causing continuous swelling, a process usually regulated by mitochondrial KATP channels [23]. This study delves into KATP, with a focus on their presence and function in mitochondria. It introduces MITOK, a novel protein complex, and details its role in ATP-sensitive K^+ transport within the mitochondrial KATP channel. The paper clarifies how MITOK and MITOSUR proteins control the mitochondrial KATP channel, emphasizing its importance in cardioprotection, cellular death regulation, and maintaining metabolic balance. The research is notable for its comprehensive molecular analysis of the mitochondrial KATP channel's functionality in the mitochondrial membrane, significantly advancing our understanding of mitochondrial physiology and related diseases. The CCDC51-depleted cells displayed unique ring-shaped mitochondria and underwent spontaneous transient depolarizations. This was accompanied by a noticeable decrease in oxygen consumption rates, pointing to reduced mitochondrial efficiency. Electron microscopy studies showed that these cells had enlarged cristae, indicative of structural changes due to altered matrix volume and osmotic balance. Furthermore, the CCDC51-lacking cells exhibited heightened ROS production, signaling compromised mitochondrial function and a shifted redox state. In cancer cells like HeLa, such mitochondrial swelling and dysfunction can profoundly affect metabolism, which relies heavily on mitochondria for both energy production and controlling cell death. The resulting oxidative stress from altered redox balance and increased ROS could interfere with cellular signaling and DNA stability, factors critical in cancer development and resistance to treatment. The study's findings that CCDC51 is essential for mitochondrial response to cellular stress have important implications in cancer cell biology. By influencing redox balance and maintaining mitochondrial structure, CCDC51 plays a key role in managing how cancer cells survive and adapt to stress, highlighting its potential as a therapeutic target in cancer treatment.

7. Exploring the Role of KATP Channel Activators in Cancer Biology

In cancer biology, activators and inhibitors of KATP channels are crucial as they can regulate cancer cell survival, metabolism, and response to therapies by modulating mitochondrial functions and cellular ion balance. Table 2 outlines a range of substances that either activate or inhibit KATP channels located in the plasma membrane and mitochondria. Certain compounds exert their effects on both types of KATP channels, whereas others are selective in their action, targeting either plasma membrane or mitochondrial channels exclusively.

Table 2. Regulators of KATP channels and their specificity for mitochondrial versus plasma membrane channels.

Action on KATP Channels	Plasma Membrane KATP Channel	Plasma Membrane and Mitochondrial KATP Channel	Mitochondrial KATP Channel
Activator	P-1075 MCC-134	Cromakalim Pinacidil P-1060 Sildenafil Isoflurane Aprikalim Minoxidil Sulfate	Diazoxide Nicorandil BMS 191095
Inhibitor	HMR1098 (1833) Glimepiridec	Glibenclamide Glipizide	5-Hydroxydecanoate MCC-134

The function of KATP channel activators is to stimulate the opening of these channels. When KATP channels open, K^+ ions flow out of the cell, leading to hyperpolarization of the cell membrane. This hyperpolarization can affect many cellular activities, including the regulation of insulin secretion in pancreatic cells, dilation of blood vessels, and protection of cardiac tissue during periods of metabolic stress. Types of KATP channel activators include diazoxide, minoxidil, Pinacidil, and Cromakalim. The exploration of KATP channel activators in cancer research has unfolded a complex landscape where drugs interact diversely with various cancer cell types. Each drug's unique impact offers a glimpse into the intricate relationship between ion channels and cancer cell behavior.

In a study by Wondergem et al., diazoxide was shown to stimulate growth in human bladder carcinoma cells, as evidenced by increased protein accumulation [100]. However, this stimulation did not translate to an increase in cell number. The research implies that diazoxide's role in cancer cell growth might be more nuanced, possibly affecting certain cellular processes without necessarily promoting cell proliferation.

Several studies have shed light on the diverse impacts of minoxidil on cancer cells. Maqoud et al. found that, in renal tumors and canine breast cancer, minoxidil led to elevated expression of the Sur2A subunit in proliferating cells, suggesting a possible role in cancer progression [102]. Meanwhile, Qiu et al. demonstrated that minoxidil could reduce invasion in human breast cancer cells in a dose-dependent manner, with its effects being amplified when used in combination with ranolazine [103]. In studies by Gu et al., minoxidil was shown to increase blood–tumor barrier (BTB) permeability in a rat brain tumor model, indicating its potential in enhancing drug delivery to tumors. This effect was further elaborated upon by Ningaraj et al., who suggested that minoxidil could improve the delivery of other anti-neoplastic agents to brain tumors, potentially enhancing their efficacy [104]. Kim et al.'s study uniquely positions Pinacidil as an apoptosis inducer in HepG2 human hepatoblastoma cells, highlighting its potential for selectively targeting cancer cells [105]. Lee et al.'s research presents Cromakalim as an anti-tumor agent, inhibiting the growth of human neuroblastoma and astrocytoma cell lines [106]. This effect, counteracted by sulfonylureas, underscores Cromakalim's specific action on the KATP channel. Malhi et al. found that Cromakalim stimulated DNA synthesis in liver cells, suggesting a role in liver regeneration and growth control, with significant implications for liver cancer therapy and liver regeneration research [107]. Table 3 presents the biological impacts of KATP channel activators on cancer cells.

Table 3. Impact of KATP Channel Activators on Cancer Cell Dynamics and Tissue Responses.

Action on KATP Channels	Drug	Treatment Concentration	Model	Results	Ref.
Activator	Diazoxide	10 μM	Human Bladder Carcinoma (HTB-9)	Stimulated growth measured by protein accumulation but did not increase cell number.	[100]
Activator	Minoxidil	0.777–77.7 mg/kg/day	Renal tumor in male rats and Breast cancer in female dogs	Elevated immunohistochemical reactivity to Sur2A-mAb in cytosol of $Ki67^+$/G3 cells in renal tumor. Elevated expression of Sur2A subunit in proliferating cells in breast cancer.	[102]
Activator	Minoxidil	2.5, 5 and 50 μM	MDA-MB-231, MDA-MB-468 (Triple-negative human breast cancer)	No effect on cell viability and proliferation. Reduced invasion in a dose-dependent manner.	[103]
Activator	Minoxidil + Ranolazine	0.625 μM Ranolazine + 2.5 μM minoxidil	MDA-MB-231, MDA-MB-468	Significant additive anti-invasive effects at low concentrations.	[103]
Activator	Minoxidil Sulfate (MS)	30 μg/kg/min for 15, 30, and 60 min	Rat brain glioma (C6)	Increased expression of caveolin-1 protein at tumor sites. Peak expression at 15 min of MS perfusion. Increased BTB permeability potentially mediated by ROS.	[104]
Activator	Pinacidil	1 mM	HepG2 human hepatoblastoma cells	Increase apoptosis.	[105]
Activator	Cromakalim	200 μM for SK-N-MC and 600 μM for U-373 MG	SK-N-MC human neuroblastoma, U-373 MG human astrocytoma cells	Inhibition of intracellular Ca^{2+} signaling. Inhibited growth of SK-N-MC and U-373 MG cell lines.	[106]
Activator	Cromakalim	5 μM	Primary rat hepatocytes, Human cancer cell lines	Increased cellular DNA synthesis in rat hepatocytes and human liver cell lines.	[107]

In conclusion, these studies collectively highlight the significant roles of KATP channel activators in cancer biology. They underscore the potential of these drugs in managing various aspects of cancer progression, from cell proliferation to metastasis control and drug delivery enhancement. The insights gained are crucial for developing novel therapeutic strategies, yet the complexity of their mechanisms and varied responses across cancer types necessitate more detailed investigations. As research delves deeper, the prospects for targeted cancer therapies appear increasingly promising.

8. Exploring the Role of KATP Channel Inhibitors in Cancer Biology

The intricate relationship between KATP channel inhibitors and cancer cell dynamics has been the subject of extensive research, revealing the multifaceted roles these compounds play in oncology. Among these, sulfonylurea (SU) inhibitors, originally developed for diabetes management, have shown surprising efficacy against various cancer types.

Glyburide, a prominent SU inhibitor, has demonstrated notable anti-cancer properties. In a study by Wondergem et al., it was found to reduce cell proliferation in human bladder carcinoma cells (HTB-9) by altering cell cycle distribution, particularly decreasing the proportion of cells in the S phase and increasing those in the G0/G1 phase [100]. This indicates that Glyburide has the potential to regulate cell growth through KATP channels, influencing the central mechanisms of the cell cycle. In another significant study by Li et al., Glyburide significantly reduced lung tumor incidence and severity in a mouse model, potentially through its inhibition of the NLRP3 inflammasome, a key player in inflammation and cancer development [108]. This dual action against both cell proliferation and inflammation underscores Glyburide's potential as a versatile anti-cancer agent. Sun et al. demonstrated that Glyburide at concentrations of 100–1000 μM in PC3 human prostate cancer cells induces PLC-dependent Ca^{2+} rises involving ER release and also triggers Ca^{2+}-independent cell death [109].

Glipizide, another SU-class drug, has shown efficacy in breast cancer treatment, especially when used in combination with Atrial Natriuretic Peptide (ANP). Mao et al. discovered that this combination more effectively inhibited breast cancer growth and metastasis in MMTV-PyMT mice than Glipizide alone [110]. Their research also highlighted Glipizide's ability to impede tumor-induced angiogenesis, a critical factor in cancer progression, by inhibiting VEGF/VEGFR2 signaling in human umbilical vein endothelial cells. Additionally, in the study by Nazim et al., Glipizide was found to enhance TRAIL-mediated apoptotic cell death in human lung adenocarcinoma cells. This was achieved by downregulating p-Akt and p-mTOR and promoting autophagy flux activation, indicating its potential to overcome TRAIL resistance in cancer cells [111]. In addition, studies by Cuiling Qi et al. have shown that Glipizide acts as a potent inhibitor of tumor angiogenesis [112]. In prostate cancer, studies by Cuiling Qi et al. revealed that Glipizide significantly reduces microvessel density in tumor tissues, highlighting its potential in anti-angiogenic therapy [113]. Long et al. synthesized glimepiride–metformin adduct (GMA) and showed that it not only inhibited the viability of breast cancer cells more effectively than either glimepiride or metformin alone but also induced G_1/S phase cell cycle arrest and apoptosis. This was achieved through the activation of AMPK and the modulation of p53, p21, cyclin D1, and CDK4 expression, highlighting GMA's potential as a therapeutic option for breast cancer in diabetic patients [114].

In addition to these compounds, Shuai Li et al. demonstrated that Gliclazide reduces colitis-associated colorectal cancer formation by decreasing colonic inflammation and regulating the AMPK-NF-κB signaling pathway, suggesting its potential as a preventive treatment for colitis-associated colorectal cancer [115].

The nitrated form of Nateglinide, NO_2-NAT, as studied by Koji Nishi et al., has shown promising results as a novel nitric oxide-based chemotherapeutic agent. It induces apoptosis in human pancreatic cancer cells through the release of nitrate and nitrite ions, thereby increasing extracellular lactate dehydrogenase leakage and annexin-positive cells [116]. This study adds to the growing body of evidence supporting the repurposing of diabetic drugs for cancer treatment, leveraging their unique mechanisms of action to target various aspects of cancer cell physiology.

Lastly, Repaglinide, a drug identified from a drug library screen, emerged as an effective FOXO3 inhibitor in neuroblastoma treatment. Salcher et al. demonstrated that Repaglinide effectively suppresses FOXO3-mediated cellular migration by inhibiting FOXO3's binding to the LUM promoter, thereby reducing lumican RNA and protein expression [117]. This finding suggests Repaglinide's potential role in targeting aggressive tumor behaviors linked to FOXO3. Figure 5 and Table 4 present the biological impacts of KATP channel inhibitors on cancer cells.

Overall, the research in this field encourages a broader perspective on existing drugs and their potential applications, advocating for continued exploration and clinical trials to fully harness their capabilities in cancer treatment. The repurposing of these drugs not only accelerates the availability of new cancer treatments but also exemplifies the efficiency and cost-effectiveness of leveraging existing pharmacological knowledge for novel therapeutic purposes.

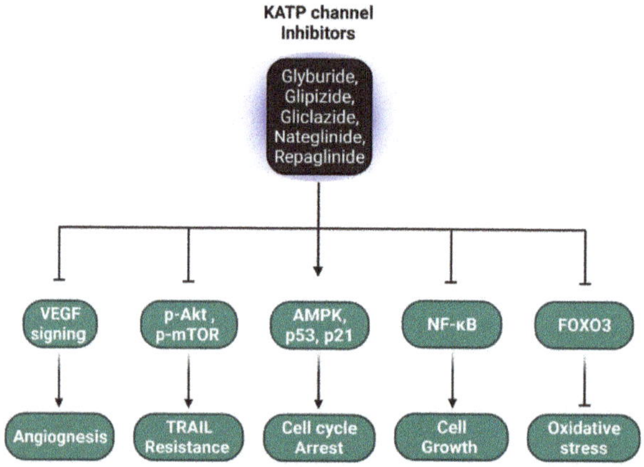

Figure 5. KATP Channel Inhibitors and Their Effects on Cancer Cell Signaling. KATP channel inhibitors, including Glyburide, Glipizide, Gliclazide, Nateglinide, and Repaglinide, modulate key signaling pathways in cancer cells. These agents impact angiogenesis through VEGF signaling, induce TRAIL resistance via the p-Akt and p-mTOR pathways, promote cell cycle arrest by activating AMPK and enhancing p53/p21, inhibit cell growth through NF-κB pathways, and affect oxidative stress management through the FOXO3 axis. The representation underscores the multifaceted roles of KATP channel inhibitors as modulators of cancer cell dynamics. Cartoon in Figure 5 was created with BioRender.com.

Table 4. Impact of KATP Channel Inhibitors on Cancer Cell Dynamics and Tissue Responses.

Action on KATP Channels	Drug	Treatment Concentration	Model	Results	Ref.
Inhibitor	Glyburide	75 and 150 μM for 48 hr	Human Bladder Carcinoma (HTB-9)	Reduced cell proliferation. Increased percentage of cells in G_0/G_1 phase; reduced percentage in S phase.	[100]
Inhibitor	Glyburide	10 μL/g body weight	B(a)p + LPS-induced mouse lung cancer	Reduced lung tumor incidence. Lower expression of NLRP3, IL-1β, and Cleaved-IL-1β proteins.	[108]
Inhibitor	Glyburide	100–1000 μM	PC3 human prostate cancer cells	Induced Ca^{2+} rises were PLC-dependent and involved Ca^{2+} release from the ER. Also caused Ca^{2+}-independent cell death.	[109]
Inhibitor	Glipizide	5 mg/kg	MMTV-PyMT mice, HUVECs	Inhibited breast cancer growth and metastasis in MMTV-PyMT mice by suppressing VEGF/VEGFR2 signaling.	[110]
Inhibitor	Glipizide	0, 25, 50, and 100 μM	Human lung adenocarcinoma cells	Triggered TRAIL-mediated apoptotic cell death. Downregulated p-Akt and p-mTOR.	[111]

Table 4. *Cont.*

Action on KATP Channels	Drug	Treatment Concentration	Model	Results	Ref.
Inhibitor	Glipizide	2, 4, and 8 μg	Chick embryo CAM and YSM models, Xenograft tumor and MMTV-PyMT transgenic mouse models	Significantly inhibited blood vessel formation and development. Suppressed tumor angiogenesis, growth, and metastasis.	[112]
Inhibitor	Glipizide	5 mg/kg	TRAMP transgenic mouse model, Human umbilical vein endothelial cells	Suppressed prostate cancer growth and metastasis. Significantly reduced microvessel density in tumor tissues without inhibiting cell proliferation.	[113]
Inhibitor	Glimepiride	0.4 mM Glimepiride alone, 0.4 mM Metformin alone and Glimepiride + Metformin	Human breast cancer cell lines (CAL-148, MDA-MB-453, MDA-MB-231, MCF-7), CAL-148 xenografts	Suppressed tumor growth in CAL-148 xenografts. Induced G_1/S phase cell cycle arrest and apoptosis. Activated AMPK, upregulated p53 and p21, downregulated cyclin D1 and CDK4.	[114]
Inhibitor	Gliclazide	6 mg/kg for 12 weeks	Colon cancer-inducing mouse	Reduced cell proliferation	[115]
Inhibitor	Nateglinide (NO_2-NAT)	10~50 μM	Human pancreatic cancer cell lines (AsPC1, BxPC3)	Enhanced activity of caspases 3 and cell death.	[116]
Inhibitor	Repaglinide	1 μM to 200 μM	Neuroblastoma cells	Binds to FOXO3 DNA binding domain, silencing FOXO3's transcriptional activity. Reduces cellular migration	[117]

9. Conclusions

In summary, the exploration of KATP channels as potential therapeutic targets in cancer treatments has revealed new horizons in oncology. The unique regulatory functions of these channels in cancer cell metabolism and electrical signaling offer innovative avenues for intervention. However, the journey from theoretical understanding to practical application in clinical settings is fraught with challenges and opportunities.

The promise of KATP channels in cancer therapy lies in their ability to modulate crucial cellular processes, which are often dysregulated in cancer cells. By targeting these channels, there is the potential to disrupt cancer cell proliferation and survival selectively. However, this approach requires a nuanced understanding of the diverse roles that KATP channels play in different types of cancer as their function can vary significantly depending on the tumor environment and cancer cell type [97].

One of the major challenges in targeting KATP channels is the risk of adverse effects on normal cells given the channels' presence and importance in various tissues. This necessitates the development of strategies that can selectively target cancer cells while minimizing harm to normal cells. Additionally, the variability in response to KATP channel-targeted therapies among patients highlights the need for personalized medicine approaches in cancer treatment.

Investigations into ATP-sensitive potassium channels within plasma membranes have greatly enriched our knowledge regarding cell function and drug action. However, exploring mitochondrial KATP channels is becoming an essential aspect of cancer research. These channels are key to regulating mitochondrial operations, influencing essential functions like ATP generation, programmed cell death, and defense mechanisms against physiological stress. Strategically influencing these channels presents a viable approach for selectively targeting cancer cells for destruction while preserving normal cells, underscoring the importance of dedicated research in this domain. Progressing research on mitochondrial KATP channels poses distinct challenges, including understanding the complex nature of mitochondrial biology, achieving targeted modulation, and crafting precise agents that specifically affect mitochondrial channels without impacting those in the plasma membrane. Furthermore, transporting drugs into mitochondria is challenging due to their protective double membrane and the requirement to traverse the cellular interior. Overcoming these hurdles necessitates a focused endeavor to clarify the characteristics of mitochondrial KATP channels, innovate drug transport mechanisms, and synthesize targeted modulators. Such progress will not only deepen our grasp of how mitochondria function in cancer but also pave the way for developing treatments that are both more effective and safer.

Funding: This research received no external funding.

Conflicts of Interest: The author declares no conflict of interest.

References

1. Li, C.G.; Cui, W.Y.; Wang, H. Sensitivity of KATP channels to cellular metabolic disorders and the underlying structural basis. *Acta Pharmacol. Sin.* **2016**, *37*, 134–142. [CrossRef] [PubMed]
2. Tinker, A.; Aziz, Q.; Li, Y.; Specterman, M. ATP-Sensitive Potassium Channels and Their Physiological and Pathophysiological Roles. *Compr. Physiol.* **2018**, *8*, 1463–1511. [CrossRef] [PubMed]
3. Leanza, L.; Biasutto, L.; Managò, A.; Gulbins, E.; Zoratti, M.; Szabò, I. Intracellular ion channels and cancer. *Front. Physiol.* **2013**, *4*, 227. [CrossRef] [PubMed]
4. Vázquez-Sánchez, A.Y.; Hinojosa, L.M.; Parraguirre-Martínez, S.; González, A.; Morales, F.; Montalvo, G.; Vera, E.; Hernández-Gallegos, E.; Camacho, J. Expression of K(ATP) channels in human cervical cancer: Potential tools for diagnosis and therapy. *Oncol. Lett.* **2018**, *15*, 6302–6308. [CrossRef] [PubMed]
5. Abu-Hamad, S.; Zaid, H.; Israelson, A.; Nahon, E.; Shoshan-Barmatz, V. Hexokinase-I protection against apoptotic cell death is mediated via interaction with the voltage-dependent anion channel-1: Mapping the site of binding. *J. Biol. Chem.* **2008**, *283*, 13482–13490. [CrossRef] [PubMed]
6. Mathupala, S.P.; Ko, Y.H.; Pedersen, P.L. Hexokinase II: Cancer's double-edged sword acting as both facilitator and gatekeeper of malignancy when bound to mitochondria. *Oncogene* **2006**, *25*, 4777–4786. [CrossRef] [PubMed]
7. Bischof, H.; Burgstaller, S.; Springer, A.; Matt, L.; Rauter, T.; Bachkönig, O.A.; Schmidt, T.; Groschner, K.; Schindl, R.; Madl, T.; et al. Potassium ions promote hexokinase-II dependent glycolysis. *iScience* **2021**, *24*, 102346. [CrossRef]
8. Zahra, K.; Dey, T.; Ashish Mishra, S.P.; Pandey, U. Pyruvate Kinase M2 and Cancer: The Role of PKM2 in Promoting Tumorigenesis. *Front. Oncol.* **2020**, *10*, 159. [CrossRef]
9. El Hiani, Y.; Ahidouch, A.; Lehen'kyi, V.; Hague, F.; Gouilleux, F.; Mentaverri, R.; Kamel, S.; Lassoued, K.; Brûlé, G.; Ouadid-Ahidouch, H. Extracellular signal-regulated kinases 1 and 2 and TRPC1 channels are required for calcium-sensing receptor-stimulated MCF-7 breast cancer cell proliferation. *Cell. Physiol. Biochem.* **2009**, *23*, 335–346. [CrossRef]
10. Faouzi, M.; Hague, F.; Potier, M.; Ahidouch, A.; Sevestre, H.; Ouadid-Ahidouch, H. Down-regulation of Orai3 arrests cell-cycle progression and induces apoptosis in breast cancer cells but not in normal breast epithelial cells. *J. Cell. Physiol.* **2011**, *226*, 542–551. [CrossRef]
11. Hammadi, M.; Chopin, V.; Matifat, F.; Dhennin-Duthille, I.; Chasseraud, M.; Sevestre, H.; Ouadid-Ahidouch, H. Human ether à-gogo K^+ channel 1 (hEag1) regulates MDA-MB-231 breast cancer cell migration through Orai1-dependent calcium entry. *J. Cell. Physiol.* **2012**, *227*, 3837–3846. [CrossRef]
12. Huang, X.; Dubuc, A.M.; Hashizume, R.; Berg, J.; He, Y.; Wang, J.; Chiang, C.; Cooper, M.K.; Northcott, P.A.; Taylor, M.D.; et al. Voltage-gated potassium channel EAG2 controls mitotic entry and tumor growth in medulloblastoma via regulating cell volume dynamics. *Genes. Dev.* **2012**, *26*, 1780–1796. [CrossRef] [PubMed]
13. Hughes, F.M., Jr.; Cidlowski, J.A. Potassium is a critical regulator of apoptotic enzymes in vitro and in vivo. *Adv. Enzym. Regul.* **1999**, *39*, 157–171. [CrossRef] [PubMed]
14. Bortner, C.D.; Cidlowski, J.A. Cell shrinkage and monovalent cation fluxes: Role in apoptosis. *Arch. Biochem. Biophys.* **2007**, *462*, 176–188. [CrossRef] [PubMed]
15. Hanahan, D.; Weinberg, R.A. Hallmarks of cancer: The next generation. *Cell* **2011**, *144*, 646–674. [CrossRef] [PubMed]
16. Huang, X.; Jan, L.Y. Targeting potassium channels in cancer. *J. Cell Biol.* **2014**, *206*, 151–162. [CrossRef] [PubMed]
17. deHart, G.W.; Jin, T.; McCloskey, D.E.; Pegg, A.E.; Sheppard, D. The alpha9beta1 integrin enhances cell migration by polyamine-mediated modulation of an inward-rectifier potassium channel. *Proc. Natl. Acad. Sci. USA* **2008**, *105*, 7188–7193. [CrossRef] [PubMed]
18. Nichols, C.G. KATP channels as molecular sensors of cellular metabolism. *Nature* **2006**, *440*, 470–476. [CrossRef]
19. Martin, G.M.; Kandasamy, B.; DiMaio, F.; Yoshioka, C.; Shyng, S.L. Anti-diabetic drug binding site in a mammalian K(ATP) channel revealed by Cryo-EM. *eLife* **2017**, *6*, e31054. [CrossRef]
20. Li, N.; Wu, J.X.; Ding, D.; Cheng, J.; Gao, N.; Chen, L. Structure of a Pancreatic ATP-Sensitive Potassium Channel. *Cell* **2017**, *168*, 101–110.e10. [CrossRef]
21. Foster, D.B.; Ho, A.S.; Rucker, J.; Garlid, A.O.; Chen, L.; Sidor, A.; Garlid, K.D.; O'Rourke, B. Mitochondrial ROMK channel is a molecular component of mitoK(ATP). *Circ. Res.* **2012**, *111*, 446–454. [CrossRef] [PubMed]
22. Bednarczyk, P.; Kicinska, A.; Laskowski, M.; Kulawiak, B.; Kampa, R.; Walewska, A.; Krajewska, M.; Jarmuszkiewicz, W.; Szewczyk, A. Evidence for a mitochondrial ATP-regulated potassium channel in human dermal fibroblasts. *Biochim. Biophys. Acta Bioenerg.* **2018**, *1859*, 309–318. [CrossRef] [PubMed]

23. Paggio, A.; Checchetto, V.; Campo, A.; Menabò, R.; Di Marco, G.; Di Lisa, F.; Szabo, I.; Rizzuto, R.; De Stefani, D. Identification of an ATP-sensitive potassium channel in mitochondria. *Nature* **2019**, *572*, 609–613. [CrossRef] [PubMed]
24. Juhaszova, M.; Kobrinsky, E.; Zorov, D.B.; Nuss, H.B.; Yaniv, Y.; Fishbein, K.W.; de Cabo, R.; Montoliu, L.; Gabelli, S.B.; Aon, M.A.; et al. ATP Synthase K^+- and H^+-Fluxes Drive ATP Synthesis and Enable Mitochondrial K^+-"Uniporter" Function: I. Characterization of Ion Fluxes. *Function* **2022**, *3*, zqab065. [CrossRef]
25. Drain, P.; Li, L.; Wang, J. KATP channel inhibition by ATP requires distinct functional domains of the cytoplasmic C terminus of the pore-forming subunit. *Proc. Natl. Acad. Sci. USA* **1998**, *95*, 13953–13958. [CrossRef] [PubMed]
26. Foster, M.N.; Coetzee, W.A. KATP Channels in the Cardiovascular System. *Physiol. Rev.* **2016**, *96*, 177–252. [CrossRef] [PubMed]
27. Kakei, M.; Noma, A.; Shibasaki, T. Properties of adenosine-triphosphate-regulated potassium channels in guinea-pig ventricular cells. *J. Physiol.* **1985**, *363*, 441–462. [CrossRef]
28. Lederer, W.J.; Nichols, C.G. Nucleotide modulation of the activity of rat heart ATP-sensitive K^+ channels in isolated membrane patches. *J. Physiol.* **1989**, *419*, 193–211. [CrossRef]
29. Lemasters, J.J. Metabolic implications of non-electrogenic ATP/ADP exchange in cancer cells: A mechanistic basis for the Warburg effect. *Biochim. Biophys. Acta Bioenerg.* **2021**, *1862*, 148410. [CrossRef]
30. Traba, J.; Del Arco, A.; Duchen, M.R.; Szabadkai, G.; Satrústegui, J. SCaMC-1 promotes cancer cell survival by desensitizing mitochondrial permeability transition via ATP/ADP-mediated matrix Ca^{2+} buffering. *Cell Death Differ.* **2012**, *19*, 650–660. [CrossRef]
31. Del Arco, A.; Contreras, L.; Pardo, B.; Satrustegui, J. Calcium regulation of mitochondrial carriers. *Biochim. Biophys. Acta* **2016**, *1863*, 2413–2421. [CrossRef] [PubMed]
32. Maldonado, E.N.; DeHart, D.N.; Patnaik, J.; Klatt, S.C.; Gooz, M.B.; Lemasters, J.J. ATP/ADP Turnover and Import of Glycolytic ATP into Mitochondria in Cancer Cells Is Independent of the Adenine Nucleotide Translocator. *J. Biol. Chem.* **2016**, *291*, 19642–19650. [CrossRef] [PubMed]
33. Tran, Q.H.; Unden, G. Changes in the proton potential and the cellular energetics of Escherichia coli during growth by aerobic and anaerobic respiration or by fermentation. *Eur. J. Biochem.* **1998**, *251*, 538–543. [CrossRef] [PubMed]
34. Schwenke, W.D.; Soboll, S.; Seitz, H.J.; Sies, H. Mitochondrial and cytosolic ATP/ADP ratios in rat liver in vivo. *Biochem. J.* **1981**, *200*, 405–408. [CrossRef] [PubMed]
35. Baukrowitz, T.; Schulte, U.; Oliver, D.; Herlitze, S.; Krauter, T.; Tucker, S.J.; Ruppersberg, J.P.; Fakler, B. PIP2 and PIP as determinants for ATP inhibition of KATP channels. *Science* **1998**, *282*, 1141–1144. [CrossRef]
36. Fan, Z.; Makielski, J.C. Anionic phospholipids activate ATP-sensitive potassium channels. *J. Biol. Chem.* **1997**, *272*, 5388–5395. [CrossRef] [PubMed]
37. Bunney, T.D.; Katan, M. Phosphoinositide signalling in cancer: Beyond PI3K and PTEN. *Nat. Rev. Cancer* **2010**, *10*, 342–352. [CrossRef]
38. Janku, F.; Yap, T.A.; Meric-Bernstam, F. Targeting the PI3K pathway in cancer: Are we making headway? *Nat. Rev. Clin. Oncol.* **2018**, *15*, 273–291. [CrossRef]
39. Liu, G.X.; Hanley, P.J.; Ray, J.; Daut, J. Long-chain acyl-coenzyme A esters and fatty acids directly link metabolism to K(ATP) channels in the heart. *Circ. Res.* **2001**, *88*, 918–924. [CrossRef]
40. Manning Fox, J.E.; Nichols, C.G.; Light, P.E. Activation of adenosine triphosphate-sensitive potassium channels by acyl coenzyme A esters involves multiple phosphatidylinositol 4,5-bisphosphate-interacting residues. *Mol. Endocrinol.* **2004**, *18*, 679–686. [CrossRef]
41. Carracedo, A.; Cantley, L.C.; Pandolfi, P.P. Cancer metabolism: Fatty acid oxidation in the limelight. *Nat. Rev. Cancer* **2013**, *13*, 227–232. [CrossRef] [PubMed]
42. Davies, N.W. Modulation of ATP-sensitive K^+ channels in skeletal muscle by intracellular protons. *Nature* **1990**, *343*, 375–377. [CrossRef] [PubMed]
43. Xu, H.; Wu, J.; Cui, N.; Abdulkadir, L.; Wang, R.; Mao, J.; Giwa, L.R.; Chanchevalap, S.; Jiang, C. Distinct histidine residues control the acid-induced activation and inhibition of the cloned K(ATP) channel. *J. Biol. Chem.* **2001**, *276*, 38690–38696. [CrossRef] [PubMed]
44. Cui, N.; Li, L.; Wang, X.; Shi, Y.; Shi, W.; Jiang, C. Elimination of allosteric modulation of myocardial KATP channels by ATP and protons in two Kir6.2 polymorphisms found in sudden cardiac death. *Physiol. Genom.* **2006**, *25*, 105–115. [CrossRef] [PubMed]
45. Wu, J.; Cui, N.; Piao, H.; Wang, Y.; Xu, H.; Mao, J.; Jiang, C. Allosteric modulation of the mouse Kir6.2 channel by intracellular H^+ and ATP. *J. Physiol.* **2002**, *543*, 495–504. [CrossRef] [PubMed]
46. Webb, B.A.; Chimenti, M.; Jacobson, M.P.; Barber, D.L. Dysregulated pH: A perfect storm for cancer progression. *Nat. Rev. Cancer* **2011**, *11*, 671–677. [CrossRef] [PubMed]
47. Béguin, P.; Nagashima, K.; Nishimura, M.; Gonoi, T.; Seino, S. PKA-mediated phosphorylation of the human K(ATP) channel: Separate roles of Kir6.2 and SUR1 subunit phosphorylation. *EMBO J.* **1999**, *18*, 4722–4732. [CrossRef]
48. Lin, Y.F.; Jan, Y.N.; Jan, L.Y. Regulation of ATP-sensitive potassium channel function by protein kinase A-mediated phosphorylation in transfected HEK293 cells. *EMBO J.* **2000**, *19*, 942–955. [CrossRef]
49. Bar-Shavit, R.; Maoz, M.; Kancharla, A.; Nag, J.K.; Agranovich, D.; Grisaru-Granovsky, S.; Uziely, B. G Protein-Coupled Receptors in Cancer. *Int. J. Mol. Sci.* **2016**, *17*, 1320. [CrossRef]

50. Light, P.E.; Sabir, A.A.; Allen, B.G.; Walsh, M.P.; French, R.J. Protein kinase C-induced changes in the stoichiometry of ATP binding activate cardiac ATP-sensitive K^+ channels. A possible mechanistic link to ischemic preconditioning. *Circ. Res.* **1996**, *79*, 399–406. [CrossRef]
51. Light, P.E.; Bladen, C.; Winkfein, R.J.; Walsh, M.P.; French, R.J. Molecular basis of protein kinase C-induced activation of ATP-sensitive potassium channels. *Proc. Natl. Acad. Sci. USA* **2000**, *97*, 9058–9063. [CrossRef] [PubMed]
52. He, S.; Li, Q.; Huang, Q.; Cheng, J. Targeting Protein Kinase C for Cancer Therapy. *Cancers* **2022**, *14*, 1104. [CrossRef]
53. Kulawiak, B.; Szewczyk, A. Current Challenges of Mitochondrial Potassium Channel Research. *Front. Physiol.* **2022**, *13*, 907015. [CrossRef] [PubMed]
54. Giorgio, V.; Guo, L.; Bassot, C.; Petronilli, V.; Bernardi, P. Calcium and regulation of the mitochondrial permeability transition. *Cell Calcium* **2018**, *70*, 56–63. [CrossRef] [PubMed]
55. Kulawiak, B.; Bednarczyk, P.; Szewczyk, A. Multidimensional Regulation of Cardiac Mitochondrial Potassium Channels. *Cells* **2021**, *10*, 1554. [CrossRef] [PubMed]
56. Borutaite, V.; Toleikis, A.; Brown, G.C. In the eye of the storm: Mitochondrial damage during heart and brain ischaemia. *FEBS J.* **2013**, *280*, 4999–5014. [CrossRef] [PubMed]
57. Lebuffe, G.; Schumacker, P.T.; Shao, Z.H.; Anderson, T.; Iwase, H.; Vanden Hoek, T.L. ROS and NO trigger early preconditioning: Relationship to mitochondrial KATP channel. *Am. J. Physiol. Heart Circ. Physiol.* **2003**, *284*, H299–H308. [CrossRef]
58. Mohelnikova-Duchonova, B.; Brynychova, V.; Oliverius, M.; Honsova, E.; Kala, Z.; Muckova, K.; Soucek, P. Differences in transcript levels of ABC transporters between pancreatic adenocarcinoma and nonneoplastic tissues. *Pancreas* **2013**, *42*, 707–716. [CrossRef]
59. Hlaváč, V.; Brynychová, V.; Václavíková, R.; Ehrlichová, M.; Vrána, D.; Pecha, V.; Koževnikovová, R.; Trnková, M.; Gatěk, J.; Kopperová, D.; et al. The expression profile of ATP-binding cassette transporter genes in breast carcinoma. *Pharmacogenomics* **2013**, *14*, 515–529. [CrossRef]
60. Wang, Z.; Xu, H.; Zhu, L.; He, T.; Lv, W.; Wu, Z. Establishment and Evaluation of a 6-Gene Survival Risk Assessment Model Related to Lung Adenocarcinoma Microenvironment. *BioMed Res. Int.* **2020**, *2020*, 6472153. [CrossRef]
61. Hlavata, I.; Mohelnikova-Duchonova, B.; Vaclavikova, R.; Liska, V.; Pitule, P.; Novak, P.; Bruha, J.; Vycital, O.; Holubec, L.; Treska, V.; et al. The role of ABC transporters in progression and clinical outcome of colorectal cancer. *Mutagenesis* **2012**, *27*, 187–196. [CrossRef]
62. Huang, L.; Li, B.; Li, W.; Guo, H.; Zou, F. ATP-sensitive potassium channels control glioma cells proliferation by regulating ERK activity. *Carcinogenesis* **2009**, *30*, 737–744. [CrossRef] [PubMed]
63. Mao, X.; He, Z.; Zhou, F.; Huang, Y.; Zhu, G. Prognostic significance and molecular mechanisms of adenosine triphosphate-binding cassette subfamily C members in gastric cancer. *Medicine* **2019**, *98*, e18347. [CrossRef] [PubMed]
64. Xiao, Y.; Yang, Y.; Wang, Y.; Li, X.; Wang, W. Five Novel Genes Related to the Pathogenesis and Progression of Pancreatic Neuroendocrine Tumors by Bioinformatics Analysis With RT-qPCR Verification. *Front. Neurosci.* **2019**, *13*, 937. [CrossRef] [PubMed]
65. Ashfield, R.; Ashcroft, S.J. Cloning of the promoters for the beta-cell ATP-sensitive K-channel subunits Kir6.2 and SUR1. *Diabetes* **1998**, *47*, 1274–1280. [CrossRef] [PubMed]
66. Hernández-Sánchez, C.; Ito, Y.; Ferrer, J.; Reitman, M.; LeRoith, D. Characterization of the mouse sulfonylurea receptor 1 promoter and its regulation. *J. Biol. Chem.* **1999**, *274*, 18261–18270. [CrossRef] [PubMed]
67. Gorogawa, S.; Fujitani, Y.; Kaneto, H.; Hazama, Y.; Watada, H.; Miyamoto, Y.; Takeda, K.; Akira, S.; Magnuson, M.A.; Yamasaki, Y.; et al. Insulin secretory defects and impaired islet architecture in pancreatic beta-cell-specific STAT3 knockout mice. *Biochem. Biophys. Res. Commun.* **2004**, *319*, 1159–1170. [CrossRef] [PubMed]
68. Kim, J.W.; Seghers, V.; Cho, J.H.; Kang, Y.; Kim, S.; Ryu, Y.; Baek, K.; Aguilar-Bryan, L.; Lee, Y.D.; Bryan, J.; et al. Transactivation of the mouse sulfonylurea receptor I gene by BETA2/NeuroD. *Mol. Endocrinol.* **2002**, *16*, 1097–1107. [CrossRef]
69. Woo, S.K.; Kwon, M.S.; Geng, Z.; Chen, Z.; Ivanov, A.; Bhatta, S.; Gerzanich, V.; Simard, J.M. Sequential activation of hypoxia-inducible factor 1 and specificity protein 1 is required for hypoxia-induced transcriptional stimulation of Abcc8. *J. Cereb. Blood Flow Metab.* **2012**, *32*, 525–536. [CrossRef]
70. Chen, C.; Hu, Q.; Yan, J.; Lei, J.; Qin, L.; Shi, X.; Luan, L.; Yang, L.; Wang, K.; Han, J.; et al. Multiple effects of 2ME2 and D609 on the cortical expression of HIF-1alpha and apoptotic genes in a middle cerebral artery occlusion-induced focal ischemia rat model. *J. Neurochem.* **2007**, *102*, 1831–1841. [CrossRef]
71. Chen, C.; Ostrowski, R.P.; Zhou, C.; Tang, J.; Zhang, J.H. Suppression of hypoxia-inducible factor-1alpha and its downstream genes reduces acute hyperglycemia-enhanced hemorrhagic transformation in a rat model of cerebral ischemia. *J. Neurosci. Res.* **2010**, *88*, 2046–2055. [CrossRef]
72. Simard, J.M.; Geng, Z.; Woo, S.K.; Ivanova, S.; Tosun, C.; Melnichenko, L.; Gerzanich, V. Glibenclamide reduces inflammation, vasogenic edema, and caspase-3 activation after subarachnoid hemorrhage. *J. Cereb. Blood Flow Metab.* **2009**, *29*, 317–330. [CrossRef] [PubMed]
73. Kurland, D.B.; Gerzanich, V.; Karimy, J.K.; Woo, S.K.; Vennekens, R.; Freichel, M.; Nilius, B.; Bryan, J.; Simard, J.M. The Sur1-Trpm4 channel regulates NOS2 transcription in TLR4-activated microglia. *J. Neuroinflammation* **2016**, *13*, 130. [CrossRef] [PubMed]
74. Laird, M.D.; Shields, J.S.; Sukumari-Ramesh, S.; Kimbler, D.E.; Fessler, R.D.; Shakir, B.; Youssef, P.; Yanasak, N.; Vender, J.R.; Dhandapani, K.M. High mobility group box protein-1 promotes cerebral edema after traumatic brain injury via activation of toll-like receptor 4. *Glia* **2014**, *62*, 26–38. [CrossRef] [PubMed]

75. Trotta, T.; Porro, C.; Calvello, R.; Panaro, M.A. Biological role of Toll-like receptor-4 in the brain. *J. Neuroimmunol.* **2014**, *268*, 1–12. [CrossRef] [PubMed]
76. Calton, E.A.; Temple, I.K.; Mackay, D.J.; Lever, M.; Ellard, S.; Flanagan, S.E.; Davies, J.H.; Hussain, K.; Gray, J.C. Hepatoblastoma in a child with a paternally-inherited ABCC8 mutation and mosaic paternal uniparental disomy 11p causing focal congenital hyperinsulinism. *Eur. J. Med. Genet.* **2013**, *56*, 114–117. [CrossRef] [PubMed]
77. Soucek, P.; Hlavac, V.; Elsnerova, K.; Vaclavikova, R.; Kozevnikovova, R.; Raus, K. Whole exome sequencing analysis of ABCC8 and ABCD2 genes associating with clinical course of breast carcinoma. *Physiol. Res.* **2015**, *64*, S549–S557. [CrossRef] [PubMed]
78. Elsnerova, K.; Bartakova, A.; Tihlarik, J.; Bouda, J.; Rob, L.; Skapa, P.; Hruda, M.; Gut, I.; Mohelnikova-Duchonova, B.; Soucek, P.; et al. Gene Expression Profiling Reveals Novel Candidate Markers of Ovarian Carcinoma Intraperitoneal Metastasis. *J. Cancer* **2017**, *8*, 3598–3606. [CrossRef]
79. Zhang, X.; Kang, X.; Jin, L.; Bai, J.; Zhang, H.; Liu, W.; Wang, Z. ABCC9, NKAPL, and TMEM132C are potential diagnostic and prognostic markers in triple-negative breast cancer. *Cell Biol. Int.* **2020**, *44*, 2002–2010. [CrossRef]
80. Demidenko, R.; Razanauskas, D.; Daniunaite, K.; Lazutka, J.R.; Jankevicius, F.; Jarmalaite, S. Frequent down-regulation of ABC transporter genes in prostate cancer. *BMC Cancer* **2015**, *15*, 683. [CrossRef]
81. Cheon, H.; Xing, J.C.; Moosic, K.B.; Ung, J.; Chan, V.W.; Chung, D.S.; Toro, M.F.; Elghawy, O.; Wang, J.S.; Hamele, C.E.; et al. Genomic landscape of TCRαβ and TCRγδ T-large granular lymphocyte leukemia. *Blood* **2022**, *139*, 3058–3072. [CrossRef] [PubMed]
82. Le Gallo, M.; O'Hara, A.J.; Rudd, M.L.; Urick, M.E.; Hansen, N.F.; O'Neil, N.J.; Price, J.C.; Zhang, S.; England, B.M.; Godwin, A.K.; et al. Exome sequencing of serous endometrial tumors identifies recurrent somatic mutations in chromatin-remodeling and ubiquitin ligase complex genes. *Nat. Genet.* **2012**, *44*, 1310–1315. [CrossRef] [PubMed]
83. Zhang, L.; Hu, D.; Huangfu, S.; Zhou, J.; Wang, W.; Liu, S.; Tang, H.; Pan, J.; Pan, Y. DNA Repair and Replication-Related Gene Signature Based on Tumor Mutation Burden Reveals Prognostic and Immunotherapy Response in Gastric Cancer. *J. Oncol.* **2022**, *2022*, 6469523. [CrossRef] [PubMed]
84. Warnecke-Eberz, U.; Metzger, R.; Hölscher, A.H.; Drebber, U.; Bollschweiler, E. Diagnostic marker signature for esophageal cancer from transcriptome analysis. *Tumor Biol.* **2016**, *37*, 6349–6358. [CrossRef] [PubMed]
85. Zhang, K.; Mu, L.; Ding, M.C.; Xu, R.; Ding, Z.J.; Liang, J. NFκB mediated elevation of KCNJ11 promotes tumor progression of hepatocellular carcinoma through interaction of lactate dehydrogenase A. *Biochem. Biophys. Res. Commun.* **2018**, *495*, 246–253. [CrossRef] [PubMed]
86. Calvo, S.E.; Clauser, K.R.; Mootha, V.K. MitoCarta2.0: An updated inventory of mammalian mitochondrial proteins. *Nucleic Acids Res.* **2016**, *44*, D1251–D1257. [CrossRef] [PubMed]
87. Human Genomics. The Genotype-Tissue Expression (GTEx) pilot analysis: Multitissue gene regulation in humans. *Science* **2015**, *348*, 648–660. [CrossRef]
88. Zeitz, C.; Méjécase, C.; Michiels, C.; Condroyer, C.; Wohlschlegel, J.; Foussard, M.; Antonio, A.; Démontant, V.; Emmenegger, L.; Schalk, A.; et al. Mutated CCDC51 Coding for a Mitochondrial Protein, MITOK Is a Candidate Gene Defect for Autosomal Recessive Rod-Cone Dystrophy. *Int. J. Mol. Sci.* **2021**, *22*, 7875. [CrossRef]
89. Takahashi, A.; Yamaguchi, H.; Miyamoto, H. Change in K^+ current of HeLa cells with progression of the cell cycle studied by patch-clamp technique. *Am. J. Physiol.* **1993**, *265*, C328–C336. [CrossRef]
90. Pardo, L.A.; Brüggemann, A.; Camacho, J.; Stühmer, W. Cell cycle-related changes in the conducting properties of r-eag K^+ channels. *J. Cell Biol.* **1998**, *143*, 767–775. [CrossRef]
91. Chandy, K.G.; DeCoursey, T.E.; Cahalan, M.D.; McLaughlin, C.; Gupta, S. Voltage-gated potassium channels are required for human T lymphocyte activation. *J. Exp. Med.* **1984**, *160*, 369–385. [CrossRef]
92. Chiu, S.Y.; Wilson, G.F. The role of potassium channels in Schwann cell proliferation in Wallerian degeneration of explant rabbit sciatic nerves. *J. Physiol.* **1989**, *408*, 199–222. [CrossRef] [PubMed]
93. Lenzi, D.; Radke, K.; Wilson, M. Clonal cells from embryonic retinal cell lines express qualitative electrophysiological differences. *J. Neurobiol.* **1991**, *22*, 823–836. [CrossRef] [PubMed]
94. Day, M.L.; Johnson, M.H.; Cook, D.I. A cytoplasmic cell cycle controls the activity of a K^+ channel in pre-implantation mouse embryos. *EMBO J.* **1998**, *17*, 1952–1960. [CrossRef] [PubMed]
95. Lee, Y.S.; Sayeed, M.M.; Wurster, R.D. Inhibition of cell growth by K+ channel modulators is due to interference with agonist-induced Ca^{2+} release. *Cell. Signal.* **1993**, *5*, 803–809. [CrossRef] [PubMed]
96. Lallet-Daher, H.; Roudbaraki, M.; Bavencoffe, A.; Mariot, P.; Gackière, F.; Bidaux, G.; Urbain, R.; Gosset, P.; Delcourt, P.; Fleurisse, L.; et al. Intermediate-conductance Ca^{2+}-activated K^+ channels (IKCa1) regulate human prostate cancer cell proliferation through a close control of calcium entry. *Oncogene* **2009**, *28*, 1792–1806. [CrossRef] [PubMed]
97. Scarth, J.A.; Wasson, C.W.; Patterson, M.R.; Evans, D.; Barba-Moreno, D.; Carden, H.; Cassidy, R.; Whitehouse, A.; Mankouri, J.; Samson, A.; et al. Exploitation of ATP-sensitive potassium ion (K(ATP)) channels by HPV promotes cervical cancer cell proliferation by contributing to MAPK/AP-1 signalling. *Oncogene* **2023**, *42*, 2558–2577. [CrossRef]
98. Ru, Q.; Tian, X.; Wu, Y.X.; Wu, R.H.; Pi, M.S.; Li, C.Y. Voltage-gated and ATP-sensitive K+ channels are associated with cell proliferation and tumorigenesis of human glioma. *Oncol. Rep.* **2014**, *31*, 842–848. [CrossRef] [PubMed]
99. Klimatcheva, E.; Wonderlin, W.F. An ATP-sensitive K^+ current that regulates progression through early G1 phase of the cell cycle in MCF-7 human breast cancer cells. *J. Membr. Biol.* **1999**, *171*, 35–46. [CrossRef]

100. Wondergem, R.; Cregan, M.; Strickler, L.; Miller, R.; Suttles, J. Membrane potassium channels and human bladder tumor cells: II. Growth properties. *J. Membr. Biol.* **1998**, *161*, 257–262. [CrossRef]
101. Wonderlin, W.F.; Woodfork, K.A.; Strobl, J.S. Changes in membrane potential during the progression of MCF-7 human mammary tumor cells through the cell cycle. *J. Cell. Physiol.* **1995**, *165*, 177–185. [CrossRef] [PubMed]
102. Maqoud, F.; Zizzo, N.; Attimonelli, M.; Tinelli, A.; Passantino, G.; Antonacci, M.; Ranieri, G.; Tricarico, D. Immunohistochemical, pharmacovigilance, and omics analyses reveal the involvement of ATP-sensitive K^+ channel subunits in cancers: Role in drug-disease interactions. *Front. Pharmacol.* **2023**, *14*, 1115543. [CrossRef]
103. Qiu, S.; Fraser, S.P.; Pires, W.; Djamgoz, M.B.A. Anti-invasive effects of minoxidil on human breast cancer cells: Combination with ranolazine. *Clin. Exp. Metastasis* **2022**, *39*, 679–689. [CrossRef] [PubMed]
104. Gu, Y.T.; Xue, Y.X.; Zhang, H.; Li, Y.; Liang, X.Y. Adenosine 5′-triphosphate-sensitive potassium channel activator induces the up-regulation of caveolin-1 expression in a rat brain tumor model. *Cell. Mol. Neurobiol.* **2011**, *31*, 629–634. [CrossRef] [PubMed]
105. Kim, J.A.; Kang, Y.Y.; Lee, Y.S. Activation of Na^+, K^+, Cl^--cotransport mediates intracellular Ca^{2+} increase and apoptosis induced by Pinacidil in HepG2 human hepatoblastoma cells. *Biochem. Biophys. Res. Commun.* **2001**, *281*, 511–519. [CrossRef] [PubMed]
106. Lee, Y.S.; Sayeed, M.M.; Wurster, R.D. In vitro antitumor activity of cromakalim in human brain tumor cells. *Pharmacology* **1994**, *49*, 69–74. [CrossRef]
107. Malhi, H.; Irani, A.N.; Rajvanshi, P.; Suadicani, S.O.; Spray, D.C.; McDonald, T.V.; Gupta, S. KATP channels regulate mitogenically induced proliferation in primary rat hepatocytes and human liver cell lines. Implications for liver growth control and potential therapeutic targeting. *J. Biol. Chem.* **2000**, *275*, 26050–26057. [CrossRef]
108. Li, M.; Liu, H.; Shao, H.; Zhang, P.; Gao, M.; Huang, L.; Shang, P.; Zhang, Q.; Wang, W.; Feng, F. Glyburide attenuates B(a)p and LPS-induced inflammation-related lung tumorigenesis in mice. *Environ. Toxicol.* **2021**, *36*, 1713–1722. [CrossRef]
109. Sun, G.C.; Liang, W.Z.; Jan, C.R. Mechanisms underlying the effect of an oral antihyperglycaemic agent glyburide on calcium ion (Ca^{2+}) movement and its related cytotoxicity in prostate cancer cells. *Clin. Exp. Pharmacol. Physiol.* **2020**, *47*, 111–118. [CrossRef]
110. Mao, G.; Zheng, S.; Li, J.; Liu, X.; Zhou, Q.; Cao, J.; Zhang, Q.; Zheng, L.; Wang, L.; Qi, C. Glipizide Combined with ANP Suppresses Breast Cancer Growth and Metastasis by Inhibiting Angiogenesis through VEGF/VEGFR2 Signaling. *Anti-Cancer Agents Med. Chem.* **2022**, *22*, 1735–1741. [CrossRef]
111. Nazim, U.M.; Moon, J.H.; Lee, Y.J.; Seol, J.W.; Kim, Y.J.; Park, S.Y. Glipizide sensitizes lung cancer cells to TRAIL-induced apoptosis via Akt/mTOR/autophagy pathways. *Oncotarget* **2017**, *8*, 100021–100033. [CrossRef]
112. Qi, C.; Zhou, Q.; Li, B.; Yang, Y.; Cao, L.; Ye, Y.; Li, J.; Ding, Y.; Wang, H.; Wang, J.; et al. Glipizide, an antidiabetic drug, suppresses tumor growth and metastasis by inhibiting angiogenesis. *Oncotarget* **2014**, *5*, 9966–9979. [CrossRef] [PubMed]
113. Qi, C.; Bin, L.; Yang, Y.; Yang, Y.; Li, J.; Zhou, Q.; Wen, Y.; Zeng, C.; Zheng, L.; Zhang, Q.; et al. Glipizide suppresses prostate cancer progression in the TRAMP model by inhibiting angiogenesis. *Sci. Rep.* **2016**, *6*, 27819. [CrossRef] [PubMed]
114. Long, L.; Hu, X.; Li, X.; Zhou, D.; Shi, Y.; Wang, L.; Zeng, H.; Yu, X.; Zhou, W. The Anti-Breast Cancer Effect and Mechanism of Glimepiride-Metformin Adduct. *Onco Targets Ther.* **2020**, *13*, 3777–3788. [CrossRef] [PubMed]
115. Li, S.; Wang, Y.; Zhang, D.; Wang, H.; Cui, X.; Zhang, C.; Xin, Y. Gliclazide Reduces Colitis-Associated Colorectal Cancer Formation by Deceasing Colonic Inflammation and Regulating AMPK-NF-κB Signaling Pathway. *Dig. Dis. Sci.* **2023**. [CrossRef] [PubMed]
116. Nishi, K.; Imoto, S.; Beppu, T.; Uchibori, S.; Yano, A.; Ishima, Y.U.; Ikeda, T.; Tsukigawa, K.; Otagiri, M.; Yamasaki, K. The Nitrated Form of Nateglinide Induces Apoptosis in Human Pancreatic Cancer Cells Through a Caspase-dependent Mechanism. *Anticancer Res.* **2022**, *42*, 1333–1338. [CrossRef] [PubMed]
117. Salcher, S.; Spoden, G.; Huber, J.M.; Golderer, G.; Lindner, H.; Ausserlechner, M.J.; Kiechl-Kohlendorfer, U.; Geiger, K.; Obexer, P. Repaglinide Silences the FOXO3/Lumican Axis and Represses the Associated Metastatic Potential of Neuronal Cancer Cells. *Cells* **2019**, *9*, 1. [CrossRef] [PubMed]

International Journal of *Molecular Sciences*

MDPI

Article

Exploiting *Glycyrrhiza glabra* L. (Licorice) Flavanones: Licoflavanone's Impact on Breast Cancer Cell Bioenergetics

Luca Frattaruolo [1,†], Graziantonio Lauria [1,†], Francesca Aiello [1], Gabriele Carullo [2], Rosita Curcio [1], Marco Fiorillo [1,*], Giuseppe Campiani [2], Vincenza Dolce [1] and Anna Rita Cappello [1,*]

1 Department of Pharmacy, Health and Nutritional Sciences, University of Calabria, Via P. Bucci, 87036 Rende, CS, Italy
2 Department of Biotechnology, Chemistry and Pharmacy, University of Siena, Via A. Moro 2, 53100 Siena, SI, Italy
* Correspondence: marco.fiorillo@unical.it (M.F.); annarita.cappello@unical.it (A.R.C.); Tel.: +39-0984-493194 (M.F.); +39-0984-493177 (A.R.C.)
† These authors contributed equally to this work.

Abstract: Research on the energy metabolism of cancer cells is becoming a central element in oncology, and in recent decades, it has allowed us to better understand the mechanisms underlying the onset and chemoresistance of oncological pathologies. Mitochondrial bioenergetic processes, in particular, have proven to be fundamental for the survival of tumor stem cells (CSC), a subpopulation of tumor cells responsible for tumor recurrence, the onset of metastasis, and the failure of conventional anticancer therapies. Over the years, numerous natural products, in particular flavonoids, widely distributed in the plant kingdom, have been shown to interfere with tumor bioenergetics, demonstrating promising antitumor effects. Herein, the anticancer potential of Licoflavanone, a flavanone isolated from the leaves of *G. glabra*, was explored for the first time in breast cancer cells. The results obtained highlighted a marked antitumor activity that proved to be greater than that mediated by Glabranin or Pinocembrin, flavanones isolated from the same plant matrix. Furthermore, the investigation of Licoflavanone's effects on breast cancer energy metabolism highlighted the inhibitory activity of this natural product on tumor bioenergetics, a mechanism that could underlie its ability to reduce tumor proliferation, invasiveness, and stemness.

Keywords: Licoflavanone; licorice; flavanones; breast cancer; anticancer agents; energy metabolism; cancer stem cells

1. Introduction

Nature has always represented an invaluable source of bioactive compounds, used over the years as remedies for various pathological conditions, drawing the attention first of traditional medicine and subsequently of phytotherapy and pharmaceutical research. The latter was also able to optimize the pharmacological features of natural compounds to maximize their therapeutic efficacy in order to support conventional therapeutic strategies.

Licorice is a plant of the Glycyrrhiza genus belonging to the Fabaceae family. This genus includes over 30 species widespread in Eurasia, Australia, and America, but the most widely used is *Glycyrrhiza glabra*.

Besides their crucial role in the food and confectionery industry, the roots of *G. glabra* are the most utilized component of licorice in traditional medicine worldwide, either independently or in combination with other herbal remedies, to treat several health conditions. They act as laxative, anti-inflammatory, anti-ulcer, antibiotic, anti-arthritic, antiviral, memory stimulant, anti-cholinergic, antitussive, anti-caries, hypolipidemic, anti-mycotic, estrogenic, antioxidant, and anticancer agents [1–3].

The biological potential of licorice roots is attributable to the variety of active compounds they contain, including hundreds of different polyphenols, classified as phenolic acids, flavonoids, flavones, chalcones, and isoflavonoids, and saponins, such as glycyrrhizin, which is considered the molecule mainly responsible for the beneficial activities of licorice root, particularly the anti-inflammatory one.

On the other hand, *G. glabra* leaves, considered a waste product for the food industry, have been shown in previous studies to contain several flavonoids and dihydrostilbenes with antioxidant, anti-genotoxic, and anti-inflammatory potential, which are either present in small traces or not at all in the roots [4,5]. Moreover, our recent study allowed us to isolate three different flavonoids from the leaves of *G. glabra*, namely Licoflavanone, Pinocembrin, and Glabranin, and to study their anti-inflammatory potential, bringing out an interesting biological potential, in particular for Licoflavanone, triggered by a modulation of the NF-kB transcription factor, which could be widely exploited in human health [6].

Indeed, pathways associated with inflammatory processes are often dysregulated in neoplastic diseases, favoring the proliferation of tumor cells as well as tumor angiogenesis, invasion and metastasis [7–9]. This premise, together with the experimental evidence that numerous flavonoids are able to determine antitumor effects thanks to their ability to modulate the redox state of the tumor cell as well as the programmed cell death processes [10], pave the way for studying the antitumor potential of flavanoids present in licorice leaves.

The objective of this study was to evaluate the antitumor activity of three different flavanones isolated from *G. glabra* leaves, Glabranin, Pinocembrin, and Licoflavanone, with the aim of providing more insights into the anticancer potential of these natural products, as well as to better understand their structure-activity relationship and the contribution of the prenyl substituent in the bioactivity of licorice flavanones. In particular, this study allowed us to evaluate and compare the ability of the three flavanones to inhibit breast cancer cell proliferation as well as modulate the cancer hallmarks associated with tumor aggressiveness and invasiveness. Furthermore, recent research showed that two flavonoids from bergamot fruit, Brutieridin and Melitidin, when combined in an enriched fraction (BMF), exhibit great potential in counteracting cancer stem cell (CSC) propagation of MCF7 breast tumor cells. The BMF was able to inhibit various characteristics of CSC behavior, such as mammosphere formation, ALDH level, mitochondrial respiration, and fatty acid oxidation, as well as several signaling pathways involved in stemness [11]. Based on these findings, this work investigated for the first time the effects of Glabranin, Pinocembrin, and Licoflavanone on cancer stem cells, a subpopulation of tumor cells with increased mitochondrial activity and high metabolic flexibility that promote phenomena such as chemoresistance, metastasis, and tumor recurrence, which are responsible in many cases for the failure of current therapeutic regimens [12].

2. Results and Discussion

2.1. *Antitumoral Potential of Glabranin, Pinocembrin, and Licoflavanone*

Here, we tested the antitumor potential of Glabranin, Pinocembrin, and Licoflavanone (Figure 1A) in both the luminal breast cancer cell line MCF-7 and the aggressive triple-negative breast cancer cell line MDA-MB-231; the effects of the three flavanones on tumor cell viability were compared to those observed in non-tumorigenic epithelial breast cells MCF-10A. After 72 h of treatment, the results showed the ability of all three compounds to elicit a stronger dose-dependent cytotoxic effect in the two breast cancer cell models than that observed in MCF-10A cells (Figures 1B and S3). Proliferation of tumor and non-tumor cell lines at 24, 48 and 72 h was assessed by MTT assay (Figure S2). The IC_{50} values for each compound were calculated in all cell lines tested (Table 1) and highlighted that MDA-MB-231 cells were the most sensitive to flavanone activity, and, among the three natural compounds, the highest activity was triggered by Licoflavanone. Moreover, our results revealed a fair selectivity of the three different molecules towards the tumor phenotype since, as shown in Figure 1C, 50 μM Glabranin and Pinocembrin as well as 25 μM Licoflavanone drastically reduced tumor cell viability without exerting any cytotoxicity on healthy cells (MCF-10A).

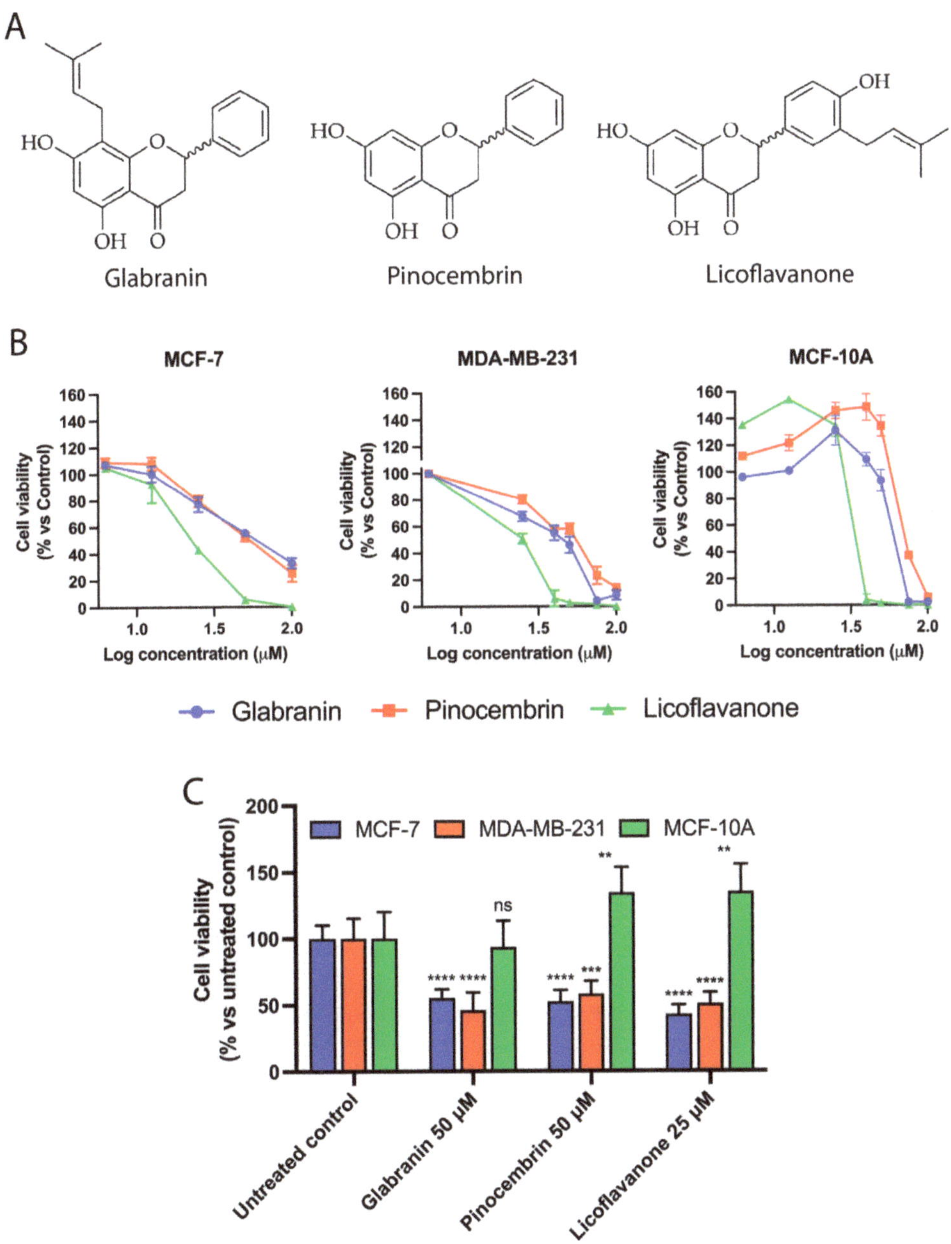

Figure 1. (**A**) Structure of Glabranin, Pinocembrin, and Licoflavanone. (**B**) Cell viability assessment of MCF-7, MDA-MB-231, and MCF-10A cells exposed to different concentrations of Glabranin, Pinocembrin, and Licoflavanone for 72 h. (**C**) Cytotoxic activity comparison between different breast cell lines. Values represent mean ± S.D. of three independent experiments, each performed with triplicate samples. ** $p < 0.01$; *** $p < 0.001$; **** $p < 0.0001$. ns: not significant.

Table 1. Cytotoxic activity of Glabranin, Pinocembrin, and Licoflavanone.

Compound	IC$_{50}$ (μM)		
	MCF-7	**MDA-MB-231**	**MCF-10A**
Glabranin	68.21 95% CI: 54.09 to 86.81	32.50 95% CI: 23.38 to 44.45	113.7 95% CI: 61.26 to 247.8
Pinocembrin	64.43 95% CI: 48.01 to 87.69	48.38 95% CI: 37.09 to 63.02	234.5 95% CI: 92.37 to 2637
Licoflavanone	19.18 95% CI: 13.21 to 27.34	10.97 95% CI: 6.751 to 16.16	41.38 95% CI: 19.66 to 88.79

2.2. Glabranin, Pinocembrin, and Licoflavanone Induce ROS Accumulation and Apoptosis

To investigate whether the cytotoxic activity of the three flavanones arises from triggering the apoptotic process, an apoptosis test was performed using the Annexin V assay as reported in the Section 3. The results showed that all three compounds enriched the apoptotic population in both breast cancer cell lines after 48 h of treatment (Figure 2A). A similar apoptotic rate was observed in MCF-7 cells treated with 50 μM Glabranin or Pinocembrin and 25 μM Licoflavanone. On the other hand, in MDA-MB-231 cells, a stronger apoptotic activity was observed after treatment with 50 μM Glabranin or Pinocembrin (Figure 2B).

Moreover, using the CM-H2DCFDA fluorescent probe, an increase in reactive oxygen species levels was detected after MDA-MB-231 cell exposure to the three different natural compounds (Figure 2C), suggesting that the three flavanones are able to trigger both oxidative stress and apoptosis in breast tumor cells. However, further studies are needed in order to assess additional oxidative stress biomarkers as well as to clarify the molecular pathways linking oxidative stress and apoptotic cell death.

These findings are consistent with the literature data, as the ability of pinocembrin to induce apoptotic death in tumor cells is well documented [13–15]; a recent study revealed the ability of Licoflavanone to also induce programmed cell death in nasopharyngeal tumor cells [16].

Our results not only corroborate the proapoptotic activity of Licoflavanone in breast cancer cell models, but also, for the first time, allow a comparison between the three different flavanones. This comparison revealed that Licoflavanone is able to elicit the same effects as pinocembrin (its not-prenylated analogue) and Glabranin (its prenylated analogue at a different position) at significantly lower concentrations.

2.3. Effect of the Three Different Natural Compounds on Cell Motility of MDA-MB-231 Cells

The ability of cancer cells to detach from the primary tumor and invade distant tissues and organs underlies the metastasizing power of malignant neoplasms. For this reason, to better characterize the antitumor potential of the three flavanones covered in this study, the cell motility of the highly aggressive MDA-MB-231 cell line was monitored by means of the wound healing assay, after 24 h of treatment with 50 μM Glabranin or Pinocembrin or 25 μM Licoflavanone. Untreated cells were used as a control. As shown in Figure 3, the obtained results highlighted the ability of all three compounds to inhibit the motility of these cells. Remarkably, the most pronounced effect was achieved by the 25 μM Licoflavanone treatment, which visibly reduced the "wound healing" more than the treatments with 50 μM Glabranin or Pinocembrin.

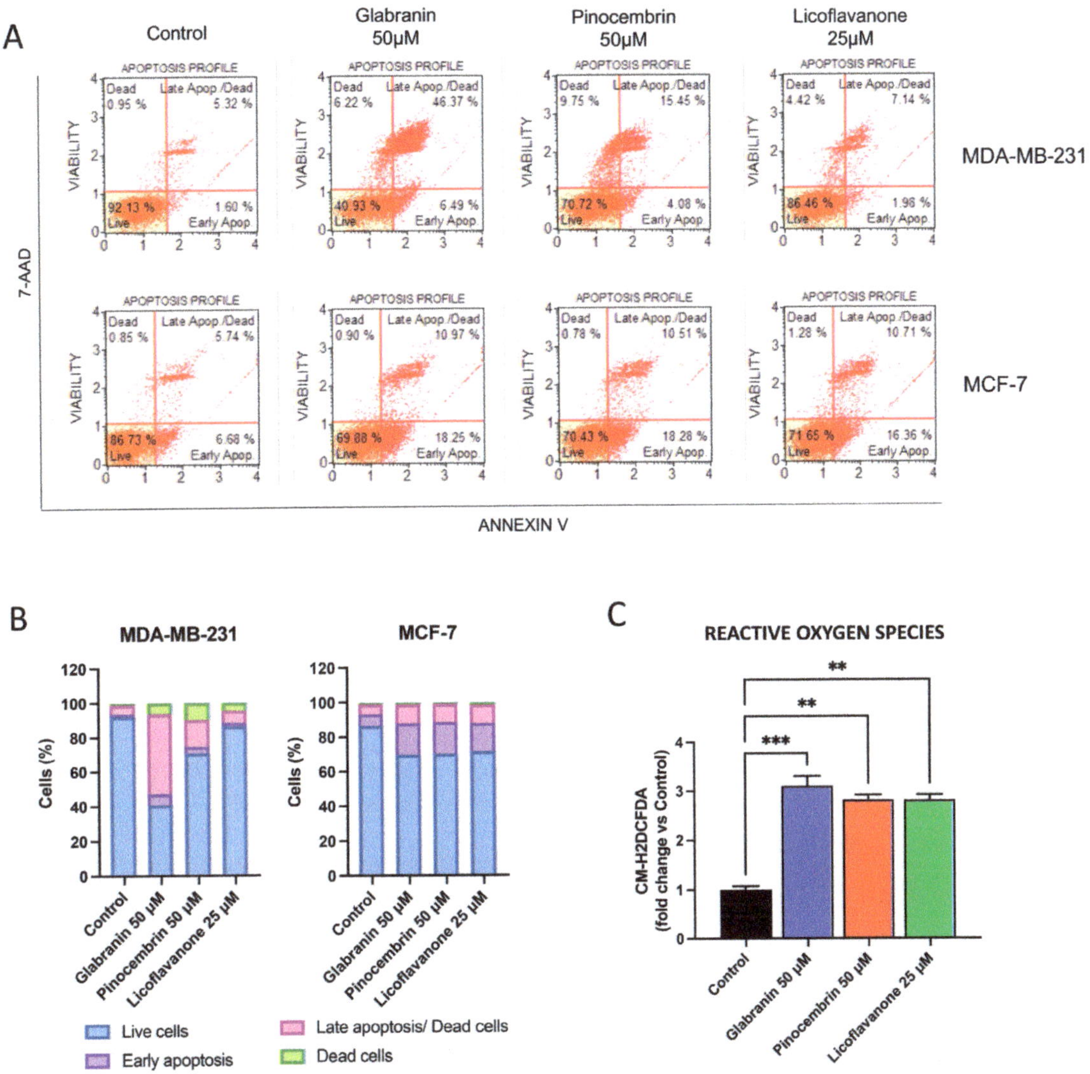

Figure 2. (**A**) Annexin V assay performed in MDA-MB-231 and MCF-7 cells exposed for 48 h to 50 μM Glabranin or Pinocembrin or 25 μM Licoflavanone. (**B**) Quantification of viable, apoptotic, and dead cell populations after 48 h of treatment. (**C**) Reactive oxygen species levels, quantified by using the CM-H2DCFDA fluorescent probe, after MDA-MB-231 cells exposure for 48 h to 50 μM Glabranin or Pinocembrin or 25 μM Licoflavanone. Values represent mean ± S.D. of three independent experiments, each performed with triplicate samples. ** $p < 0.01$; *** $p < 0.001$.

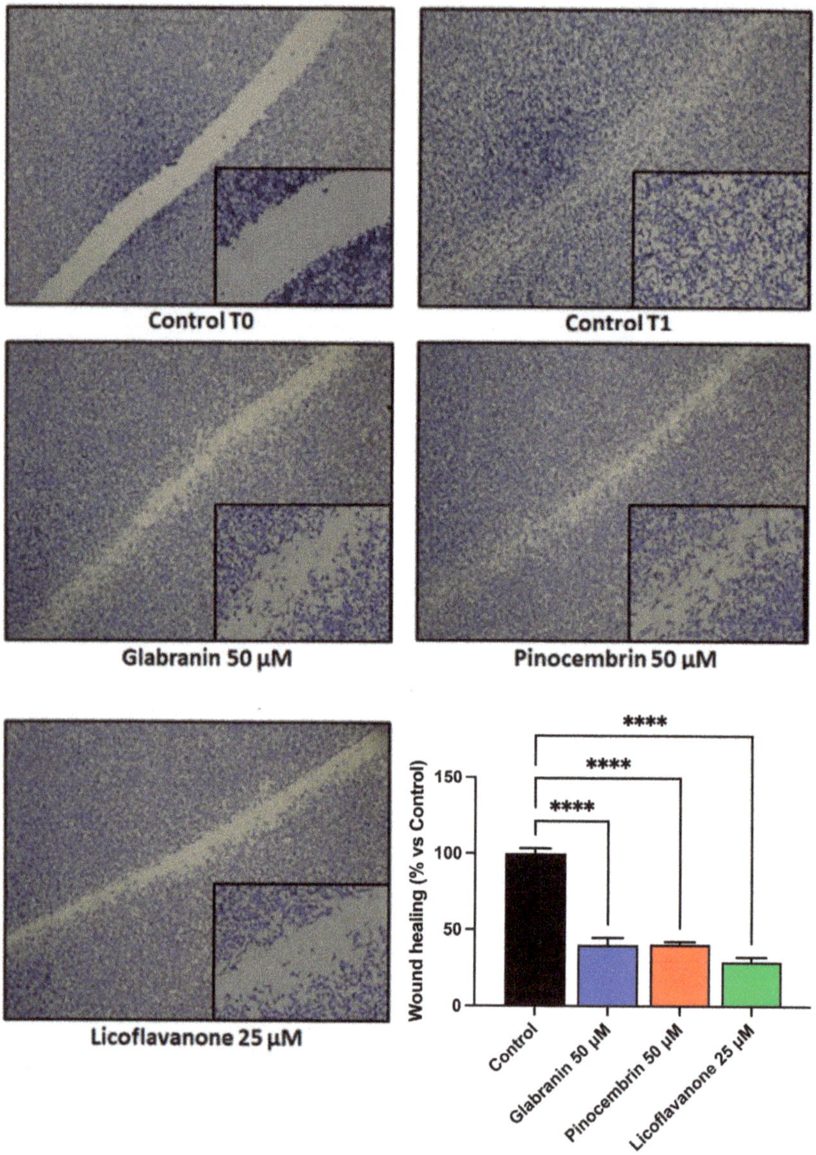

Figure 3. Effects of Glabranin, Pinocembrin, and Licoflavanone on MDA-MB-231 cell motility. Images were taken immediately after wounding (control T0) and after 24 h of treatment, using an Olympus BX41 microscope with CSV1.14 software and a CAMXC-30 for image acquisition. Images were acquired using a 2× objective, while magnifications were obtained with a 20× objective. Histograms indicate % wound healing vs. control. **** $p < 0.0001$.

2.4. Glabranin, Pinocembrin, and Licoflavanone Reduce Macrophage Activation Induced by Breast Cancer-Conditioned Media

Over the past twenty years, inflammation has gained increasing significance in cancer research. It has emerged that some tumors are directly linked to severe inflammatory processes that can promote the development of neoplasms by altering tissue structure [17]. Additionally, interest has grown in the tumor microenvironment as it plays a significant role in tumor progression. Indeed, it is known that cancer cells release various mediators with pro-inflammatory and angiogenic functions, which synergistically cooperate to orchestrate an optimal microenvironment for cancer cell survival and proliferation [18].

An important cellular component within the tumor microenvironment consists of tumor-associated macrophages (TAMs), which are known to be activated by cancer cells, thereby releasing biochemical mediators that promote cancer progression and metastatic dissemination. For this reason, TAMs represent an interesting target for potential exploitation in cancer therapy [19–21]. Here, we demonstrated the ability of Glabranin, Pinocembrin, and Licoflavanone to modulate RAW 264.7 macrophage activation by MCF-7 and MDA-MB-231 cell-conditioned media, comparing their ability to inhibit the production of nitric oxide (NO), an important inflammatory mediator. Our results demonstrated that NO production was reduced by Pinocembrin and Licoflavanone, while just a slight decrease was observed after Glabranin treatment (Figure 4). Also, in this case, the most noteworthy effect was achieved by the Licoflavanone treatment, which resulted in statistically more significant effects compared to its analogues, Pinocembrin and Glabranin.

It is necessary to underline that, in the experimental conditions used, the three polyphenols did not determine any effect on the viability of macrophages stimulated with conditioned medium. For this reason, the inhibitory effect of the three compounds on NO production cannot be correlated to their cytotoxic activity but rather can be ascribed exclusively to their anti-inflammatory action.

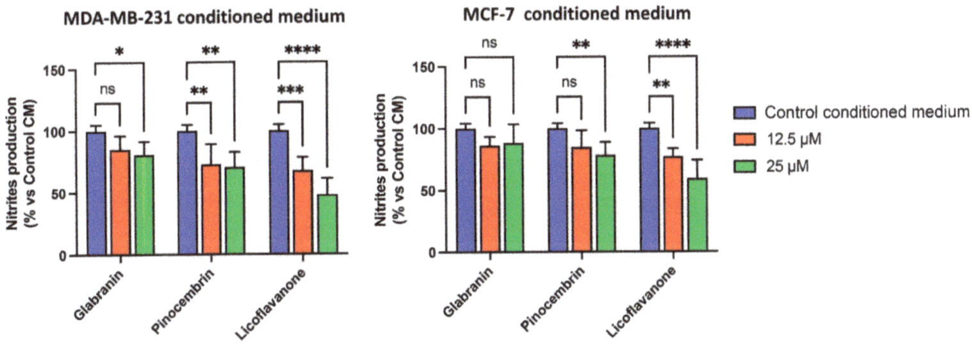

Figure 4. Effects of Glabranin, Pinocembrin, and Licoflavanone on RAW 264.7 macrophage activation induced by breast cancer-conditioned media from MDA-MB-231 or MCF-7 cells (as indicated). Data are the mean ± S.D. of three independent experiments, each performed with triplicate samples. * $p < 0.05$; ** $p < 0.01$; *** $p < 0.001$; **** $p < 0.0001$; ns: not significant.

2.5. Licoflavanone Modulates the Metabolic Profile of MCF-7 and MDA-MB-231 Cells

To evaluate if Licoflavanone modulates energy metabolism in cancer cells, the metabolic profiles of both MCF-7 and MDA-MB-231 cells were assessed after 72 h of treatment with 25 µM Licoflavanone. Specifically, using the Seahorse Extracellular Flux (XFe96) analyzer (Agilent, Santa Clara, CA, USA), the glycolytic function of breast cancer cells was evaluated through a Glycolysis Stress test, while the mitochondrial function was assessed by performing a Mito Stress test (as described in the Section 3). The results, depicted in Figure 5, displayed a strong decrease in the oxygen consumption rate linked to ATP production in both cell lines tested when compared to control cells (cells treated with vehicle alone). A significant reduction in basal respiration was also detected in MCF-7 cells. These findings on breast cancer cells treated with Licoflavanone are consistent with the literature, as the inhibitory action of various polyphenolic phytochemicals against the F_OF_1-ATPase complex has been widely reported [22–24].

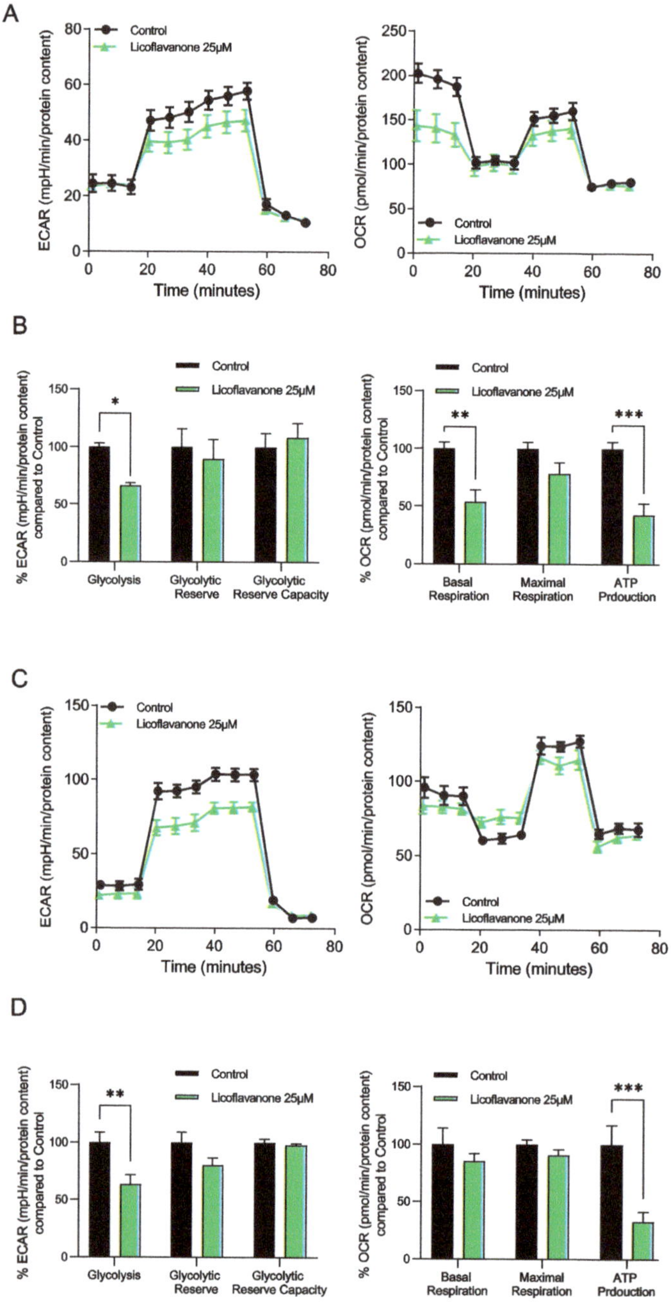

Figure 5. The ECAR (extracellular acidification rate) and the OCR (oxygen consumption rate) were determined using the Seahorse XFe96 via metabolic flux analysis. Note that both MCF-7 (**A**,**B**) and MDA-MB-231 (**C**,**D**) cell populations treated (72 h) with 25 µM Licoflavanone show a decrease in glycolysis as well as a decrease in basal respiration and mitochondrial ATP production compared to control (vehicle-alone) cells. (**A**–**C**) Representative images of the ECAR and OCR were presented. (**B**–**D**) Data represent the % average ± SD over control cells, n = 3. * $p < 0.05$, ** $p < 0.01$, *** $p < 0.001$.

2.6. Glabranin, Pinocembrin, and Licoflavanone Significantly Inhibits CSC Propagation and Survival by Reducing Stemness Marker Expression

Since Glabranin, Pinocembrin, and Licoflavanone behaved as inhibitors of cell proliferation and motility, we next examined their effects on the behavior of the CSC population, which is believed to be the tumor-initiating cells responsible for chemotherapy resistance, cancer dissemination, and tumor relapse. More specifically, MCF-7 and MDA-MB-231 cells were grown as mammospheres and treated with 25 μM and 50 μM Glabranin, Pinocembrin, and Licoflavanone. Vehicle-alone (control) cells were processed in parallel. Interestingly, Figure 6A shows that all three natural compounds halted mammosphere formation in a dose-dependent manner. In addition, expression levels of validated CSC markers, such as Snail, OCT4, SOX2, and NANOG [25–28], were determined by qPCR analysis (Figure 6B). 25 μM Licoflavanone diminished the CSC marker expression better than the other two compounds tested, indicating it as a potent inhibitor of CSC formation and propagation.

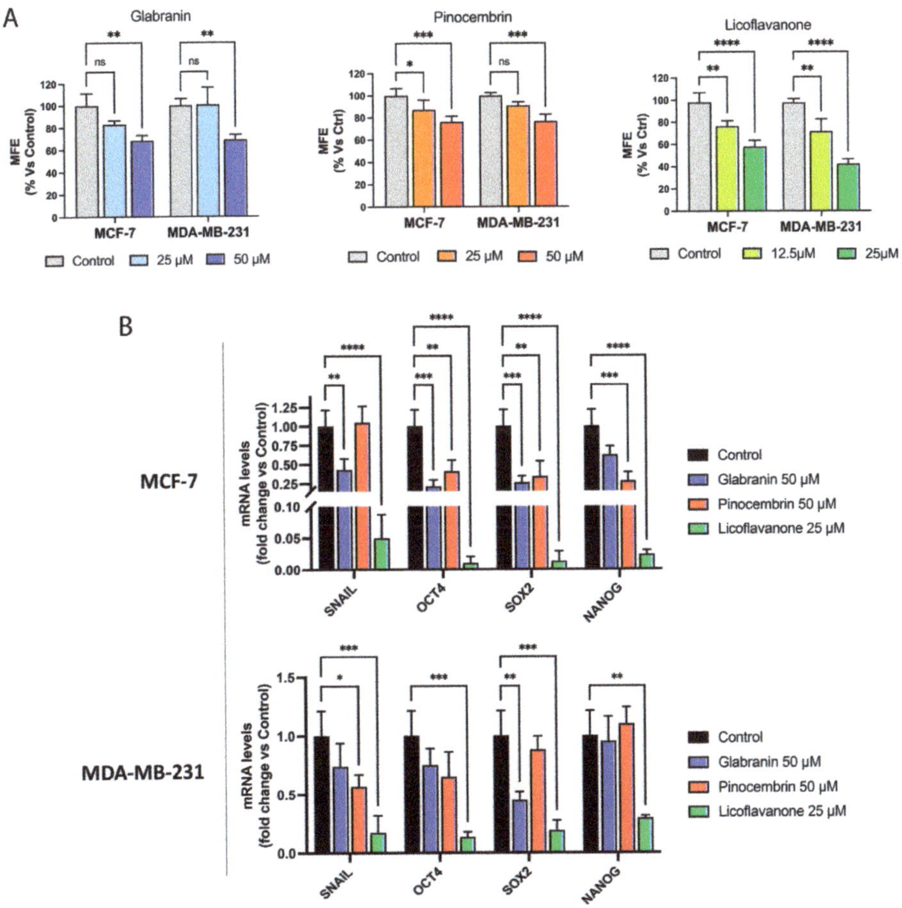

Figure 6. (**A**) Mammosphere formation efficiency (MFE) of MCF-7 and MDA-MB-231 cells treated with 50 μM Glabranin or Pinocembrin or 25 μM Licoflavanone. (**B**) qPCR analysis of mRNA levels of CSC markers (Snail, OCT4, SOX2, NANOG) in MCF-7 and MDA-MB-231 cells exposed to Glabranin, Pinocembrin, and Licoflavanone for 48 h. Values represent mean ± S.D. of three independent experiments, each performed with triplicate samples. * $p < 0.05$; ** $p < 0.01$; *** $p < 0.001$; **** $p < 0.0001$. ns: not significant.

2.7. Structural Elucidation of Licoflavanone, Glabranin and Pinocembrin

Pinocembrin, Glabranin, and Licoflavanone share the 5,7-dihydroxy-2-phenylchroman-4-one scaffold (Figure 7). Giving a glance at the in vitro results, the activity of Licoflavanone is always better than that of the other compounds. Lacking a biological target, so far, we have tried to explain this significant difference only using a structure-based approach. The nucleus A is decorated with two hydroxy groups in the C5 and C7 positions, for Pinocembrin and Licoflavanone, with Log $p = 2.843$ and 4.019, respectively, while it shows a prenyl moiety at position C8 in Glabranin with a Log $p = 4.303$ (see Supplementary Material for a complete ADMET profile, Figure S1). The nucleus B in Glabranin and Pinocembrin is free of any substituents. It is well known that the number of hydroxyl groups improves the antioxidant power of all polyphenols, especially when located in nucleus B. In this case, only in Licoflavanone is this condition satisfied by a hydroxyl group in C4′. The contemporary presence of a prenyl chain in C3′ in Licoflavavnone improves the lipophilic behavior with respect to Pinocembrin. Maybe this condition could be responsible for the better activities registered for Licoflavanone. Furthermore, Glabranin seems to be more active than Pinocembrin, from which it differs only in C8 on nucleus A; in this case, the prenyl fragment is the distinguishing element accounting for the different biological profile in the same set of in vitro experiments.

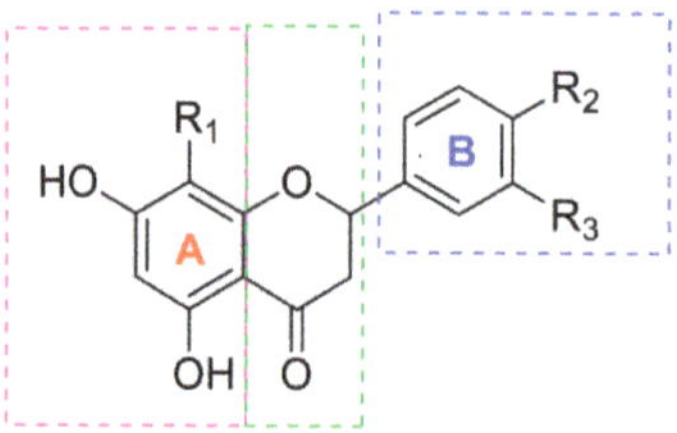

Pinocembrin R1=R2=R3=H
Glabranin R1= prenyl, R2=R3= H
Licoflavanone R1=H; R2= OH; R3= prenyl,

Figure 7. General chemical structure of the assayed compounds.

As an example of the capability of a prenyl chain to modulate biological activities, isoflavonoids, a class of secondary metabolites abundant in Leguminosae, can bind to the human estrogen receptor (hER) with affinities similar to or lower than those of estradiol. Dietary intake of these so-called phytoestrogens has been associated with positive effects on menopausal complaints, hormone-related cancers, and osteoporosis. Therefore, phytoestrogens are used as nutraceuticals in functional foods or food supplements. Most of the isoflavonoids show agonistic activity towards both hERα and hERβ, the extent of which is modulated by the substitution pattern of their skeleton (i.e., –OH, –OCH_3). Interestingly, substitutions consisting of a five-carbon prenyl group often seem to result in antiestrogenic activity. Prenylated flavonoids have been documented to be more bioactive than their flavonoid precursors, as prenylation increases the lipophilicity of flavonoids, leading to higher permeability and bioavailability in vivo [29].

Exploiting mammosphere formation, it is worth noting that dietary supplementation with Piperine and Curcumine is able to modify mammosphere formation [30].

Piperine is a *N*-acylpiperidine that is piperidine substituted by a (1E,3E)-1-(1,3-benzodioxol-5-yl)-5-oxopenta-1,3-dien-5-yl group at the nitrogen atom (PubChem).

Curcumin is a beta-diketone that is methane in which two of the hydrogens are substituted by feruloyl groups. Curcumin, also known as diferuloylmethane, is an active component in the golden spice turmeric (*Curcuma longa*) and in Curcuma xanthorrhiza oil. It is a highly pleiotropic molecule that exhibits antibacterial, anti-inflammatory, hypoglycemic, antioxidant, wound-healing, and antimicrobial activities (PubChem). Both of them show an unsaturated chain and hydroxyl group on the phenyl ring, masked as ketals in Piperine (Figure 8).

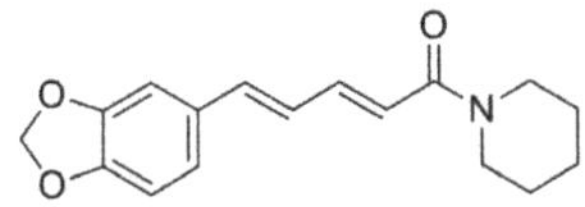

Piperine

(2E,4E)-5-(1,3-benzodioxol-5-yl)-1-piperidin-1-ylpenta-2,4-dien-1-one

Log P: 2.78
Henry's Law: 10.1
tPSA: 38.77
CLogP: 3.313

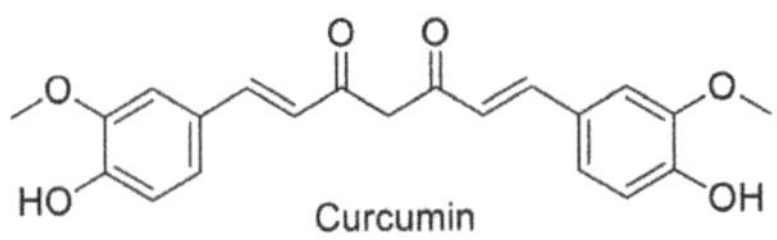

Curcumin

(1E,6E)-1,7-bis(4-hydroxy-3-methoxyphenyl)hepta-1,6-diene-3,5-dione

Log P: 2.56
Henry's Law: 19.54
tPSA: 93.06
CLogP: 2.2506

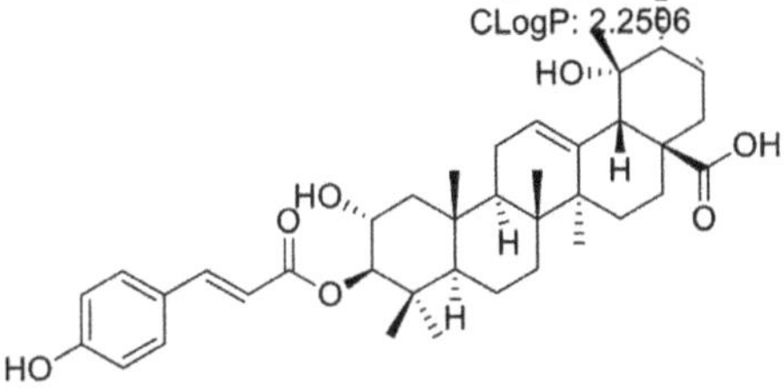

3-*O*-trans- *p*-coumaroyltormentic acid

(1R,2R,4aS,6aR,6aS,6bR,8aR,10R,11R,12aR,14bS)-1,11-dihydroxy-10-[(E)-3-(4-hydroxyphenyl)prop-2-enoyl]oxy-1,2,6a,6b,9,9,12a-heptamethyl-2,3,4,5,6,6a,7,8,8a,10,11,12,13,14b-tetradecahydropicene-4a-carboxylic acid

tPSA: 124.29
CLogP: 8.233

Figure 8. Structure of Piperine, Curcumin, and 3-*O*-trans-*p*-coumaroyltormentic acid.

Triterpene acid (3-*O*-trans-*p*-coumaroyltormentic acid), a triterpenoid isolated from Aronia extracts, effectively inhibits breast cancer cell proliferation and mammosphere formation in a dose-dependent manner. Similarly, several triterpenoids can inhibit cancer stem cells, such as ginsenoside Rg3, a triterpene saponin that inhibits CSCs of colorectal cancer, and gedunin, a natural tetranortriterpenoid that inhibits teratocarcinomal (NTERA-2) cancer stem-like cells. Cucurbitacin E, a tetracyclic triterpene, betulonic acid, a pentacyclic lupane-type triterpenoid, and plant-derived triterpenoid tingenin B inhibit cervical cancer cell lines, leukemia stem cells, and breast CSCs, respectively. Also, triterpene glycosides may be used as adjuvants for the rational design of vaccines against cancer. Phenethyl isothiocyanate, a naturally occurring isothiocyanate, and 8-bromo-7-methoxychrysin, a synthetic derivative of chrysin that is a naturally widely distributed flavonoid, have been shown to possess inhibitory activity against colon and liver CSCs [31].

All these natural compounds are endowed with an unsaturated chain in their scaffold, other than hydroxyl groups.

To better understand the structural relevance of the tested compounds, we split the 5,7-dihydroxy-2-phenylchroman-4-one scaffold into three regions (see Figure 7): nucleus A (purple), nucleus B (blue), and tetrahydro-4*H*-pyran-4-one (green). The green region does not appear to be crucial for biological activity in our in vitro experiments, whereas the blue and purple ones are necessary. Referring to the structure of Glabranin and Licoflavanone, these two portions are, respectively, 4-isopentenyl-1,3-dihydroxybenzene (purple) and 2-hydroxyisopentenyl benzene (blue), and could be considered the pharmacophore. From a medicinal chemistry point of view, applying the scaffold hopping theory, the hypothetical lead scaffold is depicted in Figure 9.

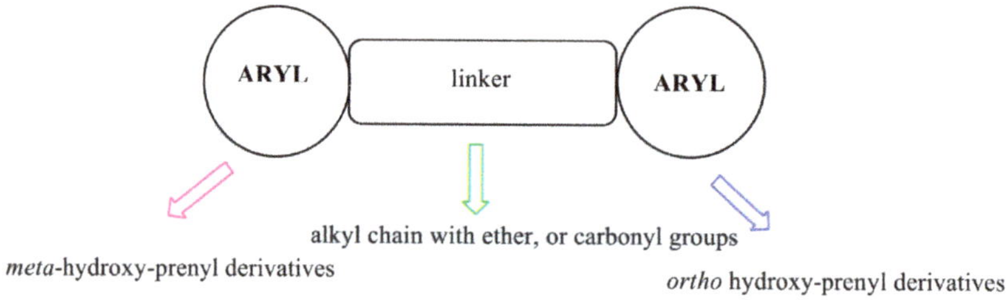

Figure 9. Hypothesis of a suitable lead scaffold.

3. Materials and Methods

3.1. Cell Cultures

Breast cell lines MCF-7, MDA-MB-231, and MCF-10A, as well as murine macrophage RAW 264.7 cell lines, were purchased from the American Culture Collection (ATCC, Manassas, VA, USA). MCF-7 and MDA-MB-231 cells were cultured in DMEM/F12 (Sigma Aldrich, St. Louis, MO, USA) supplemented with 10% Fetal Bovine Serum (FBS), 2 mM l-glutamine, and 1% penicillin/streptomycin (all from Sigma Aldrich). RAW 264.7 cells were cultured in DMEM High Glucose (Sigma Aldrich) supplemented with 10% FBS, 2 mM l-glutamine, and 1% penicillin/streptomycin. MCF-10A cells were cultured in DMEM/F12 supplemented with 5% horse serum (HS), 2 mM l-glutamine, 1% penicillin/streptomycin, 0.5 mg/mL hydrocortisone, 20 ng/mL human epidermal growth factor (hEGF), 10 mg/mL insulin, and 0.1 mg/mL cholera toxin (all from Sigma Aldrich). All cell lines were cultured at 37 °C in 5% CO_2 in a humidified atmosphere. Licoflavanone, Glabranin, and Pinocembrin were purified as previously described [6]. Treatments were performed in the above-mentioned media containing a lower amount of serum (2%).

3.2. Viability Assay

Cell viability was determined by using the 3-(4,5-dimethyl-2-thiazolyl)-2,5-diphenyl-2H-tetrazolium bromide (MTT) assay and the Sulforhodamine B (SRB) assay, as previously described [32,33]. In order to calculate IC_{50} values for each cell line, a non-linear regression analysis (GraphPad Prism 9) was performed to generate sigmoidal dose–response curves.

3.3. Apoptosis Assay

MCF-7 and MDA-MB-231 cells were seeded in 6-well plates (2×10^5 cells/well) and treated with different concentrations of compounds for 48 h. They were then subjected to apoptosis assays by means of the Muse® Annexin V & Dead Cell Kit (Merk, Milan, Italy), following the manufacturer's recommendations.

3.4. Intracellular ROS Assessment

MDA-MB-231 cells were seeded in 6-well plates (2×10^5 cells/well) and treated with the compounds for 24 h. After treatment, the intracellular ROS level in each sample was assessed using the CM-H_2DCFDA fluorescent dye, as previously reported [33]. Samples were then analyzed by flow cytometry (CytoFLEX Beckman, Beckman Coulter, Milan, Italy). Data analysis was performed using the CytExpert Beckman Coulter software v2.3 (Beckman Coulter, Milan, Italy).

3.5. Wound-Healing Scratch Assay

In order to assess the effect of compounds on tumor cell motility, MDA-MB-231 cells were treated for 24 h with 50 μM Glabranin or Pinocembrin and 25 μM Licoflavanone and then subjected to a wound healing scratch assay, as previously reported [34].

3.6. Nitric Oxide Assessment in RAW 264.7 Cells Stimulated by Tumor-Conditioned Medium

The ability of compounds to modulate the inflammatory process in RAW 264.7 cells exposed to MCF-7 and MDA-MB-231-conditioned media was evaluated by quantifying nitrite levels in macrophages medium by using the Griess reagent (Sigma Aldrich), as previously described [35]. Briefly, breast cancer cells were seeded in 24-well plates at a density of 1×10^5 cells per well and incubated overnight in DMEM/F-12 medium. The following day, in each well, the medium was replaced with a fresh medium for 24 h. Then, RAW 264.7 macrophages were treated with the conditioned media and simultaneously exposed to different concentrations of flavanones (12.5 and 25 μM). After 24 h, the nitrite concentration in each sample was assessed using the Griess assay, following the manufacturer's recommendations. Basal NO production by unstimulated RAW 264.7 cells was subtracted from the values obtained in stimulated samples.

3.7. Metabolic Flux Analysis with the Seahorse XFe96

Real-time extracellular acidification rates (ECARs) and oxygen consumption rates (OCRs) were determined using the Seahorse Extracellular Flux (XFe96) analyzer (Agilent). Briefly, 5×10^3 cells per well were seeded into XFe96-well cell culture plates and incubated for 24 h to allow cell attachment. After 24 h, cells were treated with 25 μM Licoflavanone for 72 h. Vehicle-alone (DMSO) control cells were processed in parallel then washed in pre-warmed XF assay media (or for OCR measurement, XF assay media supplemented with 10 mM glucose, 1 mM Pyruvate, and 2 mM l-glutamine). Cells were then maintained in 175 μL/well of XF assay media at 37 °C in a non-CO_2 incubator for 1 h. During the incubation time, we loaded 25 μL of 80 mM glucose, 9 μM oligomycin, and 0.5 M 2-deoxyglucose (for ECAR measurement) or 10 μM oligomycin, 10 μM CCCP, 10 μM rotenone, and 10 μM antimycin A (for OCR measurement), in XF assay media into the injection ports in the XFe96 sensor cartridge. Measurements were normalized by protein content (SRB assay). Data sets were analyzed using XFe96 v2.6 software and GraphPad Prism software, using two-way ANOVA and Student's t test calculations. All experiments were performed in quintuplicate, three times independently.

3.8. Mammospheres Formation Efficiency

The mammosphere formation efficiency of MCF-7 and MDA-MB-231 cells treated with different concentrations of flavanones (12.5 and 25 μM) was assessed as previously described [36].

3.9. qPCR Analysis of Gene Expression

MCF-7 and MDA-MB-231 cells were grown in 10 cm dishes and treated for 48 h with 50 μM of Glabranin or Pinocembrin and 25 μM Licoflavanone. Total RNA was isolated using TRIZOL reagent (Invitrogen, Monza, Italy), following the manufacturer's procedure. Reverse transcription was performed, as previously reported [37], on each RNA sample to generate complementary DNA (cDNA). Gene expression analyses of SNAIL, OCT4, SOX2, and NANOG were carried out using the Quant Studio 3 Real-Time PCR System (Life Technologies, Monza, Italy) employing the SsoAdvanced Universal SYBR Green (Biorad Laboratories Inc., Milan, Italy), following the manufacturer's guidelines. Assays were executed in triplicate, and results were normalized using 18S rRNA levels. The ΔΔCt method was used to calculate the relative mRNA levels. All the oligonucleotides used for qPCR are listed in Table 2.

Table 2. Sequence of the oligonucleotides used in qPCR analysis of gene expression.

Primer	Forward	Reverse
SNAIL	CGAGTGGTTCTTCTGCGCTA	GGGCTGCTGGAAGGTAAACT
OCT4	AGCGACTATGCACAACGAGA	CCATAGCCTGGGTACCAAA
NANOG	CTCCAACATCCTGAACCTCAGC	CGTCACACCATTGCTATTCTTCG
SOX2	GGCCTCGAGCTGGGAATCGC	GCCCACTCGGGGTCTTGCAC

3.10. Statistical Analysis

GraphPad Prism 9 was used to conduct statistical analysis of all the data. Statistical significance was evaluated by an analysis of variance (ANOVA). A p value ≤ 0.05 was considered statistically significant. Normality of each distribution was confirmed by the Shapiro–Wilk test, while equality of variance was verified by Levene's test. Tukey's post-hoc test was used to study differences between groups.

4. Conclusions

In the past decade, the mitochondrial energy metabolism of different tumor cell types has been proposed as a central element for understanding the pathological mechanisms underlying oncological pathology itself and as a possible target for the development of new therapeutic strategies aimed at eradicating it [38,39]. Moreover, mitochondrial metabolism also drives the proliferation of cancer stem cells (CSCs), a subpopulation of tumor cells accountable for tumor recurrence, metastasis onset, and the failure of conventional anticancer therapies [40]. Consequently, investigating molecules capable of influencing mitochondrial metabolism and translating findings into clinical applications could offer an effective approach for treating those tumors strictly dependent on oxidative metabolism [41]. On the other hand, the literature extensively documents that flavonoids, a family of secondary metabolites widely distributed in the plant kingdom and known for their beneficial effects on human health, can exert their actions by modulating various mitochondrial mechanisms [42].

Consistent with the existing literature, our study has uncovered the antiproliferative potential of Licoflavanone from G. glabra leaves, alongside its role in modulating breast cancer aggressiveness and invasiveness. Additionally, our findings have highlighted the heightened potency of this activity compared to Glabranin and Pinocembrin, two flavonoids derived from the same source. Furthermore, this research has shed light, for the first time, on Licoflavanone's ability to affect mitochondrial metabolism, as demonstrated by the decrease in basal respiration as well as in the oxygen consumption rate linked to ATP production.

These results suggest that the anticancer activity demonstrated by Licoflavanone could be mediated by mitochondrial modulation, as indicated by its ability to inhibit the growth of cancer stem cells, a subset of tumor cells that heavily rely on mitochondrial function for their proliferation.

Supplementary Materials: The following supporting information can be downloaded at: https://www.mdpi.com/article/10.3390/ijms25147907/s1.

Author Contributions: Conceptualization, L.F., M.F. and A.R.C.; investigation, L.F., G.L., F.A., G.C. (Gabriele Carullo), M.F. and R.C.; data curation, L.F., F.A., M.F. and A.R.C.; writing—original draft preparation, L.F., G.L., F.A. and A.R.C.; writing—review and editing, G.C. (Giuseppe Campiani) and V.D.; supervision, A.R.C. All authors have read and agreed to the published version of the manuscript.

Funding: This research received no external funding.

Institutional Review Board Statement: Not applicable.

Informed Consent Statement: Not applicable.

Data Availability Statement: The original contributions presented in the study are included in the article/Supplementary Materials; further inquiries can be directed to the corresponding authors.

Acknowledgments: The Botanical Garden of the University of Calabria is acknowledged for kindly donating licorice leaves.

Conflicts of Interest: The authors declare no conflicts of interest.

References

1. Sharifi-Rad, J.; Quispe, C.; Herrera-Bravo, J.; Belén, L.H.; Kaur, R.; Kregiel, D.; Uprety, Y.; Beyatli, A.; Yeskaliyeva, B.; Kırkın, C.; et al. *Glycyrrhiza* Genus: Enlightening Phytochemical Components for Pharmacological and Health-Promoting Abilities. *Oxidative Med. Cell. Longev.* **2021**, *2021*, 7571132. [CrossRef] [PubMed]
2. Wahab, S.; Annadurai, S.; Abullais, S.S.; Das, G.; Ahmad, W.; Ahmad, M.F.; Kandasamy, G.; Vasudevan, R.; Ali, M.S.; Amir, M. *Glycyrrhiza glabra* (Licorice): A Comprehensive Review on Its Phytochemistry, Biological Activities, Clinical Evidence and Toxicology. *Plants* **2021**, *10*, 2751. [CrossRef]
3. El-Saber Batiha, G.; Magdy Beshbishy, A.; El-Mleeh, A.; Abdel-Daim, M.M.; Prasad Devkota, H. Traditional Uses, Bioactive Chemical Constituents, and Pharmacological and Toxicological Activities of *Glycyrrhiza glabra* L. (Fabaceae). *Biomolecules* **2020**, *10*, 352. [CrossRef] [PubMed]
4. Hayashi, H.; Yasuma, M.; Hiraoka, N.; Ikeshiro, Y.; Yamamoto, H.; Yeşilada, E.; Sezik, E.; Honda, G.; Tabata, M. Flavonoid Variation in the Leaves of *Glycyrrhiza glabra*. *Phytochemistry* **1996**, *42*, 701–704. [CrossRef]
5. Siracusa, L.; Saija, A.; Cristani, M.; Cimino, F.; D'Arrigo, M.; Trombetta, D.; Rao, F.; Ruberto, G. Phytocomplexes from Liquorice (*Glycyrrhiza glabra* L.) Leaves—Chemical Characterization and Evaluation of Their Antioxidant, Anti-Genotoxic and Anti-Inflammatory Activity. *Fitoterapia* **2011**, *82*, 546–556. [CrossRef]
6. Frattaruolo, L.; Carullo, G.; Brindisi, M.; Mazzotta, S.; Bellissimo, L.; Rago, V.; Curcio, R.; Dolce, V.; Aiello, F.; Cappello, A.R. Antioxidant and Anti-Inflammatory Activities of Flavanones from *Glycyrrhiza glabra* L. (Licorice) Leaf Phytocomplexes: Identification of Licoflavanone as a Modulator of NF-kB/MAPK Pathway. *Antioxidants* **2019**, *8*, 186. [CrossRef] [PubMed]
7. Zhao, H.; Wu, L.; Yan, G.; Chen, Y.; Zhou, M.; Wu, Y.; Li, Y. Inflammation and Tumor Progression: Signaling Pathways and Targeted Intervention. *Signal Transduct. Target. Ther.* **2021**, *6*, 263. [CrossRef] [PubMed]
8. Zhang, T.; Ma, C.; Zhang, Z.; Zhang, H.; Hu, H. NF-κB Signaling in Inflammation and Cancer. *MedComm* **2021**, *2*, 618–653. [CrossRef]
9. Zinatizadeh, M.R.; Schock, B.; Chalbatani, G.M.; Zarandi, P.K.; Jalali, S.A.; Miri, S.R. The Nuclear Factor Kappa B (NF-kB) Signaling in Cancer Development and Immune Diseases. *Genes Dis.* **2021**, *8*, 287–297. [CrossRef]
10. Ponte, L.G.S.; Pavan, I.C.B.; Mancini, M.C.S.; Da Silva, L.G.S.; Morelli, A.P.; Severino, M.B.; Bezerra, R.M.N.; Simabuco, F.M. The Hallmarks of Flavonoids in Cancer. *Molecules* **2021**, *26*, 2029. [CrossRef]
11. Fiorillo, M.; Peiris-Pagès, M.; Sanchez-Alvarez, R.; Bartella, L.; Di Donna, L.; Dolce, V.; Sindona, G.; Sotgia, F.; Cappello, A.R.; Lisanti, M.P. Bergamot Natural Products Eradicate Cancer Stem Cells (CSCs) by Targeting Mevalonate, Rho-GDI-Signalling and Mitochondrial Metabolism. *Biochim. Biophys. Acta (BBA)—Bioenerg.* **2018**, *1859*, 984–996. [CrossRef] [PubMed]
12. Snyder, V.; Reed-Newman, T.C.; Arnold, L.; Thomas, S.M.; Anant, S. Cancer Stem Cell Metabolism and Potential Therapeutic Targets. *Front. Oncol.* **2018**, *8*, 203. [CrossRef] [PubMed]
13. Zheng, Y.; Wang, K.; Wu, Y.; Chen, Y.; Chen, X.; Hu, C.W.; Hu, F. Pinocembrin Induces ER Stress Mediated Apoptosis and Suppresses Autophagy in Melanoma Cells. *Cancer Lett.* **2018**, *431*, 31–42. [CrossRef] [PubMed]
14. Gong, H. Pinocembrin Suppresses Proliferation and Enhances Apoptosis in Lung Cancer Cells in Vitro by Restraining Autophagy. *Bioengineered* **2021**, *12*, 6035–6044. [CrossRef]
15. Kumar, M.A.S.; Nair, M.; Hema, P.S.; Mohan, J.; Santhoshkumar, T.R. Pinocembrin Triggers Bax-dependent Mitochondrial Apoptosis in Colon Cancer Cells. *Mol. Carcinog.* **2007**, *46*, 231–241. [CrossRef]
16. Liu, J.; Song, C.; Liang, Z.; Long, X.; Guo, M.; Xu, J. Licoflavanone Exerts Anticancer Effects on Human Nasopharyngeal Cancer Cells via Caspase Activation, Suppression of Cell Migration and Invasion, and Inhibition of m-TOR/PI3K/AKT Pathway. *Trop. J. Pharm. Res.* **2022**, *20*, 1387–1393. [CrossRef]
17. Coussens, L.M.; Werb, Z. Inflammation and Cancer. *Nature* **2002**, *420*, 860–867. [CrossRef] [PubMed]
18. Jiang, X.; Wang, J.; Deng, X.; Xiong, F.; Zhang, S.; Gong, Z.; Li, X.; Cao, K.; Deng, H.; He, Y.; et al. The Role of Microenvironment in Tumor Angiogenesis. *J. Exp. Clin. Cancer Res.* **2020**, *39*, 204. [CrossRef]
19. Mantovani, A.; Allavena, P.; Marchesi, F.; Garlanda, C. Macrophages as Tools and Targets in Cancer Therapy. *Nat. Rev. Drug Discov.* **2022**, *21*, 799–820. [CrossRef]
20. Duan, Z.; Luo, Y. Targeting Macrophages in Cancer Immunotherapy. *Signal Transduct. Target. Ther.* **2021**, *6*, 127. [CrossRef]
21. Zhou, J.; Tang, Z.; Gao, S.; Li, C.; Feng, Y.; Zhou, X. Tumor-Associated Macrophages: Recent Insights and Therapies. *Front. Oncol.* **2020**, *10*, 188. [CrossRef] [PubMed]
22. Gledhill, J.R.; Montgomery, M.G.; Leslie, A.G.W.; Walker, J.E. Mechanism of Inhibition of Bovine F_1-ATPase by Resveratrol and Related Polyphenols. *Proc. Natl. Acad. Sci. USA* **2007**, *104*, 13632–13637. [CrossRef] [PubMed]

23. Sekiya, M.; Hisasaka, R.; Iwamoto-Kihara, A.; Futai, M.; Nakanishi-Matsui, M. A Unique Mechanism of Curcumin Inhibition on F1 ATPase. *Biochem. Biophys. Res. Commun.* **2014**, *452*, 940–944. [CrossRef] [PubMed]
24. Zheng, J.; Ramirez, V.D. Inhibition of Mitochondrial Proton F0F1-ATPase/ATP Synthase by Polyphenolic Phytochemicals. *Br. J. Pharmacol.* **2000**, *130*, 1115–1123. [CrossRef] [PubMed]
25. Apostolou, P.; Toloudi, M.; Chatziioannou, M.; Ioannou, E.; Papasotiriou, I. Cancer Stem Cells Stemness Transcription Factors Expression Correlates with Breast Cancer Disease Stage. *Curr. Stem Cell Res. Ther.* **2012**, *7*, 415–419. [CrossRef] [PubMed]
26. Luo, W.; Li, S.; Peng, B.; Ye, Y.; Deng, X.; Yao, K. Embryonic Stem Cells Markers SOX2, OCT4 and Nanog Expression and Their Correlations with Epithelial-Mesenchymal Transition in Nasopharyngeal Carcinoma. *PLoS ONE* **2013**, *8*, e56324. [CrossRef]
27. Wu, C.-W.; Wang, M.-L.; Chiou, S.-H. Targeting Cancer Stem Cells: Emerging Role of Nanog Transcription Factor. *OncoTargets Ther.* **2013**, *6*, 1207–1220. [CrossRef] [PubMed]
28. Zhou, W.; Lv, R.; Qi, W.; Wu, D.; Xu, Y.; Liu, W.; Mou, Y.; Wang, L. Snail Contributes to the Maintenance of Stem Cell-Like Phenotype Cells in Human Pancreatic Cancer. *PLoS ONE* **2014**, *9*, e87409. [CrossRef] [PubMed]
29. Simons, R.; Gruppen, H.; Bovee, T.F.H.; Verbruggen, M.A.; Vincken, J.-P. Prenylated Isoflavonoids from Plants as Selective Estrogen Receptor Modulators (phytoSERMs). *Food Funct.* **2012**, *3*, 810. [CrossRef]
30. Kakarala, M.; Brenner, D.E.; Korkaya, H.; Cheng, C.; Tazi, K.; Ginestier, C.; Liu, S.; Dontu, G.; Wicha, M.S. Targeting Breast Stem Cells with the Cancer Preventive Compounds Curcumin and Piperine. *Breast Cancer Res. Treat.* **2010**, *122*, 777–785. [CrossRef]
31. Choi, H.; Kim, S.-L.; Kim, J.-H.; Deng, H.-Y.; Yun, B.-S.; Lee, D.-S. Triterpene Acid (3-O-p-Coumaroyltormentic Acid) Isolated from Aronia Extracts Inhibits Breast Cancer Stem Cell Formation through Downregulation of c-Myc Protein. *Int. J. Mol. Sci.* **2018**, *19*, 2528. [CrossRef]
32. Curcio, M.; Brindisi, M.; Cirillo, G.; Frattaruolo, L.; Leggio, A.; Rago, V.; Nicoletta, F.P.; Cappello, A.R.; Iemma, F. Smart Lipid–Polysaccharide Nanoparticles for Targeted Delivery of Doxorubicin to Breast Cancer Cells. *Int. J. Mol. Sci.* **2022**, *23*, 2386. [CrossRef]
33. Nigro, A.; Frattaruolo, L.; Fava, M.; De Napoli, I.; Greco, M.; Comandè, A.; De Santo, M.; Pellegrino, M.; Ricci, E.; Giordano, F.; et al. Bortezomib-Loaded Mesoporous Silica Nanoparticles Selectively Alter Metabolism and Induce Death in Multiple Myeloma Cells. *Cancers* **2020**, *12*, 2709. [CrossRef] [PubMed]
34. Brindisi, M.; Frattaruolo, L.; Mancuso, R.; Palumbo Piccionello, A.; Ziccarelli, I.; Catto, M.; Nicolotti, O.; Altomare, C.D.; Gabriele, B.; Cappello, A.R. Anticancer Potential of Novel α,β-Unsaturated γ-Lactam Derivatives Targeting the PI3K/AKT Signaling Pathway. *Biochem. Pharmacol.* **2021**, *190*, 114659. [CrossRef]
35. Frattaruolo, L.; Durante, M.; Cappello, M.S.; Montefusco, A.; Mita, G.; Cappello, A.R.; Lenucci, M.S. The Ability of Supercritical CO_2 Carrot and Pumpkin Extracts to Counteract Inflammation and Oxidative Stress in RAW 264.7 Macrophages Stimulated with LPS or MDA-MB-231 Cell-Conditioned Media. *Food Funct.* **2023**, *14*, 10083–10096. [CrossRef] [PubMed]
36. Brindisi, M.; Fiorillo, M.; Frattaruolo, L.; Sotgia, F.; Lisanti, M.P.; Cappello, A.R. Cholesterol and Mevalonate: Two Metabolites Involved in Breast Cancer Progression and Drug Resistance through the ERRα Pathway. *Cells* **2020**, *9*, 1819. [CrossRef] [PubMed]
37. Mazzotta, S.; Frattaruolo, L.; Brindisi, M.; Ulivieri, C.; Vanni, F.; Brizzi, A.; Carullo, G.; Cappello, A.R.; Aiello, F. 3-Amino-Alkylated Indoles: Unexplored Green Products Acting as Anti-Inflammatory Agents. *Future Med. Chem.* **2020**, *12*, 5–17. [CrossRef]
38. Martinez-Outschoorn, U.E.; Peiris-Pagés, M.; Pestell, R.G.; Sotgia, F.; Lisanti, M.P. Cancer Metabolism: A Therapeutic Perspective. *Nat. Rev. Clin. Oncol.* **2017**, *14*, 11–31. [CrossRef]
39. Galluzzi, L.; Kepp, O.; Heiden, M.G.V.; Kroemer, G. Metabolic Targets for Cancer Therapy. *Nat. Rev. Drug Discov.* **2013**, *12*, 829–846. [CrossRef]
40. Aramini, B.; Masciale, V.; Grisendi, G.; Bertolini, F.; Maur, M.; Guaitoli, G.; Chrystel, I.; Morandi, U.; Stella, F.; Dominici, M.; et al. Dissecting Tumor Growth: The Role of Cancer Stem Cells in Drug Resistance and Recurrence. *Cancers* **2022**, *14*, 976. [CrossRef]
41. Porporato, P.E.; Filigheddu, N.; Pedro, J.M.B.-S.; Kroemer, G.; Galluzzi, L. Mitochondrial Metabolism and Cancer. *Cell Res.* **2018**, *28*, 265–280. [CrossRef] [PubMed]
42. Kicinska, A.; Jarmuszkiewicz, W. Flavonoids and Mitochondria: Activation of Cytoprotective Pathways? *Molecules* **2020**, *25*, 3060. [CrossRef] [PubMed]

International Journal of
Molecular Sciences

MDPI

Review

Biomarkers in Thyroid Cancer: Emerging Opportunities from Non-Coding RNAs and Mitochondrial Space

Patricio Cabané [1,2,3], Claudio Correa [1,2], Ignacio Bode [4], Rodrigo Aguilar [4,*] and Alvaro A. Elorza [4,*]

1 Department of Head and Neck Surgery, Clinica INDISA, Santiago 7520440, Chile; patricio.cabane@indisa.cl (P.C.); c.correallanos@uandresbello.edu (C.C.)
2 Faculty of Medicine, Universidad Andres Bello, Santiago 8370071, Chile
3 Department of Basic and Clinical Oncology, Faculty of Medicine, University of Chile, Santiago 8380453, Chile
4 Institute of Biomedical Sciences, Faculty of Medicine and Faculty of Life Sciences, Universidad Andres Bello, Santiago 8370071, Chile; ignacio.bode@gmail.com
* Correspondence: rodrigo.aguilar@unab.cl (R.A.); alvaro.elorza@unab.cl (A.A.E.)

Abstract: Thyroid cancer diagnosis primarily relies on imaging techniques and cytological analyses. In cases where the diagnosis is uncertain, the quantification of molecular markers has been incorporated after cytological examination. This approach helps physicians to make surgical decisions, estimate cancer aggressiveness, and monitor the response to treatments. Despite the availability of commercial molecular tests, their widespread use has been hindered in our experience due to cost constraints and variability between them. Thus, numerous groups are currently evaluating new molecular markers that ultimately will lead to improved diagnostic certainty, as well as better classification of prognosis and recurrence. In this review, we start reviewing the current preoperative testing methodologies, followed by a comprehensive review of emerging molecular markers. We focus on micro RNAs, long non-coding RNAs, and mitochondrial (mt) signatures, including mtDNA genes and circulating cell-free mtDNA. We envision that a robust set of molecular markers will complement the national and international clinical guides for proper assessment of the disease.

Keywords: thyroid cancer; diagnosis; molecular markers; non-coding RNAs; mitochondria

1. Introduction

Thyroid cancer accounts for 1 to 4% of all malignancies worldwide. Its incidence has increased over the years, from 1.5% before 1996 to 6.8% after 1996, with an increase of three times per decade [1] (for a definition of epidemiological terms, see Table 1). In Chile, the estimated number of new cases per year is 1300 [2]. This increase in incidence has been attributed to a higher diagnosis rate, mainly due to the implementation of imaging techniques (diagnosis achieved in 50% of cases), as well as genetic and environmental factors, such as obesity and the increase in iodine consumption [1]. Histologically, thyroid cancer develops in two cell types, with more than 90% derived from follicular cells (epithelial, responsible for the uptake of iodine and production of thyroid hormones), and 3–5% derived from parafollicular cells (associated with synthesis and production of calcitonin).

According to the WHO 2022 guidelines, thyroid cancers have been categorized into three primary groups based on their level of differentiation. (1) Low grade (differentiated) cancers, which include papillary thyroid carcinoma (PTC), follicular thyroid carcinoma (FTC) and oncocytic carcinoma. The prognosis for these cancers is generally favorable. (2) High-grade cancers, which include poorly differentiated thyroid carcinoma (PDTC) and high-grade differentiated thyroid carcinoma (DHGTC). These cancers are more aggressive, presenting poorer outcomes, than low-grade cancers. (3) Anaplastic thyroid cancer (ATC), which is the most undifferentiated and aggressive form of thyroid cancer with a very poor prognosis [3]. Papillary thyroid cancer is the most common and has several histological subtypes (diffuse sclerosing, tall cell, columnar cell, solid, and hobnail among others) and clinical behavior [4]. Although we acknowledge different tumor types of thyroid carcinomas, we mostly focus on the papillary thyroid carcinoma in this review.

Table 1. Definition of epidemiological and clinical terms used in this text.

Term	Definition
Incidence	Number of new cases of disease in a population during a period
Sensitivity	The probability that the test result will be positive when disease is present
Specificity	The probability that the test result will be negative when disease is absent
Positive Predictive Value (PPV)	The probability of having the disease with a positive test result
Negative Predictive Value (NPV)	Probability of not having the disease, with a negative test
Diagnostic Yield	Proportion of true positives cases within the study cohort, with a specific test

1.1. Diagnosis and Uncertainty in Thyroid Cancer

The classic methods for diagnosing thyroid cancer are through images (ultrasound—TIRADS classification) and fine-needle aspiration (cytology) [5,6]. The latter allows classifying the probability of thyroid cancer according to the "Bethesda Criteria" from I to VI: I, non-diagnosed or inadequate; II, benign; III, atypia of undetermined significance; IV, follicular neoplasia; V, suspicious for malignancy; and VI, malignant. In the latest update (2023), each category receives a combined risk of malignancy (ROM), with a mean of 13%, 4%, 22%, 30%, 74%, and 97%, respectively [6]. Handling cases based on an indeterminate cytological study is not solely determined by the Bethesda classification. In fact, the application of this method alone has not been able to provide clinically applicable pre-surgical recommendations, either in terms of follow-up or diagnostic surgical resection. As a result, international guidelines incorporate clinical, ultrasound, and cytological characteristics, as well as molecular markers [7]. The latter tests are based on genetic mutation analysis, gene expression evaluation, and microRNA-based classifiers (specific panels are not disclosed). Genetic mutations related to the mitogen-activated protein kinase/extracellular signal-regulated kinase (MAPK/ERK) pathway are at the forefront of research in this area [8]. Clinical and molecular tools for guiding the diagnosis and proposing therapeutic options for thyroid cancer patients based on molecular characterization are limited and have not been updated so far. Some new tumorigenic and prognostic factors have been added to the study of other tumors, and more recently, to thyroid cancer [5,9,10]. The application of these markers in clinical decision-making should be studied in detail. This review provides a comprehensive overview of potential new markers with higher clinical relevance in thyroid cancer.

1.2. Current Preoperative Molecular Markers and Commercial Tests

There are molecular tests and tumor markers to study thyroid cancer, particularly the papillary thyroid carcinoma, but there is also an availability of molecular tests to study the other histological types of thyroid neoplasia [7,11,12]. Molecular genetic markers, such as mutations in MAPK pathways, including *ALK, NTRK, RET, RAS*, and $\mathrm{BRAF}^{\mathrm{V600E}}$, have been studied for the early detection of papillary cancer [13]. Mutations in *RAS*, $\mathrm{BRAF}^{\mathrm{K601E}}$, *PAX8/PPAR* and less common *PTEN* have been observed in follicular thyroid cancer [14–16]. For less differentiated tumors with a worse prognosis, such as anaplastic thyroid cancer, where *TERT* and *P53* mutations are common, the integration of these markers will provide better diagnostic and prognostic value.

The indication to perform a molecular study arises in order to safely assign a benign status for an indeterminate thyroid nodule, i.e., reported as Bethesda III or IV [17,18], leading to the avoidance of unnecessary surgical procedure. Molecular studies also allow prognostic stratification and thus modify management decisions, although in our experience routine practice is difficult to massify due to costs and variability between tests [5]. Testing for single mutations, such as $BRAF^{V600E}$ or *RET/PTC* translocations, has yielded good specificity (100%) but poor sensitivity (50–60%) [19,20], hence panels detecting gene mutation profiles or changes in expression levels have arisen. It has been proposed that, while mutation tests are good rule-in tests for thyroid cancer, gene expression classifier testing is a good rule-out test for thyroid cancer [13]. The use of *gene mutation profiling panels*, such as a panel detecting mutations found in 70% of thyroid cancers ($BRAF^{V600E}$, *HRAS* codon 61, *KRAS* codons 12/13, *NRAS* codon 61, *RET/PTC1*, *RET/PTC3*, and *PAX8/PPARG*, [9]), has yielded a sensitivity of >90% [21]. A gene classifier test, capable of classifying changes in the expression levels of up to 167 genes, has a significant negative predictive value but little positive predictive value (52%) [9].

Regarding commercially available molecular tests used in clinical practice, Table 2 summarizes the main features of Afirma®, Thyroseq®, Thyroid Print, and ThyGeNEXT®, all belonging to a group that identifies genetic anomalies through sequencing and gene expression.

Table 2. Summary of the main characteristics of genetic classifiers.

Test	Type of Test	No. of Genes [1]	Other Biomarkers	Clinical Application	Ref.
Afirma GSC/Afirma XA	RNA NGS (mRNA Expression)	1115 Genes	Mutation Hotspots + Fusions + Loss of heterozygosity	Afirma GSC is used to evaluate thyroid nodules with indeterminate cytology (Bethesda III/IV) to rule out benignity and thus help avoid unnecessary surgeries in benign cases. Therefore, it has diagnostic applications and can guide definitive treatment. Afirma XA is used for suspicious GSC samples and Bethesda V/VI.	[5,22,23]
Thyroseq V3	Targeted DNA and RNA NGS	112 Genes	>120 Fusions + 10 Copy Number Alterations + 19 Genes (Expression)	Distinguishes between malignant and benign lesions, helping to avoid unnecessary surgery during the diagnostic phase.	[24,25]
ThyGeNEXT/ ThyraMIR	Targeted NGS + miRNA Expression	10 Genes	28 Fusions + 10 miRNAs (Expression)	To improve the risk stratification and diagnostic accuracy of indeterminate thyroid nodules. It detects mutations and micro RNAs associated with thyroid cancer and helps in selecting the right treatment. However, what sets it apart from other classifiers is its utilization for long-term monitoring. It is often combined with ThyraMIR, to enhance stratification and predictive value.	[5,26,27]
Thyroid Print	Quantitative Real-Time PCR (mRNA Expression)	10 Genes	N/A	Detects changes in gene expression to classify thyroid nodules' malignancy. It provides additional information for diagnostic evaluation, which may influence treatment planning.	[28–30]

[1] Due to confidentiality policies, only the number of genes available in commercial classifiers is disclosed.

While Afirma GSC is a rule-out test focused on Bethesda III/IV samples, Afirma XA (Xpression Atlas) is used for GSC suspicious and Bethesda V/VI samples [23]. Studies have shown that complementation of the GEC (Gene Expression Classifier) with the Afirma GSC approach leads to higher specificity without compromising sensitivity [31]. GSC can also be used on its own for benign calls [32,33], and XA improves stratification [34]. When used in combination, GSC and XC presented a high positive and negative predictive value and decreased the number of surgeries in 75% of instances [22]. Thyroseq V3 (2018) is a test based on 112 thyroid-related genes, looking for point mutations, indels, gene fusions, copy number alterations, and abnormal gene expression [25]. In return, Thyroseq reports a "genomic classifier" to separate malignant from benign lesions, preventing surgery in most patients [24]. Regarding Thyroid Print, its recent validation from two multicenter and independent clinical trials has given it a specificity of 88%, a negative predictive value of 95%, and a positive predictive value of 78%. Meanwhile, a study reported a positive predictive value of 71% despite a smaller sample [30]. In Chile, Olmos et al. [29] carried out a prospective cohort study using 1272 fine-needle aspirations in a single-health center. They studied indeterminate nodules (Bethesda III and IV) using the Thyroid Print classifier and found benign nodules (comparable to Bethesda II) in 67% of cases after a 15-month follow-up. For patients with suspicious results after the test, the risk of malignancy was estimated at 71% compared to the histological result, making the risk of malignancy comparable to Bethesda [29]. Finally, the ThyGeNEXT test looks for mutations in selected genes (*ALK, BRAF, GNAS, HRAS, KRAS, NRAS, PIK3CA, PTEN, RET*, and *TERT* promoter genes) plus fusion genes (*ALK, BRAF, NTRK, PPARG, RET, PAX8, TBP, USP33*, and *THADA)* [27], although this panel is often used in combination with a panel of microRNAs (miRNAs) named ThyraMIR to improve stratification and predictive value (more below) [26].

The current molecular classifiers have theoretically higher performance in thyroid cancer diagnosis than cytology, with sensitivities ranging from 91–94% and specificities between 68% and 90%. These molecular classifiers have been shown to provide favorable outcomes in cytologically indeterminate nodules, primarily by averting diagnostic surgeries. They achieve this through high negative predictive values, indicating a low likelihood of cancer when test results are negative. However, their widespread application is hindered by the limitation of larger studies outside the United States, either due to the high acquisition costs or logistical terms of commercialization due to patents from the country of origin (USA) and other factors that could be the real causes of exemption from diagnostic surgery in their reports. Despite the use of biological markers in indeterminate nodules following Bethesda classification, there is still no genetic characterization that works independently to select a specific treatment. However, both European and American guidelines suggest interpretation at the clinician's discretion to guide management if they are available for use [5].

The large genetic panels available on the market, as well as the study of specific mutations (which may or may not be included in the panels), have not only complementary applications with cytology but also in determining the degree of aggressiveness and response to treatment. The mutations BRAF^{V600E}, *TERT*, and *RAS* are the most widely studied in relation to these clinical variables [35,36]. Genetic mutations have been observed in various types of thyroid cancer, which have affected the different clinical pillars related to this condition. The presence of BRAF^{V600E} is associated with the classic papillary type and its high cell subtype [35]. It is often linked to locoregional invasion, lymph node metastasis (especially cervical and lung), and refractoriness to radiotherapy. Mutations in *RAS* and *RET* are both related to invasive behavior (*RAS* mostly through the hematogenous route and consequently to the bone) but with differences [37]. Mutations in *RAS* can be present in different types of thyroid cancers (papillary and follicular), with the papillary type having the highest frequency at 38%. These mutations retain susceptibility to radioactive iodine therapy. Additionally, in follicular cell cancers, *RET/PTC* fusions (particularly *RET/PTC1* and *RET/PTC3*) have been identified, especially in the papillary type in pediatric and young adult populations. Their presence indicates a certain behavior but still responds well to radioiodine treatment [35,38]. On the other hand, point mutations in *RET* (specific base pair changes) have lower susceptibility to remission with I131 and are found in medullary thyroid cancer, mainly in hereditary cases, and to a lesser extent in sporadic cases [35].

Based on various histopathological findings in large patient cohorts, the use of molecular markers has been incorporated specifically after cytological diagnosis to determine aggressiveness and response to treatment. However, this is limited to anaplastic and medullary cancer. In the context of anaplastic thyroid cancer, the identification of the BRAF mutation V600E is incorporated into the initial management process to recommend the use of selective BRAF/MEK inhibitors (dabrafenib/trametinib, respectively), particularly if the cancer is not entirely unresectable [35]. When it comes to medullary cancer, detecting the germline mutation in the *RET* gene is used to determine whether it is hereditary [39].

1.3. Stratifying the Risk of Disease Recurrence

The standard treatment for differentiated thyroid carcinoma (DTC) usually involves surgery, followed by radioiodine (RI) ablation if necessary. The American Thyroid Association (ATA) suggests classifying patients into three risk groups (high, intermediate, and low) based on the risk of disease recurrence or persistence [17]. In low-risk patients, radioiodine therapy is generally not recommended as a complementary treatment. These patients have a low mortality rate, with a recurrence or persistence risk of about 3% [40]. The ATA guidelines consider the *BRAF* gene mutation as one of the factors to predict intermediate risk of recurrence if it is associated with multifocal micropapillary thyroid cancer. Other risk factors are determined exclusively from the histopathological results following surgery. However, the *BRAF* gene mutation alone cannot determine the use of I131 as it depends on the histological characterization [35]. However, studies have shown that the presence of BRAF downregulates iodine–sodium transporters, regardless of whether it is a classic subtype of papillary thyroid cancer or a cell type, making them resistant to iodine treatment. Therefore, the molecular characterization of thyroid cancer is improved by attempting radiotherapy and, if refractory, scaling up to selective NTRK inhibitors. This reflects the usefulness of incorporating biomarkers into stratification plans, contrasting with the selective use offered by ATA [41,42]. It is worth noting that the markers we described earlier are not the only ones available. New tumor factors have been incorporated into various studies, with and without applications in thyroid cancer.

2. Emerging Molecular Markers for Thyroid Cancer: Opportunities from the Non-Coding Genome

The sequencing of the human genome revealed that most RNAs in eukaryotes are "non-coding" (ncRNA), as they do not have the potential to produce proteins [43]. Thus, 75% of the information contained in DNA is transcribed to RNAs, but only 2% is translated to proteins [44]. Originally, non-coding RNAs were interpreted as transcriptional noise [45]; however, the significant role played by these RNAs has been confirmed, both in biological mechanisms [46,47] and in the development of diseases, including cancer [48,49]. With the advancements and reduced costs in omics technologies, alongside the development of lab-on-chip devices, detecting changes in gene expression or mutations is becoming increasingly accessible and affordable [50,51].

2.1. Micro RNAs

MicroRNAs (miRNAs) are non-coding RNAs that are synthesized from longer transcripts and processed into 19- to 25-nucleotide oligonucleotides through a step-wise mechanism (reviewed in [52]). By binding to target mRNAs, miRNAs repress translation and induce mRNA decay, significantly influencing the overall gene expression profile in cells. In thyroid cancer, miRNA expression profiles analyzed through quantitative PCR have been employed to stratify tumors, with diagnostic tests such as ThyraMIR and mir-THYpe being notable examples.

As mentioned before, ThyraMIR is often used as a complement to the ThyGeNEXT test [26]. ThyraMIR analyzes changes in the expression of 11 miRNAs and their association with malignancy (Table 3) [53]. In a single-health center study, ThyGeNEXT + ThyraMIR showed a 52,94% of positive predictive value [22], and 95% of diagnostic yield [54]. Although testing positive is associated with malignancy in surgical pathology, the ThyraMIR classifier failed to differentiate between benign and malignant RAS-mutated tumors [55]. As for mir-THYpe, it analyzes 11 miRNAs, where 6 are used as normalizers (let-7a, miR-103, miR-125a-5p, let-7b, miR-145, and *RNU48*) and 5 as discriminators of malignancy (Table 3) [56]. mir-THYpe reached average values of sensitivity 89.3%, specificity 81.6%, NPV 95%, and PPV 66%, as shown by a prospective, non-interventional multicenter study carried out on 440 patients. These results allowed clinicians to reduce unnecessary surgery in 52.5% of cases [57].

Table 3. miRNAs tested in commercial tests.

miRNA	ThyraMIR®	mir-THYpe®	Status in Thyroid Cancer
miR-21	+		Promoter of cancer. Higher in tumor [53,58]
miR-29	+		Suppressor of cancer. Reduced in tumor [53]
miR-31	+		Promoter of cancer. Higher in tumor [53,59]
miR-138	+		Suppressor of cancer. Reduced in tumor [53,60]
miR-139	+		Suppressor of cancer. Reduced in tumor [53]
miR-146	+	+	Promoter of cancer. Higher in tumor [53,56,59,61]
miR-152		+	Promoter of cancer. Higher in tumor [56,59]
miR-155	+	+	Suppressor of cancer. Reduced in tumor [53,56]
miR-181		+	Discriminator [56]
miR-200		+	Discriminator [56]
miR-204	+		Suppressor of cancer. Reduced in tumor [53]
miR-222	+		Promoter of cancer. Higher in tumor [53,61]
miR-375	+		Promoter of cancer. Higher in tumor [53,58]
miR-551	+		Promoter of cancer. Higher in tumor [53,59]

It is envisioned that an increased array of molecular biomarkers will enhance the reliability of thyroid cancer tests and offer clinicians more options for stratifying indeterminate thyroid nodules. With the growing number of studies investigating the molecular mechanisms underlying thyroid cancer, additional miRNAs are emerging as potential alternatives for future diagnostic tests [59]. Interestingly, DICER, the endoribonuclease responsible for generating mature miRNAs from stem-loop miRNAs [52], may harbor pathogenic somatic mutations that alter miRNA-5p to miRNA-3p production in thyroid cancer [62].

Potential miRNA candidates for diagnosis of thyroid cancer are described in Table 4. Based on the number of studies performed with each miRNA in cancer cells, the miR-1, miR-2, miR-7, and miR144 arise as the most robust and promising biomarkers to be included in future diagnostic tests. With the advancement and refinement of small RNA purification techniques, coupled with the availability of commercial adapters, quantification of miRNAs via real-time PCR or next-generation sequencing platforms has become a routine procedure [50].

Table 4. Potential miRNAs biomarkers for thyroid cancer.

miRNA	Expression in Cancer	mRNA Target	Reference
miR-1	Downregulated	*CCND2*, *CXCR4* and *MET*	[63–65]
miR-7	Downregulated	*METTL7B*, *EGFR*	[60,66,67]
miR-2	Upregulated	*CBL* and beta-catenin	[68]
miR-30	Downregulated	*BCL9*, *SNAI1*, *SMAD2*, *TGFBR1* and *VIM*	[69,70]
miR-144	Downregulated	*TGFA*, *ZEB1*, *ZEB2*, *E2F8* and *WWTR1*	[71–73]
miR-198	Downregulated	*FGFR1*, *E2F8*	[74]
miR-485	Downregulated	*RAF1*	[75]
miR-488	Downregulated	*NUP205*	[76]
miR-613	Downregulated	*SPHK2*	[77]
miR-539	Downregulated	*MMP9*	[78]
miR-761	Downregulated	*PPME*	[79]
miR-873	Downregulated	*ZEB1*, *CXCL16*, *FSTL1*	[80–82]
miR-1183	Downregulated	*SOX2*	[83]

2.2. Long Non-Coding RNAs (lncRNAs)

Long non-coding RNAs (lncRNAs) are transcripts longer than 200 nucleotides that do not encode proteins. These RNAs are often spliced, capped, and polyadenylated [47]. lncRNAs can modulate gene expression through various mechanisms, including direct binding to the DNA, interacting with epigenetic modifiers, and recruiting transcription factors to regulatory regions. Additionally, lncRNAs regulate miRNA function by capturing them and preventing them from targeting mRNAs in cells. This mechanism prevents miRNAs from blocking translation. Consequently, when lncRNA are dysregulated in disease, associated changes in gene expression may occur at both the transcriptional and post-transcriptional level [84].

Most lncRNAs exhibit cell-specific expression patterns and are typically expressed at low levels [85]. Alterations in their expression have been linked to the development and progression of various diseases, including thyroid cancer [86]. While lncRNAs have been studied in the context of thyroid cancer, their clinical application remains in the research phase. Using long non-coding RNAs (lncRNAs) as biomarkers offers several advantages over proteins, particularly in terms of quantification. Designing, acquiring, and standardizing primers for real-time PCR is often simpler and more straightforward than developing antibodies. Additionally, while messenger RNA levels do not always correlate with protein amounts due to post-transcriptional mechanisms, non-coding RNAs are generally considered more consistent as final products. Although lncRNAs can undergo modifications, such as adenosine methylation, the implications of these modifications are still being explored.

Table 5 presents potential lncRNA candidates for use as biomarkers in thyroid cancer. While all of them may be deemed promising molecules, *HOTAIR* and *MALAT1* stand out as robust candidates due to the substantial support from numerous studies across various cancers [87], along with *PTCSC3* as an RNA originally discovered in thyroid cancer [88]. *HOTAIR* is a lncRNA with an essential role in the repression of early development-related genes in adult individuals, collaborating with epigenetic complexes [89]. In papillary thyroid cancer, *HOTAIR* has been found to be upregulated, leading to increased growth, migration, and invasive properties [76,79,90]. Patients with lower levels of *HOTAIR* have better survival rates [91]. Regarding *MALAT1*, this lncRNA is widely recognized among cancer researchers. Initially discovered as one of the most overexpressed RNAs in lung cancer patients with metastasis, *MALAT1* has been found overexpressed in numerous other tumor types, including thyroid [87,90]. *MALAT11* regulates expression of target genes by directly binding to the genome and collaborating with epigenetic complexes. By functioning also as a competing endogenous RNA, it captures miRNAs in the nucleus [92,93]. Thus, *MALAT1* increases the expression of proteins associated with proliferation, migration, and angiogenesis, such as FGF2. This association links *MALAT1* to a prognosis of metastasis and early locoregional invasion [94]. In anaplastic thyroid carcinoma, *MALAT1* knockdown leads to reduced cell proliferation, invasion, and migration [95], like the effects observed with BRAF and RET gene alterations. This phenomenon has been particularly noted in medullary thyroid cancer [94]. However, its application in clinical practice is currently limited, as it has only been tested in vitro in thyroid tissue [95]. Finally, regarding *PTCSC3*, this lncRNA was initially identified as thyroid-specific [88], although subsequent research has revealed its presence in other cancers [96]. In thyroid cancer cells, it is frequently downregulated [88], and its overexpression has been associated with growth inhibition, cell cycle arrest, and increased apoptosis [97]

Table 5. Potential long non-coding RNA biomarkers for thyroid cancer.

lncRNA	Expression in Cancer	Function	Reference
DUXAP8	Upregulated	Increases proliferation, migration, and invasion.	[98,99]
FAM230B	Upregulated	Promotes migration and invasion in cancer cells through a mechanism involving the *Wnt* pathway.	[100]
HOTAIR	Upregulated	Controls early development- related genes. Increases growth, migration, and invasive.	[76,79,90,91]
LINC00460	Upregulated	Promotes cell proliferation, invasive properties, and epithelial-to-mesenchymal transition.	[75,77,78]
MALAT1	Upregulated	Increases cell proliferation, invasion, and migration.	[87,90,94,95]
NEAT1	Upregulated	Facilitates glycolytic metabolism, cell proliferation, and metastasis.	[90,101,102]
MAPKAPK5-AS1	Upregulated	Increases proliferation and invasion.	[103]
OIP5-AS1	Upregulated	Promotes cell proliferation, migration, and invasion.	[104]
PTCSC3	Downregulated	Tumor suppressor.	[88,97]
XIST	Upregulated	Inactivates X chromosome in female cells. Promotes proliferation and invasion.	[105,106]

2.3. Emerging RNA Molecules: Circular and Double-Stranded RNAs

In recent years, RNA variants that were originally disregarded as mis-splicing artifacts or by-products have been found to play significant roles in biological models. Advances in RNA-sequencing techniques and bioinformatics have revealed that circular and double-stranded RNAs participate in various biological mechanisms [107,108]. Circular RNAs are generated by back-splicing of pre-mRNAs and can function by sponging miRNAs and interacting with proteins (see [108] for review). By designing primers flanking the back-splice site, circular RNAs can be quantified specifically. Examples of circular RNAs found to be dysregulated in thyroid cancer cells include circITGA7, circRAPGEF5, circ_0058129, and circ_0005273 [74,81,83]. However, further research is required to gather robust data and propose circular RNAs as clinical biomarkers.

Double-stranded RNAs (dsRNAs), initially associated with viral infections, accumulate in vertebrate cells during the dysregulation of various cellular processes, including cancer [108] These dsRNAs originate from activated long and short interspersed elements, endogenous retroviruses, and mitochondrial transcripts. Unlike dsRNAs derived from viruses, endogenous dsRNAs often evade degradation and remain localized within the nucleus and mitochondria. Their quantification requires antibodies or dsRNA-binding proteins [109], making their incorporation into routine clinical assays more challenging compared to miRNAs or lncRNAs. Currently, no promising candidates among double-stranded RNAs have been identified as potential biomarkers for thyroid cancer diagnosis. Further research will uncover robust biomarkers that could aid in diagnosing cancer patients in the future.

3. Opportunities beyond the Nucleus: Mitochondrial Signatures

The proliferative and invasive capacity of cancer cells involves a reprogramming of the intermediary and energy metabolism of tumor cells, where mitochondria are the key players. Beyond energy generation, mitochondria are considered a powerful signaling platform for tumor anabolism and have an impact on tumor redox environment, calcium homeostasis, transcriptional and epigenetic regulation, and cell death pathways. In fact, several anti-cancer treatments disrupt mitochondrial function to trigger cancer cell death [110]. The proper work of mitochondria is sustained by two fundamental processes: first, the oxidative phosphorylation system (OXPHOS), which is the engine of energy generation in the form of ATP from the oxidation of glucose and fatty acid molecules. When mitochondria generate ATP, reactive oxygen species (ROS) are also formed as a by-product which are responsible for many of the aging-associated diseases, including cancer [111]. Second is the mitochondrial life cycle. This cycle refers to mitochondrial dynamics (MtDy), i.e., fusion and fission events of mitochondria; mitophagy, which corresponds to the selective degradation of damaged mitochondria or those that are no longer needed; and Mitochondrial Biogenesis, which involves mtDNA replication, protein synthesis and membrane biosynthesis [112].

3.1. mtDNA Signatures

Mitochondria contain multiple copies of mtDNA, which can range from tens to hundreds depending on the physiological and pathophysiological conditions of cells. The mtDNA is highly polymorphic and maternally inherited, which configures everyone with its own molecular maternal surname, called haplogroups, which correlate with the geographic origins of populations. The oldest haplogroups are from Africa and, with geographic migration and climate adaptations, the haplogroups from Europe, Asia, and America have evolved [113]. The type of haplogroup grants adaptive advantages and/or susceptibility to disease [114]. The mtDNA is a 16 kb circular DNA and encodes for 37 genes (13 mRNA, 2 rRNA, and 22 tRNA). The mitochondrial mRNAs encode for 13 core proteins of OXPHOS, which play a critical role in the proper assembly and functioning of the electron transport chain (ETC) for the generation of the mitochondrial membrane potential and, therefore, for the ATP synthesis. As a by-product of ETC functioning, ROS are generated. Since mtDNA molecules are in the same place in which ROS are produced, that is in the mitochondrial matrix, they are prone to undergo point mutations, deletions, and a reduction in their copy number. The mutation rate of mtDNA is higher compared to the nuclear genome [115] and these mutations accumulate as organisms age. The co-existence of wild type mtDNA with mutant mtDNA is known as heteroplasmy [116,117]. mtDNA alterations are associated with severe mitochondrial dysfunction and diseases. Thus, the integrity of mtDNA is pivotal for cell survival and health of the organism [118,119].

Recycling of oxidized and damaged mitochondria, (known as mitophagy) is critical for maintaining the copy number and integrity of mtDNA while keeping reduced levels of heteroplasmy [120–122]. Elevated mtDNA heteroplasmy leads to increased ROS which damages the bioenergetic capacity of mitochondria and alters mitophagy, favoring the development of diseases such as cancer [123,124]. Thus, both mtDNA and mitophagy are interconnected and dependent on each other. When mitochondria are stressed and/or mitophagy is dysfunctional, mtDNA may leak out from mitochondria and cells to reach plasma circulation, where it can be detected. The amount and features of this circulating cell-free mtDNA (ccf-mtDNA) constitute a parameter of mitochondrial dysfunction and disease.

In the context of a disease, the detection and analysis of mtDNA in terms of copy number, heteroplasmy, and haplogroups, as well as the levels of ccf-mtDNA, which are all measurable parameters, may configure a genomic signature and a powerful diagnostic tool in cancer. In fact, mtDNA copy number alterations contribute to the development of different types of carcinomas, such as lung cancer [124], breast cancer [125], hepatic cell carcinomas [126], gastric cancers [127], bladder, esophageal, kidney, and head/neck squamous carcinomas [125]. An increased mtDNA copy number may promote cancer progression by enhancing mitochondrial oxidative phosphorylation, as has also been observed in colorectal cancer [128]. Thyroid tumor cells also present an increase in the mtDNA copy number [129]. However, the relationship of mtDNA copy number with the risk of cancer is still inconclusive.

In some cancer cells, the striking accumulation of mitochondria leads to swollen cells with distinctive granular cytoplasmic eosinophilia forming an "oncocytic tumor" [130]. These tumors present two characteristic mutations: a deletion of 4977 bp called "common deletion" [131] and Complex 1 mtDNA mutations (loss of function and missense) that affect nearly 60% of patients [132–134]. Regarding papillary thyroid cancer, it was recently reported that this type of tumor also presents mitochondrial accumulation, DNA mutations, and loss of complex I integrity [135]. As for the mitochondrial accumulation, the Tall Cell subtype of Papillary Cell Carcinoma is considered "mitochondria-rich", indicating that there is a spectrum in mitochondria content that can be indicative of disease progression [135]. In thyroid cancer, an increase has also been reported in the mtDNA heteroplasmy at the level of both point mutations and deletions, mainly affecting the respiratory complex I and IV [136]. Sasarman et al. [137] also reported mutations in *MT-CYB* encoding for Cyt b (subunit of complex III) and *MT-TL1* encoding the mitochondrial $tRNA^{Leu}$ in cancer. In addition, mtDNA mutations affecting the complex I subunit, ND1 (G3842A), ND4 (A11708G), and ND5(12418insA), have been correlated with liver cancer progression, and the ND2 (T4216C) mutation with colorectal cancer [138–140].

On the other hand, the haplogroup M has been associated with breast cancer [25] while, in thyroid cancer, a preponderance has been observed a preponderance of the haplogroup D4a in Chinese patients [141]. and notably, the haplogroup K in Europeans has been shown to be protective against thyroid cancer [142]. Su et al. [143] reported three sub-haplogroups of N (A4, B4a and B4g) and eight single-nucleotide polymorphisms (mtSNPs) (A16164G, C16266T, G5460A, T6680C, G9123A, A14587G, T16362C, and G709A) associate with the occurrence of papillary thyroid cancer.

Regarding the ccf-mtDNA, accumulating evidence suggests that plasma or serum ccf-mtDNA levels are significantly different between cancer patients and healthy individuals. Thus, the level of ccf-mtDNA has been shown to be significantly higher in patients with lung cancer than in healthy patients [144]. In patients infected with hepatitis B virus (HBV), a lower content of ccf-mtDNA had a significantly increased risk of hepatocellular carcinoma as compared with HBV patients with higher ccf-mtDNA [145]. In metastatic colorectal cancer, a decrease in ccf-mtDNA has also been shown, as compared with healthy individuals [146]. Similar results were found in patients with papillary thyroid carcinoma, who presented decreased ccf-mtDNA levels in plasma [147]. Interestingly, the amount of ccf-DNA in blood has been used as a potential non-invasive biomarker for diagnostic and prognostic evaluation in a wide variety of cancers, because it has been shown to be increased or decreased in the serum of patients with various malignant tumors as compared with healthy patients [148,149].

ccf-mtDNA is widely recognized as a favorable option over nuclear-circulating DNA because it is more abundant and then easy to detect and analyze, and because changes in ccf-mtDNA are closely related to the occurrence and development of tumors in terms of copy number and integrity [150]. Thus, the detection and analysis of ccf-mtDNA may provide important information for diagnosis and prognosis in thyroid cancer patients, which may reduce the number of unnecessary thyroid surgical procedures.

3.2. Mitophagic Gene Signature

In cancer metabolism, mitophagy not only enables the removal of dysfunctional, depolarized, or damaged mitochondria, but also allows the reduction of mitochondrial biomass as an adaptive response to metabolic stress, such as hypoxia, starvation, and DNA damage that are present in the tumor. Besides providing all the essential nutrients to support tumor biology, through carbohydrate, protein, lipid, and nucleotide degradation [151], mitophagy is also involved in the control of ROS and calcium homeostasis for cell signaling and differentiation, and in the regulation of the balance between fermentative glycolysis and OXPHOS energy metabolic pathways [152,153].

In cancer patients, it has been observed that mitophagy processes are deregulated, but whether they behave as promoters of tumor formation or as suppressors seems to be highly dependent on the type of cancer and its metabolic context [151] (Table 6). In this regard, cancer stem cells, which are associated with the promotion of metastasis, therapy resistance, and tumor dormancy, make the most of mitophagy to sustain their self-renewal properties [154]. In lung or pancreatic cancer cells, the loss of the mitophagic proteins ATG7 or ATG5 significantly decreases the aggressiveness of the tumor due to the accumulation of defective mitochondria and an excessive accumulation of lipids, accounting for a greater alteration in the ß-oxidation of fatty acids [155].

Table 6. Mitophagic genes involved in cancer [1].

Mitophagic Protein	Function	Type of Cancer	Ref.
Pink/Parkin	Pro-tumorigenic	Breast, cervical, ovarian, lung, glioma, esophagus, melanoma	[156]
	Anti-tumorigenic	Liver, renal, pancreatic, endometrial	
FUNDC-1	Pro-tumorigenic	Cervical, hepatocarcinoma, breast, colorectal, leukemia, ovarian, pancreatic, Prostate, lung, and breast adenocarcinoma; and Glioblastoma	[157–159]
NIX	Pro-tumorigenic	Pancreatic	[160]
	Anti-tumorigenic	Osteosarcoma	[161]
BNIP3	Pro-tumorigenic	Lung, prostate, glioblastoma multiforme, cervical tumors, endometrial, breast carcinomas and gastric adenocarcinomas	[162–164]
	Anti-tumorigenic	Breast, Pancreatic	[165,166]
AMBRA	Pro-tumorigenic	Hepatocellular carcinoma, metastatic breast cancer, and medulloblastoma	[167]
	Anti-tumorigenic	Colorectal cancer cell, melanoma, and squamous cell carcinoma	[167]
FKBP8	Pro-tumorigenic	Hepatocellular Carcinoma	[168]
	Anti-tumorigenic	Schwannoma, melanoma	[169]
NLRX1	Pro-tumorigenic	Breast	[170]
	Anti-tumorigenic	Pancreatic	[171]
Prohibitin-2	Pro-tumorigenic	Lung, Cervical	[172,173]

[1] This table presents only mitochondrial proteins involved in mitophagy, not proteins involved in the phagophore or autophagosome formation.

Cancer cells are also characterized by the stabilization of the hypoxia-induced transcription factor HIF-1α, one of the main factors responsible for the change in energy metabolism from the oxidative metabolism to the aerobic glycolytic metabolism, also known as the Warburg effect [151]. Notably, HIF-1α also activates the transcriptional regulation of the mitophagy receptors NIX and BNIP3, which would decrease mitochondrial biomass, reducing the cells' oxygen demand and thus promoting survival under hypoxic conditions. The HIF-1α signaling pathway is more active during the proliferation and metastasis of cancer cells, which is why high HIF-1α expression is associated with a poor clinical prognosis. Results found in U87 and Glio6 glioma cells cultured under hypoxia showed that 32 genes were upregulated, including the mitochondrial nuclear-encoded genes *BNIP3*, *NIX*, and *FAM162A* [174]. BNIP3 and NIX have been involved both in apoptosis and mitophagy [175–181], and FAM162A, only in apoptosis [182]. However, it has been mentioned as belonging to the same BH3-only family as NIX and BNIP3. Toustrup et al. [183] and Sorensen et al. [184] defined 15-gene hypoxia classifiers based on gene expression to predict prognosis and therapeutic response in various cancer types, because hypoxia is a common feature in solid tumors. They assessed four head and neck squamous cell carcinomas, three esophagus cancer cell lines, three prostate cancer cell lines, and six colon cancer cell lines, and *FAM162A, BNIP3,* and *NIX* genes were overexpressed [183,184]. To date, there is no information about those genes in thyroid cancer. Interestingly, FAM162A has been shown to be highly expressed in the SiHa uterine cervix cancer (UCC) cell line when HIF-1a is overexpressed. However, far from inducing apoptosis and cell death, the UCC SiHa cells increased their proliferation and migration capacities [185]. The expression of FAM162A was investigated in 85 human tissue samples of UCC and over 70% were positive for FAM162A by immunohistochemistry as well as for HIF-1a, suggesting that FAM162A participates in a molecular mechanism of hypoxia-regulated tumor development. In fact, FAM162A-positive tumors are associated with an advanced stage of cancer, parametrial invasion, and tumor recurrence, according to the International Federation of Gynecology and Obstetrics. In addition, the overall survival rate tended to be poorer in patients with FAM162A expression than in those without FAM162A expression [186].

4. Conclusions

Promising molecular markers for thyroid cancer associated with non-coding nuclear genes and mitochondria have been reviewed and proposed. From a diagnostic perspective, identifying novel molecular markers can enhance the accuracy of preoperative fine-needle aspiration samples. Among the increasing number of alternatives, and based on the number of studies performed with each RNA, miR-1, miR-2, miR-7, and miR-144, along with the long non-coding RNAs HOTAIR, MALAT1, and PTCSC3 emerge as the most robust and promising candidates. Regarding mitochondria, measurements and genetic analysis of mtDNA, as well as the expression of mitophagic proteins FAM162A, NIX, and BNIP3, will contribute to a better understanding of the biology and development of thyroid cancer and support current cancer diagnosis and prognosis, benefiting patients. It is envisioned that these novel biomarkers will complement the commonly used cancer risk/probability classification (Bethesda). Their results can then be compared with the definitive biopsy findings of patients operated on for thyroid cancer (Bethesda V and VI) and those operated on for suspected thyroid cancer (Bethesda III and IV). Thus, based on classifications of prognosis and recurrence, the novel molecular markers reviewed here can serve as indicators of aggressiveness in patients with papillary thyroid cancer. This can complement the guidelines from the National (Chilean Department of Health) and International (ATA and TNM) clinical guides for a more accurate assessment of the disease [187,188].

Author Contributions: Conceptualization, P.C., R.A. and A.A.E.; writing, C.C., I.B., P.C., R.A. and A.A.E. All authors have read and agreed to the published version of the manuscript.

Funding: This research was funded by UNIVERSIDAD ANDRES BELLO, grant number NUCLEO UNAB DI-03-22/NUC (to P.C., R.A., A.A.E.); and ANID FONDECYT REGULAR, grant number 1240853 (to R.A.).

Institutional Review Board Statement: Not applicable.

Informed Consent Statement: Not applicable.

Data Availability Statement: Not applicable.

Conflicts of Interest: The authors declare no conflicts of interest. The funders had no role in the design of the study; in the collection, analyses, or interpretation of data; in the writing of the manuscript; or in the decision to publish the results.

References

1. Kitahara, C.M.; Sosa, J.A. Understanding the ever-changing incidence of thyroid cancer. *Nat. Rev. Endocrinol.* **2020**, *16*, 617–618. [CrossRef] [PubMed]

2. Sapunar, Z.J.; Ferrer, R.P. Epidemiología del cáncer de tiroides en un Instituto Oncológico. Efecto de las nuevas recomendaciones clínicas. *Rev. Médica Chile* **2020**, *148*, 573–581. [CrossRef] [PubMed]
3. Jung, C.K.; Bychkov, A.; Kakudo, K. Update from the 2022 World Health Organization Classification of Thyroid Tumors: A Standardized Diagnostic Approach. *Endocrinol. Metab.* **2022**, *37*, 703–718. [CrossRef] [PubMed]
4. Coca-Pelaz, A.; Shah, J.P.; Hernandez-Prera, J.C.; Ghossein, R.A.; Rodrigo, J.P.; Hartl, D.M.; Olsen, K.D.; Shaha, A.R.; Zafereo, M.; Suarez, C.; et al. Papillary Thyroid Cancer-Aggressive Variants and Impact on Management: A Narrative Review. *Adv. Ther.* **2020**, *37*, 3112–3128. [CrossRef] [PubMed]
5. Durante, C.; Hegedus, L.; Czarniecka, A.; Paschke, R.; Russ, G.; Schmitt, F.; Soares, P.; Solymosi, T.; Papini, E. 2023 European Thyroid Association Clinical Practice Guidelines for thyroid nodule management. *Eur. Thyroid J.* **2023**, *12*, e230067. [CrossRef] [PubMed]
6. Ali, S.Z.; Baloch, Z.W.; Cochand-Priollet, B.; Schmitt, F.C.; Vielh, P.; VanderLaan, P.A. The 2023 Bethesda System for Reporting Thyroid Cytopathology. *Thyroid* **2023**, *33*, 1039–1044. [CrossRef] [PubMed]
7. Abdullah, M.I.; Junit, S.M.; Ng, K.L.; Jayapalan, J.J.; Karikalan, B.; Hashim, O.H. Papillary Thyroid Cancer: Genetic Alterations and Molecular Biomarker Investigations. *Int. J. Med. Sci.* **2019**, *16*, 450–460. [CrossRef] [PubMed]
8. Schubert, L.; Mariko, M.L.; Clerc, J.; Huillard, O.; Groussin, L. MAPK Pathway Inhibitors in Thyroid Cancer: Preclinical and Clinical Data. *Cancers* **2023**, *15*, 710. [CrossRef]
9. Alexander, E.K.; Kennedy, G.C.; Baloch, Z.W.; Cibas, E.S.; Chudova, D.; Diggans, J.; Friedman, L.; Kloos, R.T.; LiVolsi, V.A.; Mandel, S.J.; et al. Preoperative diagnosis of benign thyroid nodules with indeterminate cytology. *N. Engl. J. Med.* **2012**, *367*, 705–715. [CrossRef]
10. Liu, Y.; Khan, S.; Li, L.; Ten Hagen, T.L.M.; Falahati, M. Molecular mechanisms of thyroid cancer: A competing endogenous RNA (ceRNA) point of view. *Biomed. Pharmacother.* **2022**, *146*, 112251. [CrossRef]
11. Macerola, E.; Poma, A.M.; Vignali, P.; Proietti, A.; Ugolini, C.; Torregrossa, L.; Basolo, A.; Elisei, R.; Santini, F.; Basolo, F. Predictive Biomarkers in Thyroid Cancer. *Front. Oncol.* **2022**, *12*, 901004. [CrossRef] [PubMed]
12. Silaghi, C.A.; Lozovanu, V.; Georgescu, C.E.; Georgescu, R.D.; Susman, S.; Nasui, B.A.; Dobrean, A.; Silaghi, H. Thyroseq v3, Afirma GSC, and microRNA Panels Versus Previous Molecular Tests in the Preoperative Diagnosis of Indeterminate Thyroid Nodules: A Systematic Review and Meta-Analysis. *Front. Endocrinol.* **2021**, *12*, 649522. [CrossRef] [PubMed]
13. Lee, K.; Anastasopoulou, C.; Chandran, C.; Cassaro, S. Thyroid Cancer. 1 May 2023. Available online: https://www.ncbi.nlm.nih.gov/books/NBK459299/ (accessed on 21 January 2024).
14. Matrone, A.; Citro, F.; Gambale, C.; Prete, A.; Minaldi, E.; Ciampi, R.; Ramone, T.; Materazzi, G.; Torregrossa, L.; Elisei, R. BRAF K601E Mutation in Oncocytic Carcinoma of the Thyroid: A Case Report and Literature Review. *J. Clin. Med.* **2023**, *12*, 6970. [CrossRef] [PubMed]
15. Bandargal, S.; Rajab, M.; Forest, V.I.; Pusztaszeri, M.P.; Hier, M.P.; da Silva, S.D.; Payne, R.J. Characteristics of PTEN Mutation in Thyroid Tumours: A Retrospective Chart Review. *Cancers* **2023**, *15*, 1575. [CrossRef] [PubMed]
16. Kondo, T.; Ezzat, S.; Asa, S.L. Pathogenetic mechanisms in thyroid follicular-cell neoplasia. *Nat. Rev. Cancer* **2006**, *6*, 292–306. [CrossRef] [PubMed]
17. Haugen, B.R.; Alexander, E.K.; Bible, K.C.; Doherty, G.M.; Mandel, S.J.; Nikiforov, Y.E.; Pacini, F.; Randolph, G.W.; Sawka, A.M.; Schlumberger, M.; et al. 2015 American Thyroid Association Management Guidelines for Adult Patients with Thyroid Nodules and Differentiated Thyroid Cancer: The American Thyroid Association Guidelines Task Force on Thyroid Nodules and Differentiated Thyroid Cancer. *Thyroid* **2016**, *26*, 1–133. [CrossRef] [PubMed]
18. Sahli, Z.T.; Smith, P.W.; Umbricht, C.B.; Zeiger, M.A. Preoperative Molecular Markers in Thyroid Nodules. *Front. Endocrinol.* **2018**, *9*, 179. [CrossRef] [PubMed]
19. Adeniran, A.J.; Hui, P.; Chhieng, D.C.; Prasad, M.L.; Schofield, K.; Theoharis, C. BRAF mutation testing of thyroid fine-needle aspiration specimens enhances the predictability of malignancy in thyroid follicular lesions of undetermined significance. *Acta Cytol.* **2011**, *55*, 570–575. [CrossRef] [PubMed]
20. Kim, S.K.; Hwang, T.S.; Yoo, Y.B.; Han, H.S.; Kim, D.L.; Song, K.H.; Lim, S.D.; Kim, W.S.; Paik, N.S. Surgical results of thyroid nodules according to a management guideline based on the BRAF(V600E) mutation status. *J. Clin. Endocrinol. Metab.* **2011**, *96*, 658–664. [CrossRef]
21. Nikiforov, Y.E.; Ohori, N.P.; Hodak, S.P.; Carty, S.E.; LeBeau, S.O.; Ferris, R.L.; Yip, L.; Seethala, R.R.; Tublin, M.E.; Stang, M.T.; et al. Impact of mutational testing on the diagnosis and management of patients with cytologically indeterminate thyroid nodules: A prospective analysis of 1056 FNA samples. *J. Clin. Endocrinol. Metab.* **2011**, *96*, 3390–3397. [CrossRef]
22. Kandil, E.; Metz, T.A.; Issa, P.P.; Aboueisha, M.; Omar, M.; Attia, A.S.; Chabot, B.; Hussein, M.; Moroz, K.; Shama, M.; et al. Diagnostic Performance of Afirma and Interpace Diagnostics Genetic Testing in Indeterminate Thyroid Nodules: A Single Center Study. *Cancers* **2023**, *15*, 2098. [CrossRef] [PubMed]
23. Krane, J.F.; Cibas, E.S.; Endo, M.; Marqusee, E.; Hu, M.I.; Nasr, C.E.; Waguespack, S.G.; Wirth, L.J.; Kloos, R.T. The Afirma Xpression Atlas for thyroid nodules and thyroid cancer metastases: Insights to inform clinical decision-making from a fine-needle aspiration sample. *Cancer Cytopathol.* **2020**, *128*, 452–459. [CrossRef]
24. Desai, D.; Lepe, M.; Baloch, Z.W.; Mandel, S.J. ThyroSeq v3 for Bethesda III and IV: An institutional experience. *Cancer Cytopathol.* **2021**, *129*, 164–170. [CrossRef] [PubMed]

25. Nikiforova, M.N.; Mercurio, S.; Wald, A.I.; Barbi de Moura, M.; Callenberg, K.; Santana-Santos, L.; Gooding, W.E.; Yip, L.; Ferris, R.L.; Nikiforov, Y.E. Analytical performance of the ThyroSeq v3 genomic classifier for cancer diagnosis in thyroid nodules. *Cancer* **2018**, *124*, 1682–1690. [CrossRef]
26. Alzahrani, A.S. Clinical use of Molecular Data in Thyroid Nodules and Cancer. *J. Clin. Endocrinol. Metab.* **2023**, *108*, 2759–2771. [CrossRef]
27. Alzumaili, B.; Sadow, P.M. Update on Molecular Diagnostics in Thyroid Pathology: A Review. *Genes* **2023**, *14*, 1314. [CrossRef] [PubMed]
28. Gonzalez, H.E.; Martinez, J.R.; Vargas-Salas, S.; Solar, A.; Veliz, L.; Cruz, F.; Arias, T.; Loyola, S.; Horvath, E.; Tala, H.; et al. A 10-Gene Classifier for Indeterminate Thyroid Nodules: Development and Multicenter Accuracy Study. *Thyroid* **2017**, *27*, 1058–1067. [CrossRef]
29. Olmos, R.; Dominguez, J.M.; Vargas-Salas, S.; Mosso, L.; Fardella, C.E.; Gonzalez, G.; Baudrand, R.; Guarda, F.; Valenzuela, F.; Arteaga, E.; et al. ThyroidPrint(R): Clinical utility for indeterminate thyroid cytology. *Endocr. Relat. Cancer* **2023**, *30*, e220409. [CrossRef] [PubMed]
30. Zafereo, M.; McIver, B.; Vargas-Salas, S.; Dominguez, J.M.; Steward, D.L.; Holsinger, F.C.; Kandil, E.; Williams, M.; Cruz, F.; Loyola, S.; et al. A Thyroid Genetic Classifier Correctly Predicts Benign Nodules with Indeterminate Cytology: Two Independent, Multicenter, Prospective Validation Trials. *Thyroid* **2020**, *30*, 704–712. [CrossRef]
31. Harrell, R.M.; Eyerly-Webb, S.A.; Golding, A.C.; Edwards, C.M.; Bimston, D.N. Statistical Comparison of Afirma Gsc and Afirma Gec Outcomes in a Community Endocrine Surgical Practice: Early Findings. *Endocr. Pract.* **2019**, *25*, 161–164. [CrossRef]
32. Angell, T.E.; Heller, H.T.; Cibas, E.S.; Barletta, J.A.; Kim, M.I.; Krane, J.F.; Marqusee, E. Independent Comparison of the Afirma Genomic Sequencing Classifier and Gene Expression Classifier for Cytologically Indeterminate Thyroid Nodules. *Thyroid* **2019**, *29*, 650–656. [CrossRef] [PubMed]
33. Wei, S.; Veloski, C.; Sharda, P.; Ehya, H. Performance of the Afirma genomic sequencing classifier versus gene expression classifier: An institutional experience. *Cancer Cytopathol.* **2019**, *127*, 720–724. [CrossRef] [PubMed]
34. Munoz-Zuluaga, C.A.; Heymann, J.J.; Solomon, J.P.; Patel, A.; Siddiqui, M.T.; Scognamiglio, T.; Gokozan, H.N. Use of the Afirma Xpression Atlas for cytologically indeterminate, Afirma Genomic Sequencing Classifier suspicious thyroid nodules: Clinicopathologic analysis with postoperative molecular testing. *Am. J. Clin. Pathol.* **2024**, *161*, 463–468. [CrossRef] [PubMed]
35. Boucai, L.; Zafereo, M.; Cabanillas, M.E. Thyroid Cancer: A Review. *JAMA* **2024**, *331*, 425–435. [CrossRef] [PubMed]
36. Marrero Rodríguez, M.T.; Sinconegui Gómez, B.; Cruz Cruz, A. Marcadores moleculares en el cáncer de tiroides. *Rev. Cuba. Endocrinol.* **2015**, *26*, 93–104.
37. Nguyen, B.; Fong, C.; Luthra, A.; Smith, S.A.; DiNatale, R.G.; Nandakumar, S.; Walch, H.; Chatila, W.K.; Madupuri, R.; Kundra, R.; et al. Genomic characterization of metastatic patterns from prospective clinical sequencing of 25,000 patients. *Cell* **2022**, *185*, 563–575.e511. [CrossRef] [PubMed]
38. Zeindl-Eberhart, E.; Liebmann, S.; Jungblut, P.R.; Mattow, J.; Schmid, M.; Kerler, R.; Rabes, H.M. Influence of RET/PTC1 and RET/PTC3 oncoproteins in radiation-induced papillary thyroid carcinomas on amounts of cytoskeletal protein species. *Amino Acids* **2011**, *41*, 415–425. [CrossRef] [PubMed]
39. Larouche, V.; Akirov, A.; Thomas, C.M.; Krzyzanowska, M.K.; Ezzat, S. A primer on the genetics of medullary thyroid cancer. *Curr. Oncol.* **2019**, *26*, 389–394. [CrossRef]
40. Parvathareddy, S.K.; Siraj, A.K.; Qadri, Z.; Ahmed, S.O.; DeVera, F.; Al-Sobhi, S.; Al-Dayel, F.; Al-Kuraya, K.S. Lymph node ratio is superior to AJCC N stage for predicting recurrence in papillary thyroid carcinoma. *Endocr. Connect.* **2022**, *11*, e210518. [CrossRef]
41. Biondi, B.; Cooper, D.S. Benefits of thyrotropin suppression versus the risks of adverse effects in differentiated thyroid cancer. *Thyroid* **2010**, *20*, 135–146. [CrossRef]
42. Chakravarty, D.; Santos, E.; Ryder, M.; Knauf, J.A.; Liao, X.H.; West, B.L.; Bollag, G.; Kolesnick, R.; Thin, T.H.; Rosen, N.; et al. Small-molecule MAPK inhibitors restore radioiodine incorporation in mouse thyroid cancers with conditional BRAF activation. *J. Clin. Investig.* **2011**, *121*, 4700–4711. [CrossRef]
43. Kung, J.T.; Colognori, D.; Lee, J.T. Long noncoding RNAs: Past, present, and future. *Genetics* **2013**, *193*, 651–669. [CrossRef]
44. Consortium, E.P.; Birney, E.; Stamatoyannopoulos, J.A.; Dutta, A.; Guigo, R.; Gingeras, T.R.; Margulies, E.H.; Weng, Z.; Snyder, M.; Dermitzakis, E.T.; et al. Identification and analysis of functional elements in 1% of the human genome by the ENCODE pilot project. *Nature* **2007**, *447*, 799–816. [CrossRef] [PubMed]
45. Ohno, S. Simplicity of mammalian regulatory systems. *Dev. Biol.* **1972**, *27*, 131–136. [CrossRef]
46. Andergassen, D.; Rinn, J.L. From genotype to phenotype: Genetics of mammalian long non-coding RNAs in vivo. *Nat. Rev. Genet.* **2022**, *23*, 229–243. [CrossRef]
47. Mattick, J.S.; Amaral, P.P.; Carninci, P.; Carpenter, S.; Chang, H.Y.; Chen, L.L.; Chen, R.; Dean, C.; Dinger, M.E.; Fitzgerald, K.A.; et al. Long non-coding RNAs: Definitions, functions, challenges and recommendations. *Nat. Rev. Mol. Cell Biol.* **2023**, *24*, 430–447. [CrossRef]
48. Disney, M.D. Targeting RNA with Small Molecules To Capture Opportunities at the Intersection of Chemistry, Biology, and Medicine. *J. Am. Chem. Soc.* **2019**, *141*, 6776–6790. [CrossRef] [PubMed]
49. Zhang, F.; Lupski, J.R. Non-coding genetic variants in human disease. *Hum. Mol. Genet.* **2015**, *24*, R102–R110. [CrossRef] [PubMed]
50. Dhuli, K.; Medori, M.C.; Donato, K.; Donato, K.; Maltese, P.E.; Tanzi, B.; Tezzele, S.; Mareso, C.; Miertus, J.; Generali, D.; et al. Omics sciences and precision medicine in thyroid cancer. *Clin. Ther.* **2023**, *174*, 11–20. [CrossRef]

51. Venkatesalu, S.; Dilliyappan, S.; Satish Kumar, A.; Palaniyandi, T.; Baskar, G.; Ravi, M.; Sivaji, A. Prospectives and retrospectives of microfluidics devices and lab-on-A-chip emphasis on cancer. *Clin. Chim. Acta* **2024**, *552*, 117646. [CrossRef]
52. Bofill-De Ros, X.; Vang Orom, U.A. Recent progress in miRNA biogenesis and decay. *RNA Biol.* **2024**, *21*, 1–8. [CrossRef] [PubMed]
53. Finkelstein, S.D.; Sistrunk, J.W.; Malchoff, C.; Thompson, D.V.; Kumar, G.; Timmaraju, V.A.; Repko, B.; Mireskandari, A.; Evoy-Goodman, L.A.; Massoll, N.A.; et al. A Retrospective Evaluation of the Diagnostic Performance of an Interdependent Pairwise MicroRNA Expression Analysis with a Mutation Panel in Indeterminate Thyroid Nodules. *Thyroid* **2022**, *32*, 1362–1371. [CrossRef] [PubMed]
54. Labourier, E.; Fahey, T.J., 3rd. Preoperative molecular testing in thyroid nodules with Bethesda VI cytology: Clinical experience and review of the literature. *Diagn. Cytopathol.* **2021**, *49*, E175–E180. [CrossRef] [PubMed]
55. Tumati, A.; Egan, C.E.; Lee-Saxton, Y.J.; Marshall, T.E.; Lee, J.; Jain, K.; Heymann, J.J.; Gokozan, H.; Azar, S.A.; Schwarz, J.; et al. Clinical utility of a microRNA classifier in cytologically indeterminate thyroid nodules with RAS mutations: A multi-institutional study. *Surgery* **2024**, *175*, 234–240. [CrossRef] [PubMed]
56. Santos, M.T.D.; Buzolin, A.L.; Gama, R.R.; Silva, E.; Dufloth, R.M.; Figueiredo, D.L.A.; Carvalho, A.L. Molecular Classification of Thyroid Nodules with Indeterminate Cytology: Development and Validation of a Highly Sensitive and Specific New miRNA-Based Classifier Test Using Fine-Needle Aspiration Smear Slides. *Thyroid* **2018**, *28*, 1618–1626. [CrossRef] [PubMed]
57. Santos, M.T.; Rodrigues, B.M.; Shizukuda, S.; Oliveira, A.F.; Oliveira, M.; Figueiredo, D.L.A.; Melo, G.M.; Silva, R.A.; Fainstein, C.; Dos Reis, G.F.; et al. Clinical decision support analysis of a microRNA-based thyroid molecular classifier: A real-world, prospective and multicentre validation study. *EBioMedicine* **2022**, *82*, 104137. [CrossRef] [PubMed]
58. Mian, C.; Pennelli, G.; Fassan, M.; Balistreri, M.; Barollo, S.; Cavedon, E.; Galuppini, F.; Pizzi, M.; Vianello, F.; Pelizzo, M.R.; et al. MicroRNA profiles in familial and sporadic medullary thyroid carcinoma: Preliminary relationships with RET status and outcome. *Thyroid* **2012**, *22*, 890–896. [CrossRef]
59. Rogucki, M.; Sidorkiewicz, I.; Niemira, M.; Dzieciol, J.B.; Buczynska, A.; Adamska, A.; Siewko, K.; Kosciuszko, M.; Maliszewska, K.; Wojcicka, A.; et al. Expression Profile and Diagnostic Significance of MicroRNAs in Papillary Thyroid Cancer. *Cancers* **2022**, *14*, 2679. [CrossRef]
60. Ignjatovic Jocic, V.; Jankovic Miljus, J.; Isic Dencic, T.; Zivaljevic, V.; Tatic, S.; Doric, I.; Selemetjev, S. Expression of pY397-FAK and Its miR Regulators Drive Dedifferentiation in the Thyroid Neoplasia Spectrum. *Cells* **2023**, *12*, 1721. [CrossRef]
61. Fuziwara, C.S.; Kimura, E.T. MicroRNA Deregulation in Anaplastic Thyroid Cancer Biology. *Int. J. Endocrinol.* **2014**, *2014*, 743450. [CrossRef]
62. Ricarte-Filho, J.C.; Casado-Medrano, V.; Reichenberger, E.; Spangler, Z.; Scheerer, M.; Isaza, A.; Baran, J.; Patel, T.; MacFarland, S.P.; Brodeur, G.M.; et al. DICER1 RNase IIIb domain mutations trigger widespread miRNA dysregulation and MAPK activation in pediatric thyroid cancer. *Front. Endocrinol.* **2023**, *14*, 1083382. [CrossRef] [PubMed]
63. Di, W.; Li, Q.; Shen, W.; Guo, H.; Zhao, S. The long non-coding RNA HOTAIR promotes thyroid cancer cell growth, invasion and migration through the miR-1-CCND2 axis. *Am. J. Cancer Res.* **2017**, *7*, 1298–1309. [PubMed]
64. Leone, V.; D'Angelo, D.; Rubio, I.; de Freitas, P.M.; Federico, A.; Colamaio, M.; Pallante, P.; Medeiros-Neto, G.; Fusco, A. MiR-1 is a tumor suppressor in thyroid carcinogenesis targeting CCND2, CXCR4, and SDF-1alpha. *J. Clin. Endocrinol. Metab.* **2011**, *96*, E1388–E1398. [CrossRef] [PubMed]
65. Yip, L.; Kelly, L.; Shuai, Y.; Armstrong, M.J.; Nikiforov, Y.E.; Carty, S.E.; Nikiforova, M.N. MicroRNA signature distinguishes the degree of aggressiveness of papillary thyroid carcinoma. *Ann. Surg. Oncol.* **2011**, *18*, 2035–2041. [CrossRef] [PubMed]
66. Han, J.Y.; Guo, S.; Wei, N.; Xue, R.; Li, W.; Dong, G.; Li, J.; Tian, X.; Chen, C.; Qiu, S.; et al. ciRS-7 Promotes the Proliferation and Migration of Papillary Thyroid Cancer by Negatively Regulating the miR-7/Epidermal Growth Factor Receptor Axis. *Biomed Res. Int.* **2020**, *2020*, 9875636. [CrossRef]
67. Macerola, E.; Poma, A.M.; Proietti, A.; Rago, T.; Romani, R.; Vignali, P.; Ugolini, C.; Torregrossa, L.; Basolo, A.; Santini, F.; et al. Down-regulation of miR-7-5p and miR-548ar-5p predicts malignancy in indeterminate thyroid nodules negative for BRAF and RAS mutations. *Endocrine* **2022**, *76*, 677–686. [CrossRef] [PubMed]
68. Guo, Y.; Zheng, H.; Yin, J.; Wang, H. Rs4911154 of circ-ITCH aggravated tumor malignancy of thyroid nodules via the circ-ITCH/miR-22-3p/CBL axis. *Sci. Rep.* **2021**, *11*, 18491. [CrossRef]
69. Braun, J.; Hoang-Vu, C.; Dralle, H.; Huttelmaier, S. Downregulation of microRNAs directs the EMT and invasive potential of anaplastic thyroid carcinomas. *Oncogene* **2010**, *29*, 4237–4244. [CrossRef]
70. Chen, C.; Zhou, L.; Wang, H.; Chen, J.; Li, W.; Liu, W.; Shen, M.; Liu, H.; Fu, X. Long noncoding RNA CNALPTC1 promotes cell proliferation and migration of papillary thyroid cancer via sponging miR-30 family. *Am. J. Cancer Res.* **2018**, *8*, 192–206.
71. Guan, H.; Liang, W.; Xie, Z.; Li, H.; Liu, J.; Liu, L.; Xiu, L.; Li, Y. Down-regulation of miR-144 promotes thyroid cancer cell invasion by targeting ZEB1 and ZEB2. *Endocrine* **2015**, *48*, 566–574. [CrossRef]
72. Liu, J.; Feng, L.; Zhang, H.; Zhang, J.; Zhang, Y.; Li, S.; Qin, L.; Yang, Z.; Xiong, J. Effects of miR-144 on the sensitivity of human anaplastic thyroid carcinoma cells to cisplatin by autophagy regulation. *Cancer Biol. Ther.* **2018**, *19*, 484–496. [CrossRef] [PubMed]
73. Sun, J.; Shi, R.; Zhao, S.; Li, X.; Lu, S.; Bu, H.; Ma, X.; Su, C. E2F8, a direct target of miR-144, promotes papillary thyroid cancer progression via regulating cell cycle. *J. Exp. Clin. Cancer Res.* **2017**, *36*, 40. [CrossRef]
74. Liu, W.; Zhao, J.; Jin, M.; Zhou, M. circRAPGEF5 Contributes to Papillary Thyroid Proliferation and Metastatis by Regulation miR-198/FGFR1. *Mol. Ther. Nucleic Acids* **2019**, *14*, 609–616. [CrossRef] [PubMed]

75. Li, G.; Kong, Q. LncRNA LINC00460 promotes the papillary thyroid cancer progression by regulating the LINC00460/miR-485-5p/Raf1 axis. *Biol. Res.* **2019**, *52*, 61. [CrossRef]
76. Xia, F.; Xia, W.; Yu, X. LncRNA HOTAIR Influences the Growth, Migration, and Invasion of Papillary Thyroid Carcinoma via Affection on the miR-488-5p/NUP205 Axis. *Technol. Cancer Res. Treat.* **2020**, *19*, 1533033820962125. [CrossRef] [PubMed]
77. Feng, L.; Yang, B.; Tang, X.D. Long noncoding RNA LINC00460 promotes carcinogenesis via sponging miR-613 in papillary thyroid carcinoma. *J. Cell Physiol.* **2019**, *234*, 11431–11439. [CrossRef]
78. Zou, X.; Guo, Z.H.; Li, Q.; Wang, P.S. Long Noncoding RNA LINC00460 Modulates MMP-9 to Promote Cell Proliferation, Invasion and Apoptosis by Targeting miR-539 in Papillary Thyroid Cancer. *Cancer Manag. Res.* **2020**, *12*, 199–207. [CrossRef]
79. Guo, R.; Ning, Y.; Ma, Y.; Lin, Q.; Shen, N.; Shi, P. Long non-coding RNA HOTAIR/microRNA-761 sponge regulates PPME1 and further influences cell biological functions in thyroid carcinoma. *Laryngoscope Investig. Otolaryngol.* **2021**, *6*, 438–445. [CrossRef]
80. Jiao, D.; Guo, F.; Fu, Q. MicroRNA-873 inhibits the progression of thyroid cancer by directly targeting ZEB1. *Mol. Med. Rep.* **2019**, *20*, 1986–1993. [CrossRef]
81. Tan, X.; Zhao, J.; Lou, J.; Zheng, W.; Wang, P. Hsa_circ_0058129 regulates papillary thyroid cancer development via miR-873-5p/follistatin-like 1 axis. *J. Clin. Lab. Anal.* **2022**, *36*, e24401. [CrossRef]
82. Wang, Z.; Liu, W.; Wang, C.; Ai, Z. miR-873-5p Inhibits Cell Migration and Invasion of Papillary Thyroid Cancer via Regulation of CXCL16. *Onco Targets Ther.* **2020**, *13*, 1037–1046. [CrossRef] [PubMed]
83. Zhang, W.; Zhang, H.; Zhao, X. circ_0005273 promotes thyroid carcinoma progression by SOX2 expression. *Endocr. Relat. Cancer* **2020**, *27*, 11–21. [CrossRef] [PubMed]
84. Ferrer, J.; Dimitrova, N. Transcription regulation by long non-coding RNAs: Mechanisms and disease relevance. *Nat. Rev. Mol. Cell Biol.* **2024**, *25*, 396–415. [CrossRef] [PubMed]
85. Gloss, B.S.; Dinger, M.E. The specificity of long noncoding RNA expression. *Biochim. Biophys. Acta* **2016**, *1859*, 16–22. [CrossRef] [PubMed]
86. Lu, W.; Xu, Y.; Xu, J.; Wang, Z.; Ye, G. Identification of differential expressed lncRNAs in human thyroid cancer by a genome-wide analyses. *Cancer Med.* **2018**, *7*, 3935–3944. [CrossRef] [PubMed]
87. Malakoti, F.; Targhazeh, N.; Karimzadeh, H.; Mohammadi, E.; Asadi, M.; Asemi, Z.; Alemi, F. Multiple function of lncRNA MALAT1 in cancer occurrence and progression. *Chem. Biol. Drug Des.* **2023**, *101*, 1113–1137. [CrossRef] [PubMed]
88. Jendrzejewski, J.; He, H.; Radomska, H.S.; Li, W.; Tomsic, J.; Liyanarachchi, S.; Davuluri, R.V.; Nagy, R.; de la Chapelle, A. The polymorphism rs944289 predisposes to papillary thyroid carcinoma through a large intergenic noncoding RNA gene of tumor suppressor type. *Proc. Natl. Acad. Sci. USA* **2012**, *109*, 8646–8651. [CrossRef] [PubMed]
89. Rinn, J.L.; Kertesz, M.; Wang, J.K.; Squazzo, S.L.; Xu, X.; Brugmann, S.A.; Goodnough, L.H.; Helms, J.A.; Farnham, P.J.; Segal, E.; et al. Functional demarcation of active and silent chromatin domains in human HOX loci by noncoding RNAs. *Cell* **2007**, *129*, 1311–1323. [CrossRef]
90. Islam, F.; Zhou, Y.; Lam, A.K. Long Non-Coding RNAs Profiling Using Microarray in Papillary Thyroid Carcinoma. *Methods Mol. Biol.* **2022**, *2534*, 135–148. [CrossRef]
91. Chen, X.; Jin, J.; Zheng, L.; Sheng, Y.; Sun, J. Correlations of HOTAIR expression with pathological stage, CT characteristics and prognosis of patients with papillary thyroid carcinoma. *J. BUON* **2021**, *26*, 259–265.
92. Arratia, F.; Fierro, C.; Blanco, A.; Fuentes, S.; Nahuelquen, D.; Montecino, M.; Rojas, A.; Aguilar, R. Selective Concurrence of the Long Non-Coding RNA MALAT1 and the Polycomb Repressive Complex 2 to Promoter Regions of Active Genes in MCF7 Breast Cancer Cells. *Curr. Issues Mol. Biol.* **2023**, *45*, 4735–4748. [CrossRef] [PubMed]
93. West, J.A.; Davis, C.P.; Sunwoo, H.; Simon, M.D.; Sadreyev, R.I.; Wang, P.I.; Tolstorukov, M.Y.; Kingston, R.E. The long noncoding RNAs NEAT1 and MALAT1 bind active chromatin sites. *Mol. Cell* **2014**, *55*, 791–802. [CrossRef] [PubMed]
94. Fu, S.; Wang, Y.; Li, H.; Chen, L.; Liu, Q. Regulatory Networks of LncRNA MALAT-1 in Cancer. *Cancer Manag. Res.* **2020**, *12*, 10181–10198. [CrossRef]
95. Gou, L.; Zou, H.; Li, B. Long noncoding RNA MALAT1 knockdown inhibits progression of anaplastic thyroid carcinoma by regulating miR-200a-3p/FOXA1. *Cancer Biol. Ther.* **2019**, *20*, 1355–1365. [CrossRef] [PubMed]
96. Ghasemian, M.; Poodineh, J. A review on the biological roles of LncRNA PTCSC3 in cancerous and non-cancerous disorders. *Cancer Cell Int.* **2023**, *23*, 184. [CrossRef]
97. Fan, M.; Li, X.; Jiang, W.; Huang, Y.; Li, J.; Wang, Z. A long non-coding RNA, PTCSC3, as a tumor suppressor and a target of miRNAs in thyroid cancer cells. *Exp. Ther. Med.* **2013**, *5*, 1143–1146. [CrossRef]
98. Liu, Y.; Zhang, H.; Wang, H.; Du, J.; Dong, P.; Liu, M.; Lin, Y. Long non-coding RNA DUXAP8 promotes the cell proliferation, migration, and invasion of papillary thyroid carcinoma via miR-223-3p mediated regulation of CXCR4. *Bioengineered* **2021**, *12*, 496–506. [CrossRef]
99. Pang, R.; Yang, S. lncRNA DUXAP8 inhibits papillary thyroid carcinoma cell apoptosis via sponging the miR-20b-5p/SOS1 axis. *Oncol. Rep.* **2021**, *45*, 64. [CrossRef]
100. Zhou, Q.; Feng, J.; Yin, S.; Ma, S.; Wang, J.; Yi, H. LncRNA FAM230B promotes the metastasis of papillary thyroid cancer by sponging the miR-378a-3p/WNT5A axis. *Biochem. Biophys. Res. Commun.* **2021**, *546*, 83–89. [CrossRef]
101. Liao, G.; Huang, Z.; Gan, T.; Wu, C.; Wang, X.; Li, D. Long non-coding RNA nuclear enriched abundant transcript 1 (NEAT1) modulates inhibitor of DNA binding 1 (ID1) to facilitate papillary thyroid carcinoma development by sponging microRNA-524-5p. *Bioengineered* **2022**, *13*, 13201–13212. [CrossRef]

102. Sun, W.; Wang, Z.; Qin, Y.; Ji, X.; Huang, J.; Zhang, F.; Wang, Z.; Dong, W.; He, L.; Zhang, H. NEAT1_2/RRAD/EHF Positive Feedback Loop Facilitates Aerobic Glycolysis in Papillary Thyroid Cancer Cells. *Endocrinology* **2023**, *164*, bqad085. [CrossRef] [PubMed]
103. Zhou, Y.; Liu, S.; Luo, Y.; Zhang, M.; Jiang, X.; Xiong, Y. IncRNA MAPKAPK5-AS1 promotes proliferation and migration of thyroid cancer cell lines by targeting miR-519e-5p/YWHAH. *Eur. J. Histochem.* **2020**, *64*, 3177. [CrossRef] [PubMed]
104. Zhang, X.; Li, D.; Jia, C.; Cai, H.; Lv, Z.; Wu, B. METTL14 promotes tumorigenesis by regulating lncRNA OIP5-AS1/miR-98/ADAMTS8 signaling in papillary thyroid cancer. *Cell Death Dis.* **2021**, *12*, 617. [CrossRef] [PubMed]
105. Cai, T.; He, Y.; Peng, B. IncRNA XIST Stimulates Papillary Thyroid Cancer Development through the miR-330-3p/PDE5A Axis. *Crit. Rev. Eukaryot. Gene Expr.* **2023**, *33*, 13–26. [CrossRef] [PubMed]
106. Liu, H.; Deng, H.; Zhao, Y.; Li, C.; Liang, Y. LncRNA XIST/miR-34a axis modulates the cell proliferation and tumor growth of thyroid cancer through MET-PI3K-AKT signaling. *J. Exp. Clin. Cancer Res.* **2018**, *37*, 279. [CrossRef] [PubMed]
107. Pisignano, G.; Michael, D.C.; Visal, T.H.; Pirlog, R.; Ladomery, M.; Calin, G.A. Going circular: History, present, and future of circRNAs in cancer. *Oncogene* **2023**, *42*, 2783–2800. [CrossRef] [PubMed]
108. Chen, Y.G.; Hur, S. Cellular origins of dsRNA, their recognition and consequences. *Nat. Rev. Mol. Cell Biol.* **2022**, *23*, 286–301. [CrossRef]
109. Sadeq, S.; Al-Hashimi, S.; Cusack, C.M.; Werner, A. Endogenous Double-Stranded RNA. *Noncoding RNA* **2021**, *7*, 15. [CrossRef] [PubMed]
110. Chen, D.S.; Mellman, I. Elements of cancer immunity and the cancer-immune set point. *Nature* **2017**, *541*, 321–330. [CrossRef]
111. Brillo, V.; Chieregato, L.; Leanza, L.; Muccioli, S.; Costa, R. Mitochondrial Dynamics, ROS, and Cell Signaling: A Blended Overview. *Life* **2021**, *11*, 332. [CrossRef]
112. Elorza, A.A.; Soffia, J.P. mtDNA Heteroplasmy at the Core of Aging-Associated Heart Failure. An Integrative View of OXPHOS and Mitochondrial Life Cycle in Cardiac Mitochondrial Physiology. *Front. Cell Dev. Biol.* **2021**, *9*, 625020. [CrossRef] [PubMed]
113. Chocron, E.S.; Munkacsy, E.; Pickering, A.M. Cause or casualty: The role of mitochondrial DNA in aging and age-associated disease. *Biochim. Biophys. Acta Mol. Basis Dis.* **2019**, *1865*, 285–297. [CrossRef] [PubMed]
114. Picard, M.; Wallace, D.C.; Burelle, Y. The rise of mitochondria in medicine. *Mitochondrion* **2016**, *30*, 105–116. [CrossRef] [PubMed]
115. Soltys, D.T.; Pereira, C.P.M.; Rowies, F.T.; Farfel, J.M.; Grinberg, L.T.; Suemoto, C.K.; Leite, R.E.P.; Rodriguez, R.D.; Ericson, N.G.; Bielas, J.H.; et al. Lower mitochondrial DNA content but not increased mutagenesis associates with decreased base excision repair activity in brains of AD subjects. *Neurobiol. Aging* **2019**, *73*, 161–170. [CrossRef]
116. Lakshmanan, L.N.; Yee, Z.; Ng, L.F.; Gunawan, R.; Halliwell, B.; Gruber, J. Clonal expansion of mitochondrial DNA deletions is a private mechanism of aging in long-lived animals. *Aging Cell* **2018**, *17*, e12814. [CrossRef] [PubMed]
117. Nissanka, N.; Minczuk, M.; Moraes, C.T. Mechanisms of Mitochondrial DNA Deletion Formation. *Trends Genet.* **2019**, *35*, 235–244. [CrossRef] [PubMed]
118. Busch, K.B.; Kowald, A.; Spelbrink, J.N. Quality matters: How does mitochondrial network dynamics and quality control impact on mtDNA integrity? *Philos. Trans. R. Soc. Lond. B Biol. Sci.* **2014**, *369*, 20130442. [CrossRef] [PubMed]
119. Trifunovic, A.; Wredenberg, A.; Falkenberg, M.; Spelbrink, J.N.; Rovio, A.T.; Bruder, C.E.; Bohlooly, Y.M.; Gidlof, S.; Oldfors, A.; Wibom, R.; et al. Premature ageing in mice expressing defective mitochondrial DNA polymerase. *Nature* **2004**, *429*, 417–423. [CrossRef]
120. Medeiros, T.C.; Graef, M. Autophagy determines mtDNA copy number dynamics during starvation. *Autophagy* **2019**, *15*, 178–179. [CrossRef]
121. Medeiros, T.C.; Thomas, R.L.; Ghillebert, R.; Graef, M. Autophagy balances mtDNA synthesis and degradation by DNA polymerase POLG during starvation. *J. Cell Biol.* **2018**, *217*, 1601–1611. [CrossRef]
122. Siegmund, S.E.; Yang, H.; Sharma, R.; Javors, M.; Skinner, O.; Mootha, V.; Hirano, M.; Schon, E.A. Low-dose rapamycin extends lifespan in a mouse model of mtDNA depletion syndrome. *Hum. Mol. Genet.* **2017**, *26*, 4588–4605. [CrossRef]
123. Ahlqvist, K.J.; Leoncini, S.; Pecorelli, A.; Wortmann, S.B.; Ahola, S.; Forsstrom, S.; Guerranti, R.; De Felice, C.; Smeitink, J.; Ciccoli, L.; et al. MtDNA mutagenesis impairs elimination of mitochondria during erythroid maturation leading to enhanced erythrocyte destruction. *Nat. Commun.* **2015**, *6*, 6494. [CrossRef]
124. Hosgood, H.D., 3rd; Liu, C.S.; Rothman, N.; Weinstein, S.J.; Bonner, M.R.; Shen, M.; Lim, U.; Virtamo, J.; Cheng, W.L.; Albanes, D.; et al. Mitochondrial DNA copy number and lung cancer risk in a prospective cohort study. *Carcinogenesis* **2010**, *31*, 847–849. [CrossRef] [PubMed]
125. Thyagarajan, B.; Wang, R.; Nelson, H.; Barcelo, H.; Koh, W.P.; Yuan, J.M. Mitochondrial DNA copy number is associated with breast cancer risk. *PLoS ONE* **2013**, *8*, e65968. [CrossRef] [PubMed]
126. Yamada, S.; Nomoto, S.; Fujii, T.; Kaneko, T.; Takeda, S.; Inoue, S.; Kanazumi, N.; Nakao, A. Correlation between copy number of mitochondrial DNA and clinico-pathologic parameters of hepatocellular carcinoma. *Eur. J. Surg. Oncol.* **2006**, *32*, 303–307. [CrossRef]
127. Liao, L.M.; Baccarelli, A.; Shu, X.O.; Gao, Y.T.; Ji, B.T.; Yang, G.; Li, H.L.; Hoxha, M.; Dioni, L.; Rothman, N.; et al. Mitochondrial DNA copy number and risk of gastric cancer: A report from the Shanghai Women's Health Study. *Cancer Epidemiol. Biomarkers Prev.* **2011**, *20*, 1944–1949. [CrossRef] [PubMed]

128. Sun, X.; Zhan, L.; Chen, Y.; Wang, G.; He, L.; Wang, Q.; Zhou, F.; Yang, F.; Wu, J.; Wu, Y.; et al. Increased mtDNA copy number promotes cancer progression by enhancing mitochondrial oxidative phosphorylation in microsatellite-stable colorectal cancer. *Signal Transduct. Target. Ther.* **2018**, *3*, 8. [CrossRef]
129. Mambo, E.; Chatterjee, A.; Xing, M.; Tallini, G.; Haugen, B.R.; Yeung, S.C.; Sukumar, S.; Sidransky, D. Tumor-specific changes in mtDNA content in human cancer. *Int. J. Cancer* **2005**, *116*, 920–924. [CrossRef]
130. Tallini, G. Oncocytic tumours. *Virchows Arch.* **1998**, *433*, 5–12. [CrossRef]
131. Maximo, V.; Soares, P.; Lima, J.; Cameselle-Teijeiro, J.; Sobrinho-Simoes, M. Mitochondrial DNA somatic mutations (point mutations and large deletions) and mitochondrial DNA variants in human thyroid pathology: A study with emphasis on Hurthle cell tumors. *Am. J. Pathol.* **2002**, *160*, 1857–1865. [CrossRef]
132. Gasparre, G.; Porcelli, A.M.; Bonora, E.; Pennisi, L.F.; Toller, M.; Iommarini, L.; Ghelli, A.; Moretti, M.; Betts, C.M.; Martinelli, G.N.; et al. Disruptive mitochondrial DNA mutations in complex I subunits are markers of oncocytic phenotype in thyroid tumors. *Proc. Natl. Acad. Sci. USA* **2007**, *104*, 9001–9006. [CrossRef]
133. Gopal, R.K.; Kubler, K.; Calvo, S.E.; Polak, P.; Livitz, D.; Rosebrock, D.; Sadow, P.M.; Campbell, B.; Donovan, S.E.; Amin, S.; et al. Widespread Chromosomal Losses and Mitochondrial DNA Alterations as Genetic Drivers in Hurthle Cell Carcinoma. *Cancer Cell* **2018**, *34*, 242–255.e5. [CrossRef]
134. Lyu, L.; Wang, Q.; Song, S.; Li, L.; Zhou, H.; Li, M.; Jiang, Z.; Zhou, C.; Chen, G.; Lyu, J.; et al. Oncocytic tumors are marked by enhanced mitochondrial content and mtDNA mutations of complex I in Chinese patients. *Mitochondrion* **2019**, *45*, 1–6. [CrossRef]
135. Tsybrovskyy, O.; De Luise, M.; de Biase, D.; Caporali, L.; Fiorini, C.; Gasparre, G.; Carelli, V.; Hackl, D.; Imamovic, L.; Haim, S.; et al. Papillary thyroid carcinoma tall cell variant shares accumulation of mitochondria, mitochondrial DNA mutations, and loss of oxidative phosphorylation complex I integrity with oncocytic tumors. *J. Pathol. Clin. Res.* **2022**, *8*, 155–168. [CrossRef] [PubMed]
136. Rogounovitch, T.; Saenko, V.; Yamashita, S. Mitochondrial DNA and human thyroid diseases. *Endocr. J.* **2004**, *51*, 265–277. [CrossRef] [PubMed]
137. Sasarman, F.; Antonicka, H.; Shoubridge, E.A. The A3243G tRNALeu(UUR) MELAS mutation causes amino acid misincorporation and a combined respiratory chain assembly defect partially suppressed by overexpression of EFTu and EFG2. *Hum. Mol. Genet.* **2008**, *17*, 3697–3707. [CrossRef] [PubMed]
138. Akouchekian, M.; Houshmand, M.; Akbari, M.H.; Kamalidehghan, B.; Dehghan, M. Analysis of mitochondrial ND1 gene in human colorectal cancer. *J. Res. Med. Sci.* **2011**, *16*, 50–55. [PubMed]
139. Lin, Y.H.; Lim, S.N.; Chen, C.Y.; Chi, H.C.; Yeh, C.T.; Lin, W.R. Functional Role of Mitochondrial DNA in Cancer Progression. *Int. J. Mol. Sci.* **2022**, *23*, 1659. [CrossRef]
140. Yin, P.H.; Wu, C.C.; Lin, J.C.; Chi, C.W.; Wei, Y.H.; Lee, H.C. Somatic mutations of mitochondrial genome in hepatocellular carcinoma. *Mitochondrion* **2010**, *10*, 174–182. [CrossRef] [PubMed]
141. Fang, H.; Shen, L.; Chen, T.; He, J.; Ding, Z.; Wei, J.; Qu, J.; Chen, G.; Lu, J.; Bai, Y. Cancer type-specific modulation of mitochondrial haplogroups in breast, colorectal and thyroid cancer. *BMC Cancer* **2010**, *10*, 421. [CrossRef] [PubMed]
142. Dabravolski, S.A.; Nikiforov, N.G.; Zhuravlev, A.D.; Orekhov, N.A.; Mikhaleva, L.M.; Orekhov, A.N. The Role of Altered Mitochondrial Metabolism in Thyroid Cancer Development and Mitochondria-Targeted Thyroid Cancer Treatment. *Int. J. Mol. Sci.* **2021**, *23*, 460. [CrossRef] [PubMed]
143. Su, X.; Wang, W.; Ruan, G.; Liang, M.; Zheng, J.; Chen, Y.; Wu, H.; Fahey, T.J.; Guan, M.; Teng, L. A Comprehensive Characterization of Mitochondrial Genome in Papillary Thyroid Cancer. *Int. J. Mol. Sci.* **2016**, *17*, 1594. [CrossRef]
144. Bulgakova, O.; Kussainova, A.; Kakabayev, A.; Aripova, A.; Baikenova, G.; Izzotti, A.; Bersimbaev, R. The level of free-circulating mtDNA in patients with radon-induced lung cancer. *Environ. Res.* **2022**, *207*, 112215. [CrossRef] [PubMed]
145. Li, L.; Hann, H.W.; Wan, S.; Hann, R.S.; Wang, C.; Lai, Y.; Ye, X.; Evans, A.; Myers, R.E.; Ye, Z.; et al. Cell-free circulating mitochondrial DNA content and risk of hepatocellular carcinoma in patients with chronic HBV infection. *Sci. Rep.* **2016**, *6*, 23992. [CrossRef] [PubMed]
146. Meddeb, R.; Dache, Z.A.A.; Thezenas, S.; Otandault, A.; Tanos, R.; Pastor, B.; Sanchez, C.; Azzi, J.; Tousch, G.; Azan, S.; et al. Quantifying circulating cell-free DNA in humans. *Sci. Rep.* **2019**, *9*, 5220. [CrossRef] [PubMed]
147. Perdas, E.; Stawski, R.; Kaczka, K.; Nowak, D.; Zubrzycka, M. Altered levels of circulating nuclear and mitochondrial DNA in patients with Papillary Thyroid Cancer. *Sci. Rep.* **2019**, *9*, 14438. [CrossRef] [PubMed]
148. Ellinger, J.; Albers, P.; Muller, S.C.; von Ruecker, A.; Bastian, P.J. Circulating mitochondrial DNA in the serum of patients with testicular germ cell cancer as a novel noninvasive diagnostic biomarker. *BJU Int.* **2009**, *104*, 48–52. [CrossRef] [PubMed]
149. Seefeld, M.; El Tarhouny, S.; Fan, A.X.; Hahn, S.; Holzgreve, W.; Zhong, X.Y. Parallel assessment of circulatory cell-free DNA by PCR and nucleosomes by ELISA in breast tumors. *Int. J. Biol. Markers* **2008**, *23*, 69–73. [CrossRef] [PubMed]
150. Reznik, E.; Miller, M.L.; Senbabaoglu, Y.; Riaz, N.; Sarungbam, J.; Tickoo, S.K.; Al-Ahmadie, H.A.; Lee, W.; Seshan, V.E.; Hakimi, A.A.; et al. Mitochondrial DNA copy number variation across human cancers. *eLife* **2016**, *5*, e10769. [CrossRef]
151. Vara-Perez, M.; Felipe-Abrio, B.; Agostinis, P. Mitophagy in Cancer: A Tale of Adaptation. *Cells* **2019**, *8*, 493. [CrossRef]
152. Bassnett, S. Lens organelle degradation. *Exp. Eye Res.* **2002**, *74*, 1–6. [CrossRef] [PubMed]
153. Pua, H.H.; Guo, J.; Komatsu, M.; He, Y.W. Autophagy is essential for mitochondrial clearance in mature T lymphocytes. *J. Immunol.* **2009**, *182*, 4046–4055. [CrossRef] [PubMed]

154. Pei, S.; Minhajuddin, M.; Adane, B.; Khan, N.; Stevens, B.M.; Mack, S.C.; Lai, S.; Rich, J.N.; Inguva, A.; Shannon, K.M.; et al. AMPK/FIS1-Mediated Mitophagy Is Required for Self-Renewal of Human AML Stem Cells. *Cell Stem Cell* **2018**, *23*, 86–100.e106. [CrossRef] [PubMed]
155. Kimmelman, A.C.; White, E. Autophagy and Tumor Metabolism. *Cell Metab.* **2017**, *25*, 1037–1043. [CrossRef] [PubMed]
156. Wang, M.; Luan, S.; Fan, X.; Wang, J.; Huang, J.; Gao, X.; Han, D. The emerging multifaceted role of PINK1 in cancer biology. *Cancer Sci.* **2022**, *113*, 4037–4047. [CrossRef] [PubMed]
157. Hou, H.; Er, P.; Cheng, J.; Chen, X.; Ding, X.; Wang, Y.; Chen, X.; Yuan, Z.; Pang, Q.; Wang, P.; et al. High expression of FUNDC1 predicts poor prognostic outcomes and is a promising target to improve chemoradiotherapy effects in patients with cervical cancer. *Cancer Med.* **2017**, *6*, 1871–1881. [CrossRef]
158. Li, J.; Agarwal, E.; Bertolini, I.; Seo, J.H.; Caino, M.C.; Ghosh, J.C.; Kossenkov, A.V.; Liu, Q.; Tang, H.Y.; Goldman, A.R.; et al. The mitophagy effector FUNDC1 controls mitochondrial reprogramming and cellular plasticity in cancer cells. *Sci. Signal* **2020**, *13*, eaaz8240. [CrossRef]
159. Yuan, Q.; Sun, N.; Zheng, J.; Wang, Y.; Yan, X.; Mai, W.; Liao, Y.; Chen, X. Prognostic and Immunological Role of FUN14 Domain Containing 1 in Pan-Cancer: Friend or Foe? *Front. Oncol.* **2019**, *9*, 1502. [CrossRef] [PubMed]
160. Humpton, T.J.; Alagesan, B.; DeNicola, G.M.; Lu, D.; Yordanov, G.N.; Leonhardt, C.S.; Yao, M.A.; Alagesan, P.; Zaatari, M.N.; Park, Y.; et al. Oncogenic KRAS Induces NIX-Mediated Mitophagy to Promote Pancreatic Cancer. *Cancer Discov.* **2019**, *9*, 1268–1287. [CrossRef]
161. Fei, P.; Wang, W.; Kim, S.H.; Wang, S.; Burns, T.F.; Sax, J.K.; Buzzai, M.; Dicker, D.T.; McKenna, W.G.; Bernhard, E.J.; et al. Bnip3L is induced by p53 under hypoxia, and its knockdown promotes tumor growth. *Cancer Cell* **2004**, *6*, 597–609. [CrossRef]
162. Burton, T.R.; Gibson, S.B. The role of Bcl-2 family member BNIP3 in cell death and disease: NIPping at the heels of cell death. *Cell Death Differ.* **2009**, *16*, 515–523. [CrossRef] [PubMed]
163. Giatromanolaki, A.; Koukourakis, M.I.; Sowter, H.M.; Sivridis, E.; Gibson, S.; Gatter, K.C.; Harris, A.L. BNIP3 expression is linked with hypoxia-regulated protein expression and with poor prognosis in non-small cell lung cancer. *Clin. Cancer Res.* **2004**, *10*, 5566–5571. [CrossRef]
164. Sowter, H.M.; Ferguson, M.; Pym, C.; Watson, P.; Fox, S.B.; Han, C.; Harris, A.L. Expression of the cell death genes BNip3 and NIX in ductal carcinoma in situ of the breast; correlation of BNip3 levels with necrosis and grade. *J. Pathol.* **2003**, *201*, 573–580. [CrossRef]
165. Chourasia, A.H.; Tracy, K.; Frankenberger, C.; Boland, M.L.; Sharifi, M.N.; Drake, L.E.; Sachleben, J.R.; Asara, J.M.; Locasale, J.W.; Karczmar, G.S.; et al. Mitophagy defects arising from BNip3 loss promote mammary tumor progression to metastasis. *EMBO Rep.* **2015**, *16*, 1145–1163. [CrossRef]
166. Erkan, M.; Kleeff, J.; Esposito, I.; Giese, T.; Ketterer, K.; Buchler, M.W.; Giese, N.A.; Friess, H. Loss of BNIP3 expression is a late event in pancreatic cancer contributing to chemoresistance and worsened prognosis. *Oncogene* **2005**, *24*, 4421–4432. [CrossRef] [PubMed]
167. Li, X.; Lyu, Y.; Li, J.; Wang, X. AMBRA1 and its role as a target for anticancer therapy. *Front. Oncol.* **2022**, *12*, 946086. [CrossRef]
168. Lv, S.; Zhao, X.; Zhang, E.; Yan, Y.; Ma, X.; Li, N.; Zou, Q.; Sun, L.; Song, T. Lysine demethylase KDM1A promotes cell growth via FKBP8-BCL2 axis in hepatocellular carcinoma. *J. Biol. Chem.* **2022**, *298*, 102374. [CrossRef]
169. Fong, S.; Mounkes, L.; Liu, Y.; Maibaum, M.; Alonzo, E.; Desprez, P.Y.; Thor, A.D.; Kashani-Sabet, M.; Debs, R.J. Functional identification of distinct sets of antitumor activities mediated by the FKBP gene family. *Proc. Natl. Acad. Sci. USA* **2003**, *100*, 14253–14258. [CrossRef] [PubMed]
170. Singh, K.; Roy, M.; Prajapati, P.; Lipatova, A.; Sripada, L.; Gohel, D.; Singh, A.; Mane, M.; Godbole, M.M.; Chumakov, P.M.; et al. NLRX1 regulates TNF-alpha-induced mitochondria-lysosomal crosstalk to maintain the invasive and metastatic potential of breast cancer cells. *Biochim. Biophys. Acta Mol. Basis Dis.* **2019**, *1865*, 1460–1476. [CrossRef]
171. Nagai-Singer, M.A.; Morrison, H.A.; Woolls, M.K.; Leedy, K.; Imran, K.M.; Tupik, J.D.; Allen, I.C. NLRX1 functions as a tumor suppressor in Pan02 pancreatic cancer cells. *Front. Oncol.* **2023**, *13*, 1155831. [CrossRef]
172. Zhang, H.; Yin, C.; Liu, X.; Bai, X.; Wang, L.; Xu, H.; Ju, J.; Zhang, L. Prohibitin 2/PHB2 in Parkin-Mediated Mitophagy: A Potential Therapeutic Target for Non-Small Cell Lung Carcinoma. *Med. Sci. Monit.* **2020**, *26*, e923227. [CrossRef] [PubMed]
173. Nunez-Vazquez, S.; Saura-Esteller, J.; Sanchez-Vera, I.; Guilbaud, E.; Cosialls, A.M.; Pons, G.; Ricci, J.E.; Iglesias-Serret, D.; Marchetti, S.; Gil, J. The prohibitin-binding compound fluorizoline inhibits mitophagy in cancer cells. *Oncogenesis* **2021**, *10*, 64. [CrossRef] [PubMed]
174. Nissou, M.F.; El Atifi, M.; Guttin, A.; Godfraind, C.; Salon, C.; Garcion, E.; van der Sanden, B.; Issartel, J.P.; Berger, F.; Wion, D. Hypoxia-induced expression of VE-cadherin and filamin B in glioma cell cultures and pseudopalisade structures. *J. Neurooncol.* **2013**, *113*, 239–249. [CrossRef] [PubMed]
175. Zhang, J.; Ney, P.A. Role of BNIP3 and NIX in cell death, autophagy, and mitophagy. *Cell Death Differ.* **2009**, *16*, 939–946. [CrossRef] [PubMed]
176. Sowter, H.M.; Ratcliffe, P.J.; Watson, P.; Greenberg, A.H.; Harris, A.L. HIF-1-dependent regulation of hypoxic induction of the cell death factors BNIP3 and NIX in human tumors. *Cancer Res.* **2001**, *61*, 6669–6673. [PubMed]
177. Guo, K.; Searfoss, G.; Krolikowski, D.; Pagnoni, M.; Franks, C.; Clark, K.; Yu, K.T.; Jaye, M.; Ivashchenko, Y. Hypoxia induces the expression of the pro-apoptotic gene BNIP3. *Cell Death Differ.* **2001**, *8*, 367–376. [CrossRef] [PubMed]

178. Sandoval, H.; Thiagarajan, P.; Dasgupta, S.K.; Schumacher, A.; Prchal, J.T.; Chen, M.; Wang, J. Essential role for Nix in autophagic maturation of erythroid cells. *Nature* **2008**, *454*, 232–235. [CrossRef] [PubMed]
179. Aerbajinai, W.; Giattina, M.; Lee, Y.T.; Raffeld, M.; Miller, J.L. The proapoptotic factor Nix is coexpressed with Bcl-xL during terminal erythroid differentiation. *Blood* **2003**, *102*, 712–717. [CrossRef] [PubMed]
180. Bellot, G.; Garcia-Medina, R.; Gounon, P.; Chiche, J.; Roux, D.; Pouyssegur, J.; Mazure, N.M. Hypoxia-induced autophagy is mediated through hypoxia-inducible factor induction of BNIP3 and BNIP3L via their BH3 domains. *Mol. Cell Biol.* **2009**, *29*, 2570–2581. [CrossRef]
181. Daido, S.; Kanzawa, T.; Yamamoto, A.; Takeuchi, H.; Kondo, Y.; Kondo, S. Pivotal role of the cell death factor BNIP3 in ceramide-induced autophagic cell death in malignant glioma cells. *Cancer Res.* **2004**, *64*, 4286–4293. [CrossRef]
182. Lee, M.J.; Kim, J.Y.; Suk, K.; Park, J.H. Identification of the hypoxia-inducible factor 1 alpha-responsive HGTD-P gene as a mediator in the mitochondrial apoptotic pathway. *Mol. Cell Biol.* **2004**, *24*, 3918–3927. [CrossRef] [PubMed]
183. Toustrup, K.; Sorensen, B.S.; Nordsmark, M.; Busk, M.; Wiuf, C.; Alsner, J.; Overgaard, J. Development of a hypoxia gene expression classifier with predictive impact for hypoxic modification of radiotherapy in head and neck cancer. *Cancer Res.* **2011**, *71*, 5923–5931. [CrossRef] [PubMed]
184. Sorensen, B.S.; Knudsen, A.; Wittrup, C.F.; Nielsen, S.; Aggerholm-Pedersen, N.; Busk, M.; Horsman, M.; Hoyer, M.; Bouchelouche, P.N.; Overgaard, J.; et al. The usability of a 15-gene hypoxia classifier as a universal hypoxia profile in various cancer cell types. *Radiother. Oncol.* **2015**, *116*, 346–351. [CrossRef] [PubMed]
185. Tang, B.; Qu, Y.; Zhao, F.; Mao, M.; Tang, J.; Li, X.; Ferriero, D.; Mu, D. In vitro effects of hypoxia-inducible factor 1alpha on the biological characteristics of the SiHa uterine cervix cancer cell line. *Int. J. Gynecol. Cancer* **2009**, *19*, 898–904. [CrossRef] [PubMed]
186. Cho, Y.E.; Kim, J.Y.; Kim, Y.J.; Kim, Y.W.; Lee, S.; Park, J.H. Expression and clinicopathological significance of human growth and transformation-dependent protein (HGTD-P) in uterine cervical cancer. *Histopathology* **2010**, *57*, 479–482. [CrossRef] [PubMed]
187. Basolo, F.; Torregrossa, L.; Giannini, R.; Miccoli, M.; Lupi, C.; Sensi, E.; Berti, P.; Elisei, R.; Vitti, P.; Baggiani, A.; et al. Correlation between the BRAF V600E mutation and tumor invasiveness in papillary thyroid carcinomas smaller than 20 millimeters: Analysis of 1060 cases. *J. Clin. Endocrinol. Metab.* **2010**, *95*, 4197–4205. [CrossRef]
188. Xing, M. Genetic-guided Risk Assessment and Management of Thyroid Cancer. *Endocrinol. Metab. Clin. N. Am.* **2019**, *48*, 109–124. [CrossRef]

MDPI AG
Grosspeteranlage 5
4052 Basel
Switzerland
Tel.: +41 61 683 77 34

International Journal of Molecular Sciences Editorial Office
E-mail: ijms@mdpi.com
www.mdpi.com/journal/ijms

www.ingramcontent.com/pod-product-compliance
Lightning Source LLC
Chambersburg PA
CBHW061551210926
51850CB00009B/2070
9783725851072